Men, Gender Divisions and Welfare

Men, Gender Divisions and Welfare focuses on the relationship between men and welfare. It highlights the importance of gendered power relations and explores the complexities and contradictions of these relationships. Also addressed is how these issues are becoming increasingly part of social policy debates. Key features that emerge are the persistence of men's power and control in welfare and at the same time, men's avoidance of welfare services.

The first part of *Men, Gender Divisions and Welfare* comprises theoretical and historical reviews of the relationship between men and welfare. The main body of the book draws on new empirical studies, encompassing both men and women's perspectives. Subjects discussed include how men affect the welfare of women and children, accounts of men's violence towards women they know, women and men as carers for spouses with disabilities, accounts of parenthood, and experiences of unemployed men and their employed wives. The final section focuses on relations between service providers, men and welfare.

By bringing together empirical studies, up-to-date theoretical overviews and analysis of contemporary discourses on troubled masculinities, this book will prove invaluable for those studying social policy and gender studies, as well as for health and social welfare professionals and managers.

Jennie Popay is Professor of Community Health, Public Health Research and Resource Centre, University of Salford. **Jeff Hearn** is Professorial Research Fellow, University of Manchester and Donner Professor in Sociology, Åbo Akademi University, and **Jeanette Edwards** is a Lecturer, Department of Sociology and Social Anthropology, University of Keele.

Men, Gender Divisions and Welfare

Edited by Jennie Popay,
Jeff Hearn and Jeanette Edwards

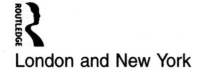

London and New York

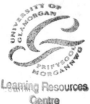
First published 1998
by Routledge
11 New Fetter Lane, London EC4P 4EE

Simultaneously published in the USA and Canada
by Routledge
29 West 35th Street, New York, NY 10001

© 1998 Jennie Popay, Jeff Hearn and Jeanette Edwards: selection
and editorial matter; individual chapters, the contributors.

Typeset in Times by BC Typesetting, Bristol
Printed and bound in Great Britain by
Creative Print and Design (Wales), Ebbw Vale

British Library Cataloguing in Publication Data
A catalogue record for this book is available from the British Library

Library of Congress Cataloging in Publication Data
A catalogue record for this book has been requested

ISBN 0–415–11970–7 (hbk)
ISBN 0–415–11971–5 (pbk)

Contents

List of illustrations

Contributors

Sue Clarke joined the Public Health Research and Resource Centre at the University of Salford as a postgraduate research student after working for a number of years in the NHS. She has been involved in a variety of research projects in the fields of social and health policy. Her main research interest is in the area of alternative and complementary medicine, with a specific focus on holistic approaches to cancer care and treatment.

Chas Critcher is Professor of Communications in the Communication, Media and Communities Research Centre at Sheffield Hallam University. He has been researching mining communities for more than a decade. He is the co-author, with David Waddington, of *Flashpoints: Studies in Public Disorder* (Routledge, 1989) and *Split at the Seams: Community, Continuity and Change after the 1984–5 Local Dispute* (Open University Press, 1991), and co-editor, with David Waddington, of *Regeneration of the Coalfield Areas: Anglo-German Perspectives* (Pinter, 1995). His other research interests include popular culture and the mass media. He is currently embarking on a study of moral panics about social problem.

Bella Dicks is Lecturer in Sociology at the University of Wales, Cardiff, at the School of Social and Administrative Studies. She is currently completing a PhD on heritage and locality based in the Rhondda Valleys. Her next research project, starting in October 1997, will be examining the authorizing of ethnographic texts through multi-media. Her research interests focus on locality and the representation of class, community and industry. She has published articles relating to coalmining communities in Yorkshire and Wales.

Jeanette Edwards is a lecturer in social anthropology, and director of the MSc in medical social anthropology at the University of Keele. One of her research interests is in kinship and, in particular, cultural understandings of what constitutes a parent in late twentieth-century Britain. She is co-author (with Sarah Franklin, Eric Hirsch, Frances Price and Marilyn Strathern) of *Technologies of Procreation: Kinship in the Age of Assisted Conception* (Manchester University Press, 1993), and author of several articles on relatedness and new reproductive technologies, and the views of community health and social service providers on the needs of women and their children.

Jalna Hanmer is Director of the Research Centre on Violence, Abuse and Gender Relations at Leeds Metropolitan University. She is currently researching a new approach to policing repeat victimization of women by known men. Her publications include *Well-founded Fear* (with Sheila Saunders, Hutchinson, 1984); *Women, Violence and Crime Prevention: A Community Study in West Yorkshire* (with Sheila Saunders, Gower, 1993); *Women, Violence and Social Control* (with Mary Maynard, Macmillan, 1987); *Women, Policing and Male Violence: International Perspectives* (with Jill Radford and Elizabeth Stanko, Routledge, 1989).

Jeff Hearn is Professorial Research Fellow in the Faculty of Economic and Social Studies, based in the School of Social Policy, University of Manchester, and is also Donner Visiting Professor in Sociology at Åbo Akademi University, Finland. His publications include *The Gender of Oppression* (Wheatsheaf, 1987); *Men, Masculinities and Social Theory* (co-editor with David Morgan, Unwin Hyman, 1990); *Men in the Public Eye* (Routledge, 1992); *'Sex' at 'Work'* (with Wendy Parkin, Prentice-Hall/ Harvester Wheatsheaf, St Martin's, 1995); *Violence and Gender Relations* (co-editor with Barbara Fawcett, Brid Featherstone and Christine Toft, Sage, 1996); *Men as Managers, Managers as Men* (co-editor with David Collinson, Sage, 1996). He has just completed *The Violences of Men* (Sage) on ESRC research on men's violence to known women, and is currently researching organizations and violence.

Ann Oakley is Professor of Sociology and Social Policy and Director of the Social Science Research Unit at the University of London Institute of Education; she is also Honorary Professor in Social Sciences in the Division of Public Health Medicine at the Institute of Child Health. She has been researching and writing in the fields of gender, the family and health for more than 30 years. Her current research interests include the evaluation of social interventions, the history of gender and methodology, and the scientific basis for screening and treatment in the field of women's health. Among her recent publications are *Social Support and Motherhood* (Blackwell, 1992); *Essays on Women, Medicine and Health* (Edinburgh University Press, 1993); *The Politics of the Welfare State* (co-editor, with Susan Williams, UCL Press, 1994); *Man and Wife* (Harper Collins, 1996); and *Who's Afraid of Feminism?* (co-editor, with Juliet Mitchell, 1997).

Gillian Parker is Professor of Community Care at the University of Leicester and Director of the Nuffield Community Care Studies Unit. Her current research interests include disability and informal care, evaluation of community care policy, the boundaries between health and social care, and the relative responsibilities of the state and the individual for paying for long-term care. Her books include *With Due Care and Attention* (Family Policy Studies Unit, 1985 and 1990); *With This Body: Caring and Disability in Marriage* (Open University Press, 1993); and *Different Types of Care, Different Types of Carer* (with Dorothy Lawton, HMSO, 1994).

Jennie Popay is Professor of Community Health at the University of Salford and Director of the Public Health Research and Resource Centre. She is also an Associate Director of Research and Development at the National Primary Care R&D Centre, a joint initiative of the Universities of Manchester, Salford and York. She has published widely in the fields of health and social policy. Her particular research interests include gender and social class inequalities in health and the sociology of knowledge, with particular reference to the relationship between lay and professional knowledge in the sphere of public health. Her recent publications include the edited collections *Dilemmas in Health Care* (with Basiro Davey, Open University Press, 1993) and *Researching the People's Health* (with Gareth Williams, Routledge, 1994).

Keith Pringle is Reader in Social Policy at the University of Sunderland. He researches in the areas of masculinity studies, childcare and comparative social policy. His publications include *Managing to Survive* (Barnado's, 1990); *Men, Masculinities and Social Welfare* (UCL Press, 1995); *Protecting Children in Europe: Towards a New Millennium* (co-edited with Margit Harder, Aalborg University Press, 1997). Currently he is completing a book on European child welfare and is engaged in a Swedish/English research project on fatherhood.

Alan S. Rigby, MSc, CStat (Senior Lecturer in Statistics and Epidemiology, Chartered Statistician) works in the Department of Paediatrics, Sheffield Children's Hospital, University of Sheffield. He has been involved in a number of research projects related to child health. Currently he is involved in two main research projects. The first is looking at the current allocation of health visitor resources in Sheffield, with a view to developing a 'weighting' formula to provide a more equal distribution of resources. This work is funded by the NHS National R&D Programme on Mother and Child Health (lead researcher, David Hall, Community Paediatrics, University of Sheffield). The second project is a descriptive study of neonatal encephalopathy. Other research interests include developing genetic models of inheritance for various childhood diseases.

Julie Seymour is Lecturer in Social Research in the School of Comparative and Applied Social Sciences at the University of Hull. The research reported on in her chapter with Gillian Parker was carried out whilst she was employed as a Research Fellow at the Social Policy Research Unit at the University of York. Her research interests include the distribution of resources in households and the associated negotiations between household members with a particular emphasis on gender, disability and social exclusion and research methodology. Recent publications include *Joint Accounts: Methodology and Practice in Research Interviews with Couples* (with Gill Dix and Tony Eardley, University of York, 1995). She is currently writing a book on research methodology.

David Waddington is Reader in Communications in the Communication, Media and Communities Research Centre at Sheffield Hallam University. He has been researching mining communities for more than a decade. He is the co-author, with Chas Critcher, of *Flashpoints: Studies in Public Disorder* (Routledge 1989) and

Split At The Seams: Mining Communities in the Aftermath of the Strike (Open University Press, 1993), and co-editor, with Chas Critcher, of *Regeneration of the Coalfield Areas: Anglo-German Perspectives* (Pinter, 1995). His work on public order includes *Contemporary Issues in Public Order* (Routledge, 1992) and *Policing and Public Order* (co-editor, with Chas Critcher, Avebury, 1996).

Fiona Williams is Professor of Social Policy in the Department of Sociology and Social Policy at the University of Leeds. She is best known for *Social Policy, a Critical Introduction: Issues of Race, Gender and Class* (Polity Press, 1989), but she has also published and edited work on learning disability, community care, feminism and postmodernism, and comparative social policy. She has recently completed editing, with Jennie Popay and Ann Oakley, *Welfare Research: A Critique of Theory and Methods* (UCL Press, forthcoming).

Acknowledgements

The original idea for this book arose out of discussions among the researchers involved in the Management of Personal Welfare Research Programme which was jointly funded by the ESRC and the Rowntree Foundation between 1991 and 1995. We are grateful to the ESRC and Rowntree for their financial support for the cross-programme workshops, without which the 'added value' arising from discussions and debate would not have happened. We are also grateful for the support given to us by Margaret Edmonds at the ESRC and Janet Lewis at Rowntree, despite our somewhat unconventional approach to programme co-ordination! Ann Oakley and Jennie Popay were the co-ordinators for the programme and produced the proposal for this book. The editors would like to thank Ann Oakley in particular for her contribution to the early stages of the book's development, after the formal end of the research programme. Ann kept the idea for the book alive, negotiating with publishers and commenting on early drafts of chapters. Our thanks are also due to Heather Gibson and her colleagues at Routledge for having faith in the project.

The book draws heavily on the studies funded within the Management of Personal Welfare Research Programme. In particular, the following studies are reported on here: Responses to Contemporary Change in Britain's Mining Communities (X206252004); The Negotiation of Coping, Disablement, Caring and Marriage (L206252002); Social Support and the Health and Welfare of Vulnerable Children: A Consumer Study (L206252005); Social Support and the Health and Welfare of Vulnerable Children: A Provider Study (X206252006); Violence, Abuse and the Stress–Coping Process: Project 1 – Women and Project 2 – Men (L206252003).

Finally, like all books, this would not have been produced without considerable administrative support, in this case from the staff at the Public Health Research and Resource Centre at the University of Salford. We are particularly grateful to Carla Warburton, who helped get the final manuscript into shape, and to Angela Greenall, Nic Parker, Chris Saunders and Paula Simcock, who typed many versions of chapters, sent endless e-mails and made many phone calls – all with endless patience and good humour. And last our thanks to Tom – who played many hours of basketball and computer games on his own.

Introduction

The trouble with men

Jeff Hearn, Jeanette Edwards, Jennie Popay and Ann Oakley

This is a book about men, gender divisions and welfare. Its particular focus is on the 'trouble with men' in and around formal and informal welfare services. It examines the various ways that men are often troublesome but also themselves sometimes troubled, and how these troubles are becoming increasingly part of debates on social policy. While the book draws primarily on UK data, questions that we discuss are of growing interest internationally.

The idea of producing *Men, Gender Divisions and Welfare* emerged out of discussions between members of the research teams working on The Management of Personal Welfare Research Programme. This was a programme of seven research projects funded, from 1991 to 1995, by the Economic and Social Research Council (ESRC) and the Joseph Rowntree Foundation.

Following a background consultancy report commissioned by the ESRC (Titterton, 1989), the Programme was initially conceptualized by the funders within the framework of a stress–coping–social support paradigm of welfare. As the Initiative progressed, this framework came under a good deal of criticism, not least in terms of its relation to gender divisions and gendered power (Hanmer and Hearn, forthcoming; Williams, forthcoming). The Programme comprised research on the connections between the personal welfare of people facing especially difficult problems in their lives, and the operation of personal welfare services and systems (see Williams *et al.*, forthcoming).

The specific projects within the Programme ranged across a wide spectrum of welfare issues and problems. However, all were in some way concerned with particularly difficult, even dire, situations, and with groups likely to be especially vulnerable to stress and lacking in support. Their main areas of study were the health and welfare of families living in poverty, from the perspectives of service providers and service users, the personal welfare of families with severely disabled children, the experience and negotiation of coping with caring for spouses with disabilities, men's violence to known women (women's and men's experiences), and personal and community responses to pit closure in mining communities.

A wide range of disciplines and methodologies were also to be found amongst the researchers and the approaches adopted in the projects. Disciplinary backgrounds included cultural studies, social anthropology, social policy, social psychology, sociology and women's studies. Research methods used included action research, community case studies, indepth interviews, document analysis, participant observation, questionnaire interviews, secondary data analysis, as well as a variety of other qualitative methods, statistical analyses and triangulations of methods. Feminist perspectives ran through the entire project, and all benefited from an interest in and an awareness of feminist issues in methodology.

These projects have thus in different ways addressed significant questions about how and why some people are able to cope with personal difficulties, whilst others are less able to do so. In turn, the concept of coping itself came under scrutiny. Many of the projects looked at the complexity of coping, and asked at what personal cost was coping achieved. One major element in understanding the problems that people have to face, and how it is that they seem more or less to cope, is gender – from the gendered terrain of caring, to the relationships, supportive or otherwise, between men and women, and between service users and service providers. Indeed, as the Programme proceeded it became clearer that not only were gender relations of special significance in determining welfare experiences and outcomes but that a persistent and pervasive part of this picture was 'the trouble with men'. The projects upon which this book draws have mainly focused on heterosexual relationships in the home, and there is clearly an absence of lesbians' and gay men's voices in this volume. An important task which needs to be addressed is the relationships between lesbians and gay men, welfare, social policy, and health and social services.

Several of the studies focused on men as the cause of trouble; for example, in situations of violence and abuse. Others focused on the troubles faced by men; for example, unemployment. All explored the implications of these gendered patterns for the health and welfare of women. Some studies noted that men were not only absent as clients or customers of health and social services but also absent from debates around appropriate and relevant services. Furthermore, all showed how in late twentieth-century Britain the model of male breadwinner and female carer continues to dominate the rhetoric of social policy and public administration despite evidence to the contrary from everyday lives. Social and economic changes, such as those occurring in men's employment and unemployment patterns, the interventions and restructurings of the welfare state, and women's changing ideas and practices around, amongst other things, marriage, motherhood and employment have not fundamentally changed dominant gendered social structures and divisions of labour, and the hierarchies implicit in them.

Eight of the chapters draw directly on the empirical results of research projects funded by the ESRC. An additional four chapters draw more generally on recent empirical, policy, political and theoretical studies; these address the relationship of men and welfare, young men, fatherhood, and men and childcare. While all the chapters highlight the importance of gendered power relations in understanding men's relations to welfare, they also show, in very different ways, the complexities and contradictions of these relations. Thus, men may be carers or avoid caring, they may be privileged or disadvantaged in the use of welfare services, they may be employed or unemployed, they may continue to be violent or may attempt to move away from violence, and they may be engaged in long-term relations with children or may flee from them. Furthermore, these and other possibilities are not mutually exclusive. Men may indeed be simultaneously present and absent from welfare.

One of the problems of placing the focus on men is that there is a long tradition in both social science and everyday conversation of explaining men and indeed masculinity as just naturally being that way, beyond social influence or control, and more generally as if determined by biology. The problems of men's violence, delinquency, competition, uncooperativeness and lack of involvement have and continue to be explained by reference to biology. The definition of men and masculinity in these terms can have a number of implications. It can be used to take responsibility away from boys and men just as it can be damaging for girls and women. However, men are generally slower than women to see this particular construction as troublesome; it is not nearly so from a position of privilege as it is from a position of disadvantage.

In recent years the increased interest in looking more closely at men has come from a wide variety of quarters – from mainstream politics, from social policy makers, from the mass media, as well as from feminist, gay and 'men's movements'. All of these initiatives are themselves immensely varied, and none more so than those of the men's movements, which range from pro-feminist to clearly anti-feminist. From feminist perspectives it might be argued that men already get too much attention, and that perhaps we ought to be wary of giving them more. For example, how do we make sense of recent concerns in the press and in political and educational circles about girls overtaking boys in school examination results? Is this justified? Is it important? What other agendas might this convey or obscure? It seems that worries are soon voiced when boys and men are dislodged from their positions of privilege. Thus it is easy to see this recent focus on men and boys as part of a backlash against the gains made through feminism and equal opportunities. On the other hand, feminism has always addressed the trouble with men. Focusing on the power of the powerful is a necessary task in critical theory, research and practice. What is perhaps slightly different is the question of combining this critique with the analysis of men in relation to welfare, where at least some of those men are likely to be relatively less powerful.

There has been in the past enormous attention on men (almost at times exclusively) in the social sciences, where men's voices and experiences have often come to stand for all. In recent years there has been a major expansion of explicitly gendered, critical academic studies on men. Some of these have been developed through feminist research, some have been part of gay studies and some have derived largely from men's responses to feminism. Together these critical studies on men have begun to demonstrate the social and political character of men and masculinity. They have pointed to the simultaneous power of and difference between men. It is clear, for example, that not all men are equally or axiomatically privileged. The social construction of men and masculinity has also been analysed in terms of both relations with women and relations between men. It is for these kinds of reasons that the notion of masculinities in the plural has effectively superseded that of masculinity in the singular. However, both concepts – masculinity and masculinities – can be somewhat problematic. Both can be vague and carry quite different connotations in different theoretical or political contexts (see Cornwall and Lindisfarne, 1994). Thus it might be more accurate to talk of either men's practices or of discourses of masculinities.

These general issues have special significance in the field of social welfare. Assumptions are constantly being made about men in families, employment and social policy. Certain categories of men (typically white, employed, able-bodied, heterosexual men, not, for example, black men, young men or gay men) may come to stand for everyman. This serves to neglect both the negative impact on welfare of some men and the positive contribution to welfare of others. Such assumptions have implications for policy development and indeed for the personal well-being of women, men and chidren. Indeed, the very idea of welfare itself continues to carry, reproduce and be underlain by many gendered premises; welfare is thus a gendered concept. More generally still, it could be argued that associating masculinity or masculinities only with men is problematic: genders are as much to do with processes of becoming, revealing and hiding, as they are with fixed social attributes.

In this book we attempt to examine these issues in the light of both empirical research and theoretical study. The book is arranged in three sections: 'Theory, discourse and policy', 'Women and men on men and welfare', and 'Service providers, men and welfare'. The first section consists of three chapters that set out the broad contexts of the troublesome relationship between men and welfare. The first of these, by Jeff Hearn, considers the welfare of men in a broad theoretical framework, drawing on, amongst other things, critical studies on men, historical perspectives on welfare and comparative studies of the gendered welfare state. The next two chapters are more contemporary in focus, and specifically address the current discourses of troubled masculinities that are operating in and around social policy. The first of these, by Jeff Hearn, is primarily on the construction of (the trouble with) young men; the next, by Fiona Williams, deals with the construction of (the trouble with) fatherhood.

The second section focuses on what women and men say about men's relationship to welfare. In different ways these six chapters look at the often troublesome effects, for women and children, of the presence of men in and around families. The first two chapters of this section detail *women*'s relation to and commentaries on the men in their lives. First, Ann Oakley and Alan Rigby directly pose the question: Are men good for the welfare of women and children?

They suggest that often the presence of men/fathers in households does indeed bring disbenefits to women and children. The next chapter by Jalna Hanmer looks at women's experiences of men being 'out of control' and considers in particular the social processes that sustain men's violence against women and children and the place of family members, friends and formal agencies within these.

The next two chapters address some of the troubles that arise with and indeed sometimes for men in welfare, and how *men* report on their own experiences of this. Chapter 6 by Jeff Hearn analyses some of the problems that can arise in men giving support to each other. While this might seem at first sight to be a good thing, complications and ambiguities arise when the problem is that of violence to women. The next chapter in this section by Gillian Parker and Julie Seymour addresses a rather different set of complications, namely the question of spouse carers set within the context of the marriage relationship. Their specific concern is with husbands who are caring for their wives, and through this focus they develop a re-examination of feminist analysis of informal care.

The final two chapters in this section comprise studies of the responses of *women* and *men* living together to issues around men and welfare. Chapter 8 by Sue Clarke and Jennie Popay is on the meanings that men and women attach to the experience of parenting, fathering and mothering. The next chapter by David Waddington, Chas Critcher and Bella Dicks uses material from a study of mining communities facing pit closure. Its particular focus is the situation and experience of women who are themselves in paid employment but whose husbands are unemployed.

The concluding section is concerned with the relation of the providers of welfare services to men and welfare. Jeanette Edwards begins by noting the relative silence about men within studies of the health and welfare of women and children. In particular she examines the perceptions of service providers in health and social services, and their interaction, or lack of interaction, with men as service users. The next chapter by Bella Dicks, David Waddington and Chas Critcher is again based on the results of a study of mining communities. Here they extend their earlier analysis by bringing together the tripartite relation of redundant men, overburdened women and the work of local welfare service providers, organizations and professionals. The final chapter is by Keith Pringle on the problems and possibilities for men's involvement in and relationship to children and childcare. This considers men in both public and private spheres, in both professional and domestic locations.

As the contributors to this book illustrate, troubled relationships between men and welfare are not confined to any one sphere or locality, they extend across the public and the private realms, and are to be found in a wide variety of forms throughout welfare and the welfare state.

REFERENCES

Cornwall, A. and Lindisfarne, N. (eds) (1994) *Dislocating Masculinity: Comparative Ethnographies*, London: Routledge.

Hanmer, J. (forthcoming) 'Gender and welfare research', in F. Williams, J. Popay and A. Oakley (eds) *Welfare Research: A Critique of Theory and Method*, London: UCL Press.

Titterton, M. (1989) *The Management of Personal Welfare*, Glasgow: Department of Social Administration and Social Work, University of Glasgow.

Williams, F. (forthcoming) 'Social difference or social divisions?', in F. Williams, J. Popay and A. Oakley (eds) *Welfare Research: A Critique of Theory and Method*, London: UCL Press.

Williams, F., Popay, J. and Oakley, A. (eds) (forthcoming) *Welfare Research: A Critique of Theory and Method*, London: UCL Press.

Part I

Theory, discourse and policy

Chapter 1

The welfare of men?

Jeff Hearn

Do welfare and welfare systems serve the welfare of men? What is the relationship of men and welfare? To explore such questions, it is not enough to rely on the discipline of Social Policy. We need to consider this question within a broad political economy framework, that includes the analysis of production and reproduction, economic life, state development, citizenship and civil society.

In this chapter I consider to what extent welfare and welfare systems might be understood as serving the welfare of men, and how the relationship of men and welfare more generally might be conceptualized. The discussion of these questions is developed through, first, examining the rethinking of welfare and work; then, the impact of feminism on the analysis of social policy; third, the review of recent debates on critical studies on men and masculinities; fourth, the relevance of these various previous debates for rethinking the relationship of men and welfare; and finally, some brief comments on contemporary developments around the place of men in social policy.

RETHINKING WELFARE AND WORK

The British welfare state, that is the Beveridgean welfare state, and the discipline of Social Administration grew up hand in hand in the post-war period. Their primary focus appeared to be the agendered citizen, even though they were implicitly gendered, being based on assumptions of the nuclear family and the unpaid work of women (see Wilson, 1977). This welfare state was based on contributions from what would be assumed to be lifelong employment, and this meant that those who were not able to achieve this – in practice, often women with family responsibilities – received reduced benefits and provisions (Laybourn, 1995: 254). As such, British welfare policy, despite its appearance of universal care from cradle to grave was fundamentally residual rather than institutional in character (Wilensky and Lebeaux, 1958). In keeping with the political traditions of Toryism and Liberalism, it was founded on the calculation of individual needs rather than social insurance guaranteeing all citizens equal rights to a decent standard of living (Tyyskä, 1995).

During the 1970s Social Administration slowly transformed itself into the discipline of Social Policy. Social Policy was much more concerned with social division and much more influenced by neo-Marxist political economy than Social Administration. Unfortunately, the traditions of political economy, both classical and modern, did not, at least not initially, do much to emphasize the significance of gendered power relations in society. Their focus was primarily on public domain activities, and often only implicitly on men there. For example, in his landmark work on *The Political Economy of the Welfare State*, Gough (1983) retained malestream (O'Brien, 1981) terminology in speaking of work as occupying economically productive or unproductive sectors. Similarly, in such models the analysis of gender relations was often implicitly relegated to the world of social consumption, social expenses (O'Connor, 1974) and collective consumption (Castells, 1977), or simply went unnoticed. Such distinctions, perhaps unwittingly or perhaps not, transplant the discriminations of patriarchal societies into supposedly radical political economic analysis.

RETHINKING WORK AND WELFARE

Increasingly, attempts have been made to rethink the political economic analysis of society to avoid the pitfalls of merely reproducing dominant definitions and ideologies of the political and the economic. To some extent this is an outgrowth of a long-established concern within welfare economics. Indeed, at the start of the twentieth century Arthur Cecil Pigou, the founder of welfare economics, noted that if a woman, employed as a housekeeper by a bachelor, marries him then national income would fall since her previously paid work would now be unpaid and thus not counted in national accounting (*Human Development Report 1995*, 1995: 87).

Of particular importance has been the impact of feminist theory and practice on the theory and practice of economics itself, and the growth of a relatively small but influential feminist economics. The domestic labour debate of the mid-1970s (Gardiner, 1975; Himmelweit and Mohun, 1977) was a major accomplishment in bringing domestic, private and unpaid labour at least partially into the analysis of political economy. This development was itself open to criticism in using economic categories in ways that are inapplicable to activities that are more than the economic (see Delphy, 1977, 1984). Feminist scholarship and politics around the economic, both domestic and beyond, has above all problematized what is meant by work, in line with broader feminist analysis in politics, sociology and development studies. It has stressed the importance of counting what has previously counted for nothing (Waring, 1988). It has led to a rethinking of state budgets in terms of how they contribute to women's welfare (*Women's Budget Statement*, 1990–91), and by implication men's welfare too. Although economics as a discipline has been resistant to feminist influence, feminist economics is now here to stay (Nelson, 1996).

Also important for social policy is the broadening of the concepts of work and labour beyond what has been called productive labour to include reproductive labour. This point has been argued strongly in a number of contexts, including Canadian feminist political economy (for example, O'Brien, 1978, 1981, 1990; Cummings, 1980). Yet another strand of work is discernible from feminist materialist anthropology, which (following an Engelsian tradition) ranks reproduction as important as if not more important than production (Mackintosh, 1977; Edholm *et al.*, 1977; Harris and Young, 1981). I have found all these perspectives immensely helpful in my own work on the structuring of reproduction in patriarchy (Hearn, 1983, 1987, 1992).

These questions have also been taken up in the realm of international politics. For example, the UN has been prominent in refining the measurement of economic activity; for example, through the distinction between productive activities that are market-orientated and included in national income accounts (System of National Accounts) (SNA), and those that are not (non-SNA). These have been measured through time-use studies, in which activities that could be performed by a third person (for example, cooking a meal) are counted as economic, and those that have to be performed by oneself (such as eating the meal or sleeping) are counted as personal and non-economic. In the most recent survey of thirteen individual countries, only 34 per cent of women's work time was spent on SNA activities and 66 per cent was spent on non-SNA activities, while for men the figures were reversed, 66 per cent of work being spent on SNA activity and 34 per cent on non-SNA activity (*Human Development Report 1995*, 1995: Table 4.2).[1]

The broad, global rethinking of work, economic activity, welfare, gender relations and gender empowerment has set a new scene for understanding not only women and welfare but also men and welfare.

FEMINISM AND SOCIAL POLICY

It is not an overstatement to argue that feminist theory and practice have transformed contemporary understandings of welfare and social policy. This comes from the insistent consciousness-raising of feminist politics and practice; feminist initiatives and politics in, around and against the state; focused feminist studies of the state of welfare and the welfare state; and feminist theory more generally, with its own multiple implications for the understanding and change of welfare and social policy.

Feminist work in and around social policy has increasingly named women in a number of different relations to welfare, the welfare state and its various institutional derivatives. There is now a very large body of work of this kind that makes the case for feminist analysis of social policy. Key works include those by Wilson (1977), McIntosh (1978), Barrett and McIntosh (1982), Finch and Groves (1983), Graham (1984), Dale and Foster (1986), Pascall (1986, 1997), Pateman (1988), Williams (1989), Dominelli (1991), MacLean and Groves (1991), Bock and Thane (1994), Hallett (1996). Accordingly, women have been the focus of much recent research on welfare: as recipients and users of health and welfare services, as the providers of welfare in both the private and public domains, as the target of preventive health and welfare campaigns, and as the victims and survivors of various kinds of diswelfare – violence, abuse, mental illness and so on.

Tyyskä (1995: 19–20) has argued that there are two other apparently contradictory strands in feminist approaches to welfare. The first has focused on the critique of the welfare state in view of its patriarchal and/or capitalist assumptions and policies; the second has treated the notion of community caring with suspicion, highlighting how this can be a way of shifting financial and other material burdens from the state to the unpaid work of women.

Partly because of such debates and contradictions, feminist studies of welfare have tended gradually to broaden their analysis from an initial focus on women as a general category of recipients of welfare to the plight of particular groups of women, to the position of women throughout the welfare system, to the examination of gendered processes throughout welfare, and most recently the intersection of gendered processes with other processes, such as those of racialization.

Sainsbury (1994) has argued that '[a] weakness of early feminist studies was a generic view of the welfare state and a lack of attention to differences in state formation. . . . Gradually feminists have extended the horizons of their theorizing and comparisons, and in the process the welfare state has been superseded by welfare states' (p. 2). She continues, stating that two broad approaches to the gendering of welfare states can be discerned:

> [t]he first has been to problematize several basic concepts in the mainstream literature by inquiring how they are gendered. In effect, this approach seeks to utilize mainstream theories and conceptions, and when necessary to refashion them, so as to encompass both women and men (Orloff, 1993; O'Connor, 1993). The second approach argues that mainstream theories are fundamentally lacking. Because crucial elements are missing, alternative theories and models are required (Lewis and Ostner, 1991; Lewis, 1992).
>
> (1994: 2–3)

To some extent these feminist critiques have been developed in response to non-gendered comparative studies of welfare, most prominently that of Esping-Andersen (1990). His classification of welfare states has been based on the extent to which the commodity status of labour is eroded through welfare. Accordingly he distinguished Conservative, Social Democratic and Labour Regime Welfare Regimes. A number of feminist analysts have questioned this approach's neglect of gender relations. For example, Leibfried (1993) and Langan and Ostner (1991) have put forward modified welfare models that spell out gender implications more fully. Interestingly, these (partially) gendered welfare state models (Duncan, 1995) are themselves open to criticism for adding on gender to a fundamentally non-gendered approach (Leira, 1992; Lewis, 1992; Borchorst, 1990, 1994). Meanwhile, as Sainsbury has noted, attempts have been made to argue for and reformulate our understanding of welfare and welfare states by placing gender and gender relations at the centre of analysis. Lewis (1992), for example, distinguishes strong, modified and weak breadwinner states, exemplified by Ireland, France and Sweden respectively (also see Julkunen, 1996; Rubery *et al.*, 1996).

An alternative approach has been proposed by Hirdmann (1988, 1990, cited in Duncan 1994, 1995; Rantalaiho, 1996) in terms of differing gender contracts. The gender system is a general concept that refers to the whole organization of society through cultural superstructure, social integration and socialization; it is equivalent to patriarchy (Walby, 1986, 1990; Hearn, 1987, 1992) or the male-dominated gender order (Stacey, 1986) or the masculine gender system (Waters, 1989). The gender contract is a middle-range concept that in effect puts the gender system into operation – it is the set of rules that operate around what people of different sexes should do, think, be. Using the example of Sweden, Hirdmann distinguishes a housewife contract, a transitional contract and an equality contract in the development of welfare from the 1930s up to the 1980s. Most importantly she argues that the gender contract is not a temporary settlement or compromise between capital and labour, but one between men and women.

Other feminist analyses have focused more fully on gendered differentiation within welfare. For example, Fraser has distinguished different constructions of needs and identities by welfare systems within male-dominated, capitalist society. She thereby summarizes:

> the separate and unequal character of the two-tiered, gender-linked, race- and culture-biased US social welfare system in the following formulas: participants in the masculine subsystem are positioned as *rights-bearing beneficiaries* and *purchasing consumers* of services, thus as possessive individuals. Participants in the feminine subsystem, on the other hand, are positioned as *dependent clients*, or *the negatives of possessive individuals*.
>
> (Fraser, 1989: 153)

With all these and similar analyses of welfare states, we can ask the simple question – what are they saying explicitly or implicitly about men, and indeed masculinities? Generally, these conceptualizations of welfare are saying something about men in three main ways: in families (particularly the heterosexual family), in paid work (particularly full-time employment), and in the state (particularly as managers and decision-makers about welfare). Less usual in these gendered models of welfare are commentaries on men managing the institutions of capital, and men outside the heterosexual family (for example, gay or lone young men).

Although it has been relatively unusual for the focus of feminist analyses of social policy to be primarily on men, recent feminist studies increasingly re-include men, but this time as gendered controllers and citizens (see, for example, Bryson *et al.*, 1994; Daly, 1994). This brings us directly to the question – how is it that men, and masculinities, have come to be increasingly recognized as just as gendered as women and femininities?

CRITICAL STUDIES ON MEN

The recent growth of interest in the study and theorizing of men and masculinities has derived from a number of directions. First, there have been feminist critiques of men. These are inevitably diverse. They include liberal feminist critiques of men's unfairness and privilege; Marxist and socialist feminist critiques of men's economic class advantage; radical and lesbian feminist critiques of men's sexuality and violence; and black feminist critiques of (white) men's sexism and racism.

Second, there has been a very different set of critiques from (male) gay liberation and (male) gay scholarship, and to an extent queer theory and queer politics. These are premised on the assumption of desire for men and the desirability of men rather than the direct critique of men (see Edwards, 1994). What is being critiqued in gay perspectives is not men in general or even men's power but dominant heterosexual men and related masculinities. Queer theory and politics have problematized dichotomous thinking to sex, gender and sexualities even more profoundly, and have argued for activist, constructionist and fluid approaches (for example, Beemyn and Eliason, 1996).

Third, there have been some men's specific and explicit responses to feminism. This includes those with a specifically pro-feminist or anti-sexist orientation; but there is also other work that is more ambiguous in relation to feminism or even is anti-feminist in its perspective. The idea of 'men's studies' is one such ambiguous development, not least because it is unclear how such studies relate to feminism, and whether they are meant to refer to studies by men or of men.[2]

These three kinds of critique of men together make up what has come to be called Critical Studies on Men. Such studies have effectively brought the question of theorizing men and masculinities into sharper relief. Paradoxically, this makes men and masculinities *explicit objects* of theory and critique, and makes men and masculinities *problematic*. These critical studies are relevant to retheorizing welfare and social policy in several ways. First, they have prompted a series of political, theoretical and epistemological set of questions about how to study welfare and social policy. Second, there are questions around the general phenomena of welfare and social policy. Third, there are questions around specific forms of welfare and specific social policies.

In developing Critical Studies on Men, a number of concepts have been specifically developed. First and most obviously, there is the concept of 'men'. Men are a social category, whether this applies to particular men, all men, or the possibility of this category in the first place. Second, the concept of 'masculinity' may be thought of as a shorthand for the indications, the set of signs, that someone is a man, a member of the category of men. Third, the concept of 'masculinities' has been developed (Carrigan *et al.*, 1985; Connell, 1995) to refer to diverse forms of masculinity. In particular, it refers to the way in which particular forms of masculinity persist not just in relation to femininity, but also to other forms of masculinity. Accordingly, different forms of masculinity exist in relations of power, that may be characterized as hegemonic or subordinated in relation to one another.

Having said that, the emphasis upon masculinities does carry with it a number of limitations and these need to be acknowledged. First, there is the danger of the emphasis upon masculinities being a means of forgetting women, of losing women from analysis and politics. Second, the emphasis upon masculinities may divert attention from other social divisions and oppressions, and the interrelations of social divisions and oppressions. Third, the concept of 'masculinities' may be just too imprecise. It may refer to institutional patterns, behaviours, identities, experiences, appearance, practices, subjectivities. The concept is premised on the assumption of a pattern or gloss that can be reasonably summarized (McMahon, 1993; Hearn, 1996).

Among the many areas of current debate that have developed in recent years around the theorizing of men and masculinities, just three that have been particularly significant are introduced here:

the concept of 'patriarchy'; unities and differences between men and between masculinities; and sexuality and subjectivity. In each case tensions between generalizations about men and masculinity and specificities of particular men and particular masculinities may be identified.

Following its central political and theoretical place within Second Wave feminism, the concept of 'patriarchy' was subject to a number of feminist and pro-feminist critiques in the late 1970s (for example, Rowbotham, 1979; Atkinson, 1979). It was suggested that the concept was too monolithic, ahistorical, biologically overdetermined, and dismissive of women's resistance and agency. Despite these critiques, the concept has not been dismissed. Instead, there has been greater attention to, first, the historicizing and periodizing of patriarchy; and second, the presence of multiple arenas, sites and structures of patriarchy. On the first count, particular attention has been paid to the historical movement from private patriarchy, where men's power is located primarily in the private domain as fathers and husbands, to public patriarchy (or patriarchies), where men's power is located primarily in the public domain as capitalist and state managers and workers. The significance of public patriarchy lies partly in the fact that organizations become the prime social unit of men's domination. In the context of welfare and social policy this is particularly important as public domain welfare organizations are often arenas of contestation between men and women. On the second count, there have been attempts to specify the various sites or bases of patriarchy. These include analyses by Walby (1986, 1990) specifying the following sets of patriarchal structures: capitalist work, the family, the state, violence, sexuality and culture. I have specified a slightly different set of structures: reproduction of labour power, procreation, regeneration/ degeneration, violence, sexuality and ideology (Hearn, 1987, 1992).

A second major area of debate has been around unities and differences between men and masculinities. Just as one of the major areas of theory and practice within feminism has been around the extent to which there are commonalities and differences between women, so too men can be usefully analysed in terms of commonalities and differences. In some ways these debates mirror debates on the concept of 'patriarchy', particularly the diversity of 'patriarchies' and patriarchal arenas. One way of understanding such unities or potential unities is through the concept of gender class – whether seen in terms of biological reproduction (Firestone, 1970;

O'Brien, 1981), sexuality (MacKinnon, 1982, 1983) or household relations and work (Delphy, 1977, 1984). All of these and indeed other social relations might be seen as possible social bases of the gender class of men (Hearn, 1987, 1992). However, the idea of a unity of men is *also* a myth. Indeed, one of the ways that men's collective power is maintained is through the assumption of hegemonic forms of men and masculinities as the most important or sole form. The focus on the assumption of white, heterosexual, able-bodied men to the exclusion of other kinds of men remains a major issue for both practical politics and theoretical analysis. Instead of there being just one kind of men, dominant or otherwise, different kinds of masculinities are reproduced, often in relation to other social divisions. In many social arenas there are tensions between the collective power of men and masculinities and differentiations among men and masculinities. Of especial importance are the differentiations between men and between masculinities, defined in part by other social divisions, such as age, class, disability, race and sexuality (Collinson and Hearn, 1994). Social policy and welfare more generally are both constructed through such divisions, and act as and reproduce social divisions between different men and masculinities.

A third area of debate on theorizing men and masculinities has been around sexuality and subjectivity, or more precisely sexualities and subjectivities. The tension between unities and differences, as described above, can be extended to the realm of sexuality. This derives from the increasing interest that has been given to the experience of masculinity and the interrelation of masculinity and identity. These debates on men's sexualities and subjectivities have various relevances for the analysis of welfare and social policy. First and most obviously, welfare and social policy provide significant social *contexts* for men's sexualities and subjectivities. Second, welfare and social policy provide *resources* for the elaboration of men's sexualities and subjectivities, for example, social policies and practices may be used for individual and collective defence by men. Third, there are the *specific enactments or instances* of men's sexualities and subjectivities. Within these contexts, resources and instances, there are recurring tensions – between the domination of heterosexuality and homosociality/homosexuality; asexuality and the sexualization/the eroticization of dominance and hierarchy; coherent identity and fragmented identity; and essentialized experience and deconstruction.

RETHINKING MEN AND SOCIAL POLICY

In the remainder of this chapter, I bring together the preceding discussions on welfare and on men – in rethinking the relationship of men and social policy. This does not just apply to the delivery of welfare services, but also to the dominant notions and forms of welfare. Different feminist perspectives on welfare and social policy in turn have different implications for the analysis of men and masculinities. For example, approaches that argue for the critique of the patriarchal and/or capitalist welfare state as opposed to women's interests are implicitly at least also presenting an account of men. In particular, these include men's relationship to experiences of power in and around the state, whether it is characterized as patriarchal (Pateman, 1988), fraternal (Pringle and Watson, 1990) or a system of masculine dominance (Burstyn, 1983). In emphasizing the patriarchal interests of the (welfare) state, men are implicitly understood as, first, having patriarchal interests as a collectivity, and, second, as occupying different positions in relation to the state – as managers, policy-makers, clients and so on. In emphasizing the capitalist interests of the (welfare) state, another set of distinctions are suggested – most obviously in terms of men's different locations in the capitalist class system, though here again men's differential relation to the state is important. In contrast to both of these approaches, some feminist perspectives have focused on the structuring of care and caring. The critique of community care directs attention not only to women's paid/unpaid care but also men's paid/unpaid care, and men's avoidance and control of care.

While welfare, of women, men and children, is affected by all structures of society, the dominant construction of welfare through the state and the welfare state is much more specific. Dominant constructions of welfare and social policy are centred on the organization of broadly reproductive processes. Policy as a broad social phenomenon is both, a major way of organizing reproduction (in the widest sense of that term), and a way of organizing the public domains, as maintained by the public–private division (or difference). In addition, and perhaps most significantly, social policy represents the public organization of reproduction – of that which occurs materially largely in the private domains, that is then subsequently organized in public. Indeed, such material activity is generally assumed to pre-exist in the private domains. Thus even though more value is usually given by men to public institutions rather than the private domains, the assumption remains within liberal democratic thinking that the public institutions are organizing preexisting private domains.

Social policy is thus concerned with the public rule over the private, the placing of reproduction in the private domains into the control of the institutions of the public domains, and thus men. Social policy and the very category 'welfare' are the public organization of reproductive labour. The phenomenon of social policy is itself a representation of organized gender divisions. Without the public–private division/difference there would be no social policy. In trying to understand the structuring of welfare within patriarchy, four dominant institutions are fundamentally important: namely, hierarchic heterosexuality; fatherhood in the heterosexual family; the professions; and the state. Social policy is especially concerned with a variety of activities and constructions between those institutions across the public–private division/difference.

The full range of experiences that occur within the private domains, including those of life, death, pain, sorrow, and sexual and emotional life more generally, are the focus of reproductive labour and emotional labour. Whereas with most of what is called 'productive labour', people work on objects to produce objects, with reproductive labour and emotional labour people are both the subjects and the objects of the labour. People work involves a social process *throughout*. Women have often been prominent in first of all making reproductive and emotional labour more public, and then transfer some of it and some of its organization and management from the private to the public domains (Hearn, 1982). Much of this process of publicization (Brown, 1981) has meant that reproductive labour becomes more fully under the control of men as a gender class; it is in a sense incorporated by men. In some cases this process has involved the specific exclusion of women, as, for example, with men's control of the professions. Having said that, these movements from the private to the public are extremely complex. For one thing, there is no absolute divide between the private and the public domains (Bose, 1987; Hearn, 1992, 1994). More specifically, the processes of movement from private to public may include the establishment of feminist action; initial incorporation through serving an individual man or an established profession; setting the *status quo* through the development of the patriarchal feminine and the professional code; division of the profession in gender segregation; and men's takeover through managerialism, men in management and full professionalization (Hearn, 1982). Having said that, the establishment and development of professions can also be subject to contrasting processes of feminization. For example, medicine, still a male bastion in some societies, may be providing posts for increasing numbers of women, especially at the lower levels of the profession.

Throughout the history of welfare, men have often acted in their own collective interests as husbands, fathers, workers and managers and have on occasion acted against those interests, and placed women's interests as a higher priority. The history of the development of welfare can be re-read not just as the extension of agendered citizenship or women's citizenship but also as a story in which men have a number of different locations, positions and interests – as citizens, politicians, workers, managers, professionals, recipients. This mirrors recent feminist Nordic analyses of welfare and the welfare state in terms of women's differential locations (for example, Hernes, 1988a, 1988b; Borchorst, 1990, 1994). In much of this work the emphasis has been on the tripartite relation of women as professionals, workers and clients/recipients. Re-applying this kind of perspective to men involves both synthetic analyses of broad patterns of relationships of different men (that is, men in different social locations as, for example, fathers, husbands, workers, managers) in relation to the welfare system, and more particular analyses of the variability of those relations to welfare, over time, between societies, and by other social divisions, such as age, class, disability, race, sexuality.

Sometimes these distinctions are clearest when one looks back at historical change around welfare. For example, there has been extensive study of the eighteenth- and nineteenth-century construction of the heterosexual or homosexual man, inside or outside marriage (Weeks, 1977; Mort, 1987; Hearn, 1992; Collier, 1995). Religion, medicine, science, law and, more specifically, welfare reform were all important in stipulating the 'correct' form of the family (as in the Marriage Act of 1836 and five subsequent Matrimonial Causes Acts up to 1895) or the assumed nature of male and female sexualities (as in the Contagious Diseases Acts of 1864, 1866 and 1869 and their repeal). Sexualities and their construction, and in this context men's sexualities, continue to be of immense importance in the definitions and delivery of welfare, often unevenly between and among women and men.

Meanwhile, another closely connected set of social relations were developed for men in the second half of the nineteenth century. First, the respectable working man was argued to be *prudent*, an obligation which required him to take a range of active steps to secure himself, his family and his dependants against future misfortune: joining insurance schemes provided by trade associations or friendly societies, personal involvement in the selection of benefits and the making of regular payments and so forth (Defert, 1991; Rose, 1996: 341). These associative relations were soon displaced by private insurance schemes run for profit, and then at the turn of the century the state intervened with national schemes of compulsory social insurance (Rose, 1996: 341). Throughout the twentieth century the place and norm of the working man and the so-called 'family wage' have continued to be crucial in the governance of welfare. In the strategies of government that developed over the twentieth century, the domains of the economic and the social were distinguished, but governed according to the principle of optimization. Economic activity, in the form of wage labour, was given a new set of *social* responsibilities, seen as a mechanism which would link males into the social order, and which would establish a proper relationship between the familial, the social and the economic orders (Rose, 1996: 338).

Another set of considerations affecting the relationship of men and welfare derived from the movement to modern welfare and the creation of mass male armies, first with the Boer War and then with the First World War. Boer War recruitment revealed the parlous state of men's health. The late nineteenth century also showed military interest in the control of soldiers' drinking and the creation of institutional eating facilities for them. The external threats of the First World War brought not only an urgent concern for the state of economic, industrial and chemical resources (Gummett, 1980), but also a parallel concern for human resources, and particularly the health of men as workers and soldiers. As Harris (1961: 7) puts it: 'the . . . search for a supply of efficient labour has been one of the few continuous threads in the history of welfare'. The Factory Inspectorate, the Health of Munitions Workers Committee Report of 1916 and the Ministry of Munitions all argued for the beneficial effects of planned nourishment and nutrition. The first Director of the Welfare Section of the Ministry, B. Seebohm Rowntree, noted that 'workers who are in good health are more efficient workers' (quoted in Harris, ibid.). In

1919 the Ministry of Health was introduced very much as a response to these problems of men as bodies. And meanwhile in the post-First World War period, public housing was expanded to provide homes fit for heroes. All of these changes in the late nineteenth century and the early twentieth century have contributed to the strong historical associations of men, manhood and the modern nation-state. For some men at least, these connections involved particular senses of imperialist manhood/nationhood, mediated by age, class, ethnicity and sexuality (see Mangan and Walvin, 1986).

These arguments on men and welfare can be related to debates around the connection of national crises, and particularly war, and the collective willingness or ability to develop the welfare state (Peacock and Wiseman, 1961; Fennell, 1990). For example, Wilensky (1975) traces the inception of the Swedish welfare state in the 1930s to responses to unrest and crisis. While such connections can be re-interpreted within a neo-Marxist view as part of ruling-class concessions to working-class demands, it is more interesting to consider the gendered character of state welfare concessions in the face of internal threat. Welfare reform, and especially that around income maintenance, can sometimes be understood partly as a pre-emptive response by the state – that is, men in the state – to the actual and potential unrest of men, particularly young men. In such developments it is men who overwhelmingly retain control of the state in general and the military in particular, and all the more so at times of crisis, which themselves may tend to involve younger, often working-class men as actual or potential insurgents, police or soldiers. The power of men in the state, army, police and criminal justice sector, with their apparatuses and machinery of violence and potential violence, may contrast abruptly with the power of individual men, small groups of men and even non-state collectivities of men, with their direct interpersonal violence and potential violence. Accordingly, as well as placing women's action and activity as central in welfare reform, it is possible to also distinguish the relative parts played by different groups of men as state politicians, state managers, workers, actual or potential insurgents and indeed beneficiaries.

The impact of the Second World War on the development of new forms of citizenship, of state planning and welfare priorities has been well established (Thane, 1982). These processes are clearly gendered – with men's movement to and return from war; women's involvement in munitions, engineering and other new work and their loss of such employment; and the evacuation of women and children to new living areas and then their subsequent return (Riley, 1983).[3] While broad correlations can be drawn between expenditure on the military and on welfare – the welfare–warfare state – there are also important exceptions to this trend (Wilensky, 1975). Indeed, heavy military burdens can themselves drain energy, expertise and resources away from domestic welfare programmes, which can in turn lead to further social antagonisms and backlash against welfare, so slowing down welfare state development (Wilensky, 1972). Either way, these macro-arguments on welfare are at least in part about the differential place of men in and around the state – as state decision-makers, military managers, soldiers, workers, welfare recipients. Furthermore, all of these historical changes in men's relation to sexuality and violence, the nation, the family, health, income maintenance, the military and civil unrest were important in the development of modern state forms and patterns of governmentality. These developments did not comprise a coherent programme of 'state intervention', but rather a diverse series of liberal interventions based in governmental knowledge of human conduct, the creation of active subjects, the authority of expertise and reflexivity on the question of rule itself (Rose, 1993).

Just as women have a contradictory relation to welfare, so too do men. Social policy and welfare systems can be a means of providing benefits and services to women formerly unavailable to them; however, at the same time, such systems can be a means of control or constraint on women by reinforcing patriarchal assumptions and practices. Similarly, men have a contradictory relation to welfare, though in a different way from women. On the one hand, social policy and welfare systems can involve the redistribution of resources from men's control, even if men are in operational control of the system; on the other, such systems can increase men's control of women, even if women are in operational control of the system. For example, income maintenance can provide a means of livelihood, albeit characteristically close to subsistence, for women and children from the (patriarchical) state rather than directly from (patriarchal) capitalist or other sources; at the same time, those very systems of income maintenance have frequently involved relative discrimination and disadvantage against women – both in their public, state definitions and delivery, and their private distribution within families.

Furthermore, while women do the majority of care work, both paid and unpaid, there has been considerable debate on the extent of care done by men, particularly older men (for example, Arber and Gilbert, 1989; Chapter 7 this volume). The relationship of men to the provision of welfare services can also be contradictory. In some situations, men may receive preferential treatment over women; for example, at times of family crisis or when it is assumed that men cannot cope. On the other hand, men may tend to use some welfare services less than women. This is most clearly seen in the field of health, both physical and mental. Briscoe (1989, cited in Lloyd and Wood, 1996: 9) suggests that, from an early age, girls become orientated towards the tendency to seek medical care for a variety of complaints, whereas boys learn to disregard pain and avoid doctors; hence an association is formed between being feminine and being more concerned with health. This kind of pattern is itself highly complicated, by, for example, class variations among girls and women's use of medical services, and some boys and men's involvement with sport and fitness.

For these reasons men may have quite diverse relations with welfare and welfare services – sometimes as those needing care from others, for example, around depression or addiction; sometimes as those needing control, for example, around violence; sometimes as those absent from or avoiding contact, from care and/or control (Hearn, 1998). Indeed, all of these relations can occur simultaneously for particular welfare agencies and individual men. What is perhaps most interesting is that patriarchical relations can persist and be reproduced through the combination of men's control of welfare, men's need for and sometimes avoidance of care (both of themselves and by others), men's need for and sometimes avoidance of control (both of themselves and by others). To put this more directly, men's power can also involve damage to men, not least in violence between men, accidents, suicide and lower life expectancy. These processes may damage individual men, and even whole categories of men, but paradoxically may assist the maintenance of men's collective power.

Throughout all these discussions of the shifting relations of men and welfare, it is important to ask the simple question – which men are we talking about? Sometimes it is men in the state; sometimes it is employed breadwinning, family men; sometimes it is men who are not employed. In particular, we can usefully ask how these specific relations of men to welfare, whether as policy-makers, beneficiaries or whatever, apply to black men, men of colour, immigrant men and ethnic minority men. There is clearly no one answer to this kind of question. However, at the very least it is necessary to consider how men's relation to welfare is determined, affected or mediated by legal nationality and by racism in and around the state and in society more generally. Such issues of 'race', racism and nationality may also be intimately bound up with those of sexuality. The state frequently defines citizens, and especially new and potential citizens, in reference to their sexuality, actual or perceived, and their marital status. Marriage is after all a state institution; and the nation-state is dominantly, but not exclusively, heterosexual. Thus men, and especially black and (potential) immigrant men, along with their relatives, may be defined by the state in relation to the presence or absence of heterosexual marriage. Gay marriage is not an easy route to citizenship for men who are not legally national citizens; similarly, gay men who are not married, like lesbians in the same situation, usually find it extremely difficult, if not impossible, to receive pensions and housing rights on the death of their partners.

Social policy is of course organized through a number of different policy areas, with their own particular institutional traditions, organizational arrangements, rules and procedures. Each of these provides not just services but also organizational spaces for workers, managers and policy-makers. Men figure differentially in these different policy arenas in these various locations. These social policy institutions and service delivery systems also provide the social spaces for different kinds of men, different kinds of masculinities – for the reproduction and occasionally opposition to masculinism. Just as it has become commonplace to speak of 'femocrats' (Yeatman, 1990; Watson, 1990; Franzway et al., 1989) who are simultaneously feminists and bureaucrats, so one might identify 'mascocrats' who are simultaneously masculinists and bureaucrats. Less common are men who are both bureaucrats and anti-masculinist/pro-feminist. These are just some of the ways for men to do masculinity, to be men, in the public domains. Other masculinities may be constructed by men in receipt of welfare services or in other related contexts, such as through the criminal justice system. These structures of welfare of course provide all kinds of possibilities for men to ally themselves with one another, and indeed to oppose, compete with and distance themselves from one another. Alliances, oppositions, continuities and discontinuities between men can also operate *across* the boundaries between the public and private domains.

CONTEMPORARY DEVELOPMENTS

All of the policy areas of social policy – housing, health, education, income support, disability, social services, criminal justice and so on – are relevant for the understanding of men and masculinities. Likewise, men and masculinities are relevant for the understanding of each of those policy areas. The trouble with men remains a practical, political and theoretical issue in each policy area. It raises questions of historical and contemporary dominance by men, men's responses to women's initiatives, men's differential locations and actions in these arenas, and then more sporadically the existence and possibilities for anti-sexist, pro-feminist action there.

Inevitably, men's relationship to welfare is also subject to changing social policies at both governmental and local levels. In particular, recent changes in patterns of governance have included the privatization of welfare services, the introduction of internal markets, the reduction of administrative discretion, the restriction of welfare payments (to the unemployed, young adults, students and others), and the fragmentation of state structures, along with increasing centralization of state financial and policy control. These developments can be seen as linked with other shifts, such as the impact of globalization and the separation of the nation and the economy (Rose, 1996). Some commentators have described the development of advanced liberal government (Rose, 1993), in which there is a new relation between expertise and politics, based on calculative regimes of accounting and financial management; a new pluralization of social technologies; and a new specification of the subject of government as self-monitoring, active agents. In this move from modern to postmodern governmentality, men are constructed in a changing relation to welfare – both as managers and purveyors of expertise around welfare and as self-monitoring customers and clients of welfare systems. The patriarchal/fratriarchal breadwinner state is being transmuted to a more complex, dispersal of the state constructions in which men have a more variable series of locations. This dispersal of the state raises the possibility of a whole range of mini-patriarchies and mini-fratriarchies that in turn construct men in diverse ways, through state bureaucracies, markets, community initiatives, third sector organizations, quangos and other interventions.

Twenty or even fifteen years ago, information on the specific location of men in relation to welfare was very limited (Hearn, 1980). Now there is a literature on almost all areas of social policy, which both chronicles relevant events of the past and present and puts forward possibilities for further future action – on men and/or by men (Pringle, 1995). There has been a particularly major development of commentaries and suggestions for actions in education and youth work (for example, Equal Opportunities Commission, 1982; Askew and Ross, 1988; Lloyd, 1985; Mahoney, 1985; Mac an Ghaill, 1994; Salisbury and Jackson, 1996); social work, social services, probation and the criminal justice system (for example, Kadushin, 1976; Hearn, 1990; Cavanagh and Cree, 1996; Potts, 1996; Wild, 1998). Of special importance is the recognition of the urgency of ending the social problem of men's violence and abuse to women, children and indeed other men.

Men's practice in and around welfare can be understood collectively, by immediate social group, and individually. One can also ask the question, what do men do politically in the face of all these issues? While men's practice in and around welfare can broadly reinforce or oppose masculinization, it may often be more accurate to consider the contradictions that bear on men. Indeed, contradictions and processes of re-incorporation operate in whatever arena men may try to act to change their politics and themselves. These questions of practice apply in private and the domestic area in public working lives, in trade-union and political activity, in campaigns around reproductive politics; in anti-sexist men's activities; in men's relation to women, children and one another. This can mean men both gaining new experiences and losing certain powers, and as such changing men's relationship to welfare and social policy.

ACKNOWLEDGEMENT

I am grateful to David Collinson for discussions on some of the theoretical issues raised in this chapter, and to Jeanette Edwards and Jennie Popay for comments on an earlier draft.

NOTES

1 Interestingly, according to the United Nations Development Programme 1995 Report (*Human Development Report 1995*, 1995: Table 3.5), the UK ranks nineteenth in the world, between Hungary and Bulgaria, on the measure of gender empowerment (GEM). The measure is compiled from the aggregation of four sub-measures; of percentage of seats held in Parliament by women (7.4% in the UK), percentage of administrators and managers who are women (22.7%), percentage of professional and technical workers who are women (39.6%), and women's share of earned income (30.8% [*sic.*]).

2 A contrast can be drawn in the US context between those studies that are broadly pro-feminist (for example, Brod, 1987), those that are ambiguous in relation to feminism (for example, Bly, 1990), and those that are anti-feminist (for example, Baumli, 1985). For discussions of the critique of men's studies, see Hearn, 1989, and several of the contributions in Hearn and Morgan, 1990.

3 This pattern was not repeated throughout Europe. For example, Finnish women were not restored to their homes after the Second World War (Rantalaiho, 1996: 26).

REFERENCES

Arber, S. and Gilbert, N. (1989) 'Men: the forgotten carers?', *Sociology*, 23(1): 111–18.

Askew, S. and Ross, C. (1988) *Boys Don't Cry*, Milton Keynes: Open University Press.

Atkinson, P. (1979) 'The problem with patriarchy', *Achilles Heel*, 2: 18–22.

Barrett, M. and McIntosh, M. (1982) *The Anti-Social Family*, London: Verso.

Baumli, Francis (ed.) (1985) *Men Freeing Men*, New Atlantic: Jersey City.

Beemyn, Brett and Eliason, Mickey (eds) (1996) *Queer Studies: A Lesbian, Gay, Bisexual and Transgender Anthology*, New York: New York University Press.

Bly, Robert (1990) *Iron John: A Book About Men*, New York: Addison-Wesley.

Bock, G. and Thane, P. (eds) (1994) *Maternity and Gender Policies: Women and the Rise of the European Welfare States 1880–1950*, London: Routledge.

Borchorst, A. (1990) *The Scandinavian Welfare States: Patriarchal, Gender Neutral or Women-Friendly?* Aarhus: Institute for Political Science, University of Aarhus.

—— (1994) 'Scandinavian welfare states – patriarchal, gender neutral or women friendly?', *International Journal of Contemporary Sociology*, 31(1).

Bose, L. (1987) 'Dual spheres' in B.B. Hess and M.M. Ferree (eds) *Analyzing Gender: A Handbook of Social Science Research*, Newbury Park, CA: Sage.

Briscoe, M.E. (1989) 'Sex differences in mental health', *Update* (1 November): 834–9.

Brod, Harry (ed.) (1987) *The Making of Masculinities: The New Men's Studies*, London: Allen & Unwin.

Brown, C. (1981) 'Mothers, fathers and children: from private to public patriarchy' in L. Sargent (ed.) *Women and Revolution: The Unhappy Marriage of Marxism and Feminism*, New York: Maple.

Bryson, L., Bittman, M. and Donath, S. (1994) 'Men's welfare state, women's welfare state: tendencies to convergence in practice and theory?', in D. Sainsbury (ed.) *Gendering Welfare States*, London: Sage.

Burstyn, V. (1983) 'Masculine dominance and the state', in R. Miliband and J. Savile (eds) *The Socialist Register 1983*, London: Merlin.

Carrigan, T., Connell, R.W. and Lee, J. (1985) 'Toward a new sociology of masculinity', *Theory and Society*, 14(5): 551–604.

Castells, M. (1977) *The Urban Question: A Marxist Approach*, London: Edward Arnold.

Cavanagh, K. and Cree, V. (eds) (1996) *Working with Men*, London: Routledge.

Collier, R. (1995) *Masculinity, Law and the Family*, London: Routledge.

Collinson, D. and Hearn, J. (1994) 'Naming men as men: implications for work, organizations and management', *Gender, Work and Organization* 1(1): 2–22.

Connell, R.W. (1995) *Masculinities*, Cambridge: Polity.

Cummings, J.E. (1980) 'Sexism in social work: some thoughts on strategy for structural change', *Catalyst*, 8.

Dale, J. and Foster, P. (1986) *Feminists and State Welfare*, London: Routledge & Kegan Paul.

Daly, M. (1994) 'Comparing welfare states: towards a gender friendly approach', in D. Sainsbury (ed.) *Gendering Welfare States*, London: Sage.

Defert, D. (1991) 'Popular life and insurance technology', in G. Burchell, C. Gordon and P. Miller (eds) *The Foucault Effect: Studies in Governmentality*, Hemel Hempstead: Harvester Wheatsheaf.

Delphy, C. (1977) *The Main Enemy*, London: Women's Research and Resources Centre.

—— (1984) *Close to Home: A Materialist Analysis of Women's Oppression*, London: Hutchinson.

Dominelli, L. (1991) *Women across Continents: Feminist Comparative Social Policy*, London: Harvester Wheatsheaf.

Duncan, S. (1994) 'Theorising differences in patriarchy', *Environment and Planning* 26: 1177–94.

—— (1995) 'Theorizing European gender systems', *Journal of European Social Policy*, 5(4): 263–84.

Edholm, F., Harris, O. and Young, K. (1977) 'Conceptualising women', *Critique of Anthropology*, 3: 101–30.

Edwards, T. (1994) *Erotics and Politics*, London: Routledge.

Equal Opportunities Commission (1982) *What's In It for the Boys?* Manchester/London: EOC/ILEA.

Esping-Andersen, G. (1990) *The Three Worlds of Welfare Capitalism*, Cambridge: Polity.

Fennell, G. (1990) 'The Second World War and the welfare state in Britain: sociological interpretations of historical development', in L. Jamieson and H. Corr (eds) *State, Private Life and Political Change*, London: Macmillan.

Finch, J. and Groves, D. (1983) *A Labour of Love*, London: Routledge & Kegan Paul.

Firestone, S. (1970) *The Dialectic of Sex*, London: Jonathan Cape.

Fraser, N. (1989) *Unruly Practices*, Cambridge: Polity.

Franzway, S., Court, D. and Connell, R.W. (1989) *Staking a Claim: Feminism, Bureaucracy and the State*, Cambridge: Polity.

Gardiner, J. (1975) 'Women's domestic labour', *New Left Review*, 89.

Gough, I. (1983) *The Political Economy of the Welfare State*, London: Macmillan.

Graham, H. (1984) *Women, Health and the Family*, Brighton: Harvester Wheatsheaf.

Gummett, P. (1980) *Scientists in Whitehall*, Manchester: Manchester University Press.

Hallett, C. (1996) *Women and Social Policy*, Hemel Hempstead: Harvester Wheatsheaf.

Harris, N. (1961) 'The decline of welfare', *International Socialism* (Winter).

Harris, O. and Young, K. (1981) 'Engendered structures: some problems in the analysis of reproduction', in J.S. Kahn and J.R. Llobera (eds) *The Anthropology of Pre-Capitalist Societies*, London: Macmillan.

Hearn, J. (1980) 'Men's politics and social policy', *Bulletin on Social Policy*, 5: 53–7.

—— (1982) 'Notes on patriarchy, professionalisation and the semi-professions', *Sociology*, 16(2): 184–202.

—— (1983) *Birth and Afterbirth: A Materialist Account*, London: Achilles Heel.

—— (1987) *The Gender of Oppression: Men, Masculinity and the Critique of Marxism*, Brighton: Wheatsheaf.

—— (1989) 'Reviewing men and masculinities – or mostly boys' own papers', *Theory, Culture and Society*, 6: 665–89.

—— (1990) 'Child abuse and men's violence', in Violence Against Children Study Group (ed.) *Taking Child Abuse Seriously*, London: Unwin Hyman.

—— (1992) *Men in the Public Eye: The Construction and Deconstruction of Public Men and Public Patriarchies*, London: Routledge.

—— (1994) 'Men in the public domains', in S. Edgell, S. Walklate and G. Williams (eds) *Debating the Future of the Public Sphere*, Aldershot: Avebury.

—— (1996) 'Is masculinity dead? A critique of the concept of masculinity/masculinities', in M. Mac an Ghaill (ed.) *Understanding Masculinities: Social Relations and Cultural Arenas*, Buckingham: Open University Press.

—— (1998) 'It's time for men to change', in J.Wild (ed.) *Working with Men for Change*, Basingstoke: Taylor & Francis.

Hearn, J. and Collinson, D.L. (1994) 'Theorizing unities and differences between men and between masculinities', in H. Brod and M. Kaufman (eds) *Theorizing Masculinities*, Thousand Oaks, CA: Sage.

Hearn, Jeff and Morgan, David (eds) (1990) *Men, Masculinities and Social Theory*, London: Unwin Hyman.

Hernes, H. (1988a) 'Scandinavian citizenship', *Acta Sociologica*, 31(3): 199–215.

—— (1988b) 'The welfare state citizenship of Scandinavian women', in K.B. Jones and A.G. Jónasdóttir (eds) *The Political Interests of Gender*, London: Sage.

Himmelweit, S. and Mohun, S. (1977) 'Domestic labour and capital', *Cambridge Journal of Economics*, 1(1).

Hirdmann, Y. (1988) 'Genussystemet – reflexioner kring kvinnors sociala underordning', *Kvinnovetenskaplig Tidskrift*, 3: 49–63.

—— (1990) Genussystemet in *Demokrati och Makt i Sverige*, Stockholm: Statens Offentliga Utredningar.

Human Development Report 1995 (1995) New York/Oxford: Oxford University Press for the United Nations Development Programme.

Julkunen, Raija (1996) 'Women's rights in Finland', *Finfo*, 6/96: 3–10.

Kadushin, K. (1976) 'Men in a woman's profession', *Social Work*, 21(6): 440–7.

Langan, M. and Ostner, I. (1991) 'Gender and welfare: towards a comparative framework', in G. Room (ed.) *Towards a European Welfare State*, Bristol: SAUS, University of Bristol.

Laybourn, K. (1995) *The Evolution of British Social Policy in the Welfare State*, Keele: Keele University Press.

Leibfried, S. (1993) 'Towards a European welfare state', in C. Jones (ed.) *New Perspectives on the Welfare State in Europe*, London: Routledge.

Leira, A. (1992) *Welfare States and Working Mothers: The Scandinavian Experience*, Cambridge: Cambridge University Press.

Lewis, J. (1992) 'Gender and the development of welfare regimes', *Journal of European Social Policy*, 2(3): 159–73.

Lewis, J. and Ostner, I. (1991) 'Gender and the evolution of European social policies', Paper at CES Workshop on Emergent Supranational Social Policy: The EC's Social Dimension in Comparative Perspective, Center for European Studies: Harvard University.

Lloyd, T. (1985) *Working With Boys*, Leicester: National Youth Bureau.

Lloyd, T. and Wood, T. (1996) 'The evidence', in T. Lloyd and T.Wood (eds) *What Next for Men?*, London: Working with Men.

Mac an Ghaill, M. (ed.) (1994) *The Making of Men: Masculinities, Sexualities and Schooling*, Milton Keynes: Open University Press.

McIntosh, M. (1978) 'The state and the oppression of women', in A. Kuhn and A.M. Wolps (eds) *Feminism and Materialism*, London: Routledge & Kegan Paul.

MacKinnon, C.A. (1982) 'Feminism, Marxism, method and the state in an agenda for theory', *Signs* 7(3): 515–44.

—— (1983) 'Feminism, Marxism, method and the state: toward feminist jurisprudence', *Signs* 8(4): 635–58.

Mackintosh, M. (1977) 'Reproduction and patriarchy: a critique of Meillassoux's *Femmes, Greniers et Capitaux*, *Capital and Class*, 2: 119–27.

MacLean, M. and Groves, D. (eds) (1991) *Women's Issues in Social Policy*, London: Routledge.

McMahon, A. (1993) 'Male readings of feminist theory: the psychologization of sexual politics in the masculinity literature', *Theory and Society*, 22(5): 675–96.

Mahoney, P. (1985) *Schools for the Boys?* London: Hutchinson.

Mangan, J.A. and Walvin, J. (eds) (1986) *Manliness and Morality: Middle-class Masculinity in Britain and America 1800–1940*, Manchester: Manchester University Press.

Mort, F. (1987) *Dangerous Sexualities: Medico-Moral Politics in England since 1830*, London: Routledge & Kegan Paul.

Nelson, J.A. (1996) *Feminism, Objectivity and Economics*, London: Routledge.

O'Brien, M. (1978) 'The dialectics of reproduction', *Women's Studies International Quarterly*, 1: 233–9.

—— (1981) *The Politics of Reproduction*, London: Routledge & Kegan Paul.

—— (1990) *Reproducing the World*, Boulder, CO: Westview.

O'Connor, J. (1974) *The Fiscal Crisis of the State*, New York: St Martin's Press.

O'Connor, J.S. (1993) 'Gender, class and citizenship in the comparative analysis of welfare state regimes: theoretical and methodological issues', *British Journal of Sociology*, 44(3): 501–18.

Orloff, A.S. (1993) 'Gender and the social rights of citizenship: state policies and gender relations in comparative research', *American Sociological Review*, 58(3): 303–28.

Pascall, G. (1986) *Social Policy: A Feminist Analysis*, London: Tavistock.

—— (1997) *Social Policy: A New Feminist Analysis*, London: Routledge.

Pateman, C. (1988) 'The patriarchal welfare state', in A. Gutman (ed.) *Democracy and Welfare State*, Princeton, NJ: Princeton University Press.

Peacock, A.T. and Wiseman, J. (1961) *The Growth of Public Expenditure in the United Kingdom*, Princeton, NJ: Princeton University Press.

Potts, D. (1996) *Why Do Men Commit Most Crime? Focusing on Masculinity in a Prison Group*, Wakefield: West Yorkshire Probation Service.

Pringle, K. (1995) *Men, Masculinities and Social Welfare*, London: UCL Press.

Pringle, R. and Watson, S. (1990) 'Fathers, brothers, mates: the fraternal state in Australia', in S. Watson (ed.) *Playing the State: Australian Feminist Interventions*, London: Verso.

Rantalaiho, L. (1996) 'Contextualizing gender', in L. Rantalaiho and T. Heiskanen (eds) *Gendered Practices in Working Life*, London: Macmillan.

Remy, J. (1990) 'Patriarchy and fratriarchy as forms of andocracy', in J. Hearn and D. Morgan (eds) *Men, Masculinities and Social Theory*, London: Unwin Hyman.

Riley, D. (1983) *War in the Nursery*, London: Virago.

Rose, N. (1993) 'Government, authority and expertise in advanced liberalism', *Economy and Society*, 22(3): 283–99.
—— (1996) 'The death of the social? Refiguring the territory of government', *Economy and Society*. 25(3): 327–56.
Rubery, Jill, Smith, Mark and Turner, Eloise (1996) *Bulletin on Women and Employment in the EU*, No.9 (October).
Rowbotham, S. (1979) 'The trouble with patriarchy', *New Statesman*, 98: 970.
Sainsbury, D. (ed.) (1994) *Gendering Welfare States*, London: Sage.
Salisbury, J. and Jackson, D. (1996) *Challenging Macho Values: Practical Ways of Working with Adolescent Boys*, London: Falmer.
Stacey, M. (1986) 'Gender and stratification: one central issue or two', in R. Crompton and M. Mann (eds) *Gender and Stratification*, Cambridge: Polity.
Thane, P. (1982) *The Foundation of the Welfare State*, London: Longman.
Tyyskä, V. (1995) *The Politics of Caring and the Welfare State*, Helsinki: Suomalainen Tiedeakatermia.
Walby, S. (1986) *Patriarchy at Work*, Cambridge: Polity.
—— (1990) *Theorizing Patriarchy*, Oxford: Basil Blackwell.
Waring, M. (1988) *Counting for Nothing: What Men Value and What Women are Worth*, Wellington, NZ: Allen & Unwin.
Waters, M. (1989) 'Patriarchy and viriarchy', *Sociology*, 23(2): 193–211.
Watson, S. (ed.) (1990) *Playing the State: Australian Feminist Interventions*, London: Verso.
Weeks, J. (1977) *Coming Out: Homosexual Politics in Britain from the Nineteenth Century to the Present*, London: Quartet.
Wild, J. (ed.) (1998) *Working with Men for Change*, Basingstoke: Taylor & Francis.
Wilensky, H.L. (1972) 'Intelligence, crises and foreign policy: reflections on the limits of rationality', in R.H. Blum (ed.) *Surveillance and Espionage in a Free Society*, New York: Praeger.
—— (1975) *The Welfare State and Equality*, Berkeley, CA: University of California Press.
Wilensky, H.L. and Lebeaux, C.N. (1958) *Industrial Society and Social Welfare*, New York: The Free Press.
Williams, F. (1989) *Social Policy: A Critical Introduction*, Cambridge: Polity.
Wilson, E. (1977) *Women and the Welfare State*, London: Tavistock.
Women's Budget Statement 1990–91 (1990) Canberra: Australian Government Publishing Service.
Yeatman, A. (1990) *Bureaucrats, Technocrats, Femocrats*, Sydney: Allen & Unwin.

Chapter 2

Troubled masculinities in social policy discourses
Young men

Jeff Hearn

The topic of men and the associated concept of 'masculinity' are now, just about, on political and policy agendas. Of course in many ways this is not new; it is just that now politicians, policy-makers, social policy managers, and increasingly practitioners are naming men and masculinities as an object of concern. This might be as something that needs to be attended to, to be dealt with, to be treated as a problem, to be changed, to be defended, or even just to be talked about and debated.

In contemporary UK and other similar societies, previously established ways of being men are being, if not destabilized, then at least questioned. This appears to be linked to a number of signi-ficant long-term social and economic changes; for example, rising male unemployment, greater paid employment of women, increas-ing rates of divorce and separation, increases in lone motherhood, the gradual democratization of parent–child relations, the high-lighting of the problem of men's violence, and shifts in racial, ethnic, national, religious and sexual identities. The attempt to reconstitute a sense of what it means to be a man is in progress in a wide range of political arenas – in social policies; in political debates; in personal quests and narratives; in law and legal con-testations; through academic research and writing; through femin-ism and backlashes to it; through cultural representations; and through the diverse organizations that represent men, such as divorced and separated fathers, anti-sexist, gay and bisexual men, as well as the multitude of organizations composed of or dominated by men that do not quite explicitly say they are men's mouthpieces for men.

These concerns with troubled masculinities have attracted atten-tion from across the political spectrum. However, that attention has not been evenly spread. Particular concern has been expressed from liberal feminist and socialist feminist commentators (Hewitt, Harman, Coote, Campbell, Melanie Phillips, Angela Phillips), from the older men formerly of the left but now of the centre (Halsey, Dennis and Erdos), and from the new right (Murray) (see Chapter 3, this volume). These and other commentaries are both divergent and convergent in different respects. They are clearly opposed, yet sometimes there are surprising similarities and over-laps. In addition, there have been a number of interventions from policy-makers and managers within the administration of the state; for example, police officers and medical officers. Often these commentaries have been pessimistic or at least driven by a notion of threat. Geoff Dench (1994: 190) has summarized some of these as follows:

> A fast growing library of studies, starting with Murray's develop-ment of Gilder's ideas (1984), and progressing in UK through Anderson (1991), Dennis and Erdos (1992 & 1993) have all iden-tified a core of irresponsible and purposeless men at the centre of our current social malaise. The culture of sex and violence (Greenstein, 1993), a rising tide of male early mortality and sui-cide (Hacker, 1991; Thomas, 1993), high long-term male un-employment rates, the deterioration in academic performance of boys even in science subjects, possibly some of the loss of busi-ness confidence at the heart of the recession, and arguably the for-mation of right-wing nationalist movements across Europe giving a sense of belonging to otherwise unattached and unlovable young men, have all been linked in some way to the erosion of the male breadwinner vocation.

Some, for example Harriet Harman (1993a, 1993b), have argued that time is running out for men and that men do not generally realize the seriousness of the situation, and yet have still remained relatively optimistic about the possibilities for change and for men sharing domestic responsibilities with women. In some cases the commentators have simply analysed; others have urged men to change before it is too late for them, for women or for society; others have concentrated on managing and controlling the problem.

There are perhaps three main elements to these developing poli-tical discourses of masculinity:

1 the naming of 'masculinity' or 'masculinities';
2 the identification of masculinity or masculinities as problematic or potentially problematic – constructing the problem in terms of what we call 'troubled masculinities';
3 the conscious understanding of the possibility of devising relevant policies to respond to these troubled masculinities, and thus constituting the right for intervention.

Sometimes, there is a fourth element:

4 the devising and implementation of relevant specific policies.

My starting point in addressing these questions draws on recent theoretical and empirical studies that have investigated men and masculinities from critical, feminist and pro-feminist perspectives (see pp. 17–20). The notion of 'masculinity/masculinities' and the production and practice of particular masculinities are both constructed through diverse historical and cultural contexts, structures and processes. Masculinity, less still masculinities, are not a single essential and coherent attribute attached to all men everywhere. Indeed in some senses, masculinities do not exist in any firm or absolute sense (Hearn, 1996). Rather, masculinities change over generations, according to the social positionings of age, class, disability, ethnicity, race, sexuality and other social divisions and differences, and reproduced through the variety of social practices that men do as fathers, sons, workers, husbands, partners, lovers and so on. Masculinities signify that a person is a man, whether in individual, collective or institutional contexts. This chapter is concerned primarily with how notions of masculinities, and particularly troubled masculinities, have figured in recent years in discourses, especially political and policy discourses, in and around social policy.

One further word of introduction is necessary around the idea of 'troubled masculinities'. In what sense are masculinities assumed to be troubled? There are perhaps five main ways in which this could be said to be the case. First, masculinities are troubled by other forces beyond themselves – by women, by technology, by rapid economic change and so on. Second, masculinities are troubled through internal contradictions and inconsistencies: they are subject to their own troubled processes, such as the contradiction between the search for control and the search for risk. Third, they are troubled in the related sense of not being simple or coherent phenomena; they are metaphorically troubled waters. Fourth, men may experience their own or other men's masculinities as 'troubling', discomforting, uneasy, uncertain. And fifth, the existence of these various forms of troubled masculinities may itself be seen as 'troubling', for policy-makers, political commentators and academic analysts alike.

This chapter thus explores these troubled masculinities, or more precisely discourses of troubled masculinities, through their construction within particular organizational contexts and policy arenas in which women, men and sometimes children, operate. In examining these issues, I mainly discuss one particular construction of troubled masculinities; namely, that of young men. This focus is important both politically and analytically; it is also linked to the concerns of the following chapter on fatherhood (also see Sarre, 1996), not least in the sense that young men may or may not be or become fathers. Both young men and fathers/fatherhood, and especially young fathers, are constructions that are often assumed to be especially troubled and indeed troubling.

TROUBLED MASCULINITIES IN POLICY ARENAS

Discourses and debates around masculinity and troubled masculinities do not occur in a vacuum; they find effects and evidence, and they gather their material in and around specific substantive policy arenas and organizational contexts. The various general discourses on masculinity are themselves grounded, if only to a limited extent, in reports of what is happening or assumed to be happening out there in society. These usually centre upon *particular* policy questions or social problem definitions; it is through these policy arenas that more general discourses of troubled masculinities can be recognized.

In many instances the focus of these debates on troubled masculinity is on boys, young men and young adult men, including young fathers and potential or former fathers. This is particularly so with regard to the analysis of men (or boys) and education, men and crime, men in the family, and men and work. These four arenas are closely interconnected, so that sub-debates on any one of these arenas tend to bear directly on the others.

EDUCATION

The education and educational attainment of boys and young men is increasingly being presented as a major problem – not just for the boys and young men themselves, but for society more generally. For many years girls were more successful than boys in academic attainment in schools until their early teenage years, when boys began to achieve more in this respect. Angela Phillips summarizes some of the evidence here:

> With the introduction of comprehensive education the overall attainment level of all children has risen (contrary to common myth). More working-class children finish their education with useful educational qualifications. But progress has been much faster for girls. In 1987, 17.9 per cent more 16-year-old girls achieved higher-grade exam results than they had done in 1967. They were now 6.6 percentage points ahead of the boys. Boys still did better at maths but that gap in attainment had halved. Between 1977 and 1987 the percentage of girls with higher-grade passes had risen by 35 per cent in maths, 84 per cent in physics and 89 per cent in chemistry.
>
> By 1991 the examinations had been changed, taking account of new teaching methods brought in over the past decade. The areas of maths and science in which boys had always excelled were not being taught in ways that would appeal more to girls. Now girls were ten percentage points ahead in overall attainment and were almost level in maths. Boys are still far more likely to specialize in science and technology, but in the compulsory, combined science exam boys and girls are now level-pegging. At the advanced level exams, taken at the age of 18, girls, overall, now do better than boys.
>
> This evidence shows clearly that, at least in school, girls more than hold their own. In just 25 years of feminist activity, the general academic attainment levels of girls and boys have reversed. It is no longer possible to argue that boys are innately superior, though there is one area in which boys are still ahead. It is in the expensive, elite, boys' public schools where a select group of young men expect to get high grades and go on to the best universities, from where they will step directly on to the ladders of power several rungs higher than everyone else. These boys are not representative of a higher male intellect;

they are actually bucking the general trend for higher attainment among girls.

(Phillips, 1993: 22–3)

In the last few years, there has been further research and publicity on girls' relatively higher performance compared with boys. In 1994, 43 per cent of girls gained five or more GCSEs at grades A to C as compared with 34 per cent of boys (Pratt, 1996). A recent report for the Equal Opportunities Commission has found girls outperforming boys at GCSE in English, Modern Languages, Technology, History, Geography and Art; and at A level in Geography, Social Studies, Art, Chemistry and Biology (Arnot *et al.*, 1996; also see Judd, 1996). In November 1996 the Labour Party published a policy discussion document on these questions, with the somewhat ambiguous sub-title 'Closing the Gender Gap' (Morris, 1996).

The concern that has been expressed about boys' academic performance can be understood in several ways (Hofkin, 1995): at its simplest, boys are underachieving compared with girls; less generously, boys have yielded what was once and sometimes still is seen as their natural advantage; more pragmatically, links are being sought between the low educational attainment of some boys and the low employment rates of some young men. Perhaps most significantly, there is for some boys and young men an *antagonism* between educational attainment, even attentiveness, and the performance and achievement of particular and valued masculinities. More subtly, some boys negotiate an image of cool cleverness that allows them to do their school work without their becoming the object of banter from other boys (Bleach *et al.*, 1996, cited in Jackson, 1996).

There are thus, not surprisingly, a variety of ways of making sense of this problem of boys and young men. It can be seen primarily as a matter of schooling – of producing effective measures for the control and then education of young people in schools. This blurs into questions of producing appropriate cultural change in schools and of changing macho values that are dominant in many school environments, whether from staff or students. This problem can be approached from a variety of perspectives, from sexist to anti-sexist (see Salisbury and Jackson, 1996). Sometimes such debates are given special poignancy through a focus on what is done about particular boys or young men who are violent or disruptive in schools. For example, in May 1996 there was considerable publicity about the strike threat of Nottingham teachers after their school's attempt to suspend a disruptive 13-year-old boy student had been overturned on appeal.

More broadly, the relative low level of educational attainment of some boys and young men can be seen as a matter of concern for economic or moral reasons. In the first case, human capital is being underdeveloped; in the second, social justice is lacking. What is perhaps ironic is that it is men's, and indeed boys', social power in some respects that may account for the lack of achievement of some boys in education. The persistence of men's will to power and domination may itself underwrite the choice of some boys and young men, individually and collectively, not to devote themselves to schooling and learning. Whereas this may not have been a problem in the past because of the structure of labour markets, the nature of school cultures and the security of that domination, this may now not be so automatic. Having said that, reports on educational achievement need to be treated with great caution – they are after all generalizations; they may obscure both major differences between boys and between boys by class, locality and culture; and indeed the construction of this debate in these terms as a problem of (young) men may also obscure the possibility that it is not so much boys and young men that have changed as it is that some girls and some women are now more ready to assume that they should have access to education and jobs rather than femininity alone. As Madeleine Arnot, one of the leading researchers into the performance of girls and boys in schools, has recently expressed it: 'We have a success story here. This is an excellent sign of the work schools have done to improve girls' performance so that they are now catching up' (quoted in Judd, 1996: 1). Most importantly, young women's initial advantage begins to slow down when they have children and enter the labour market.

The rise of this whole *debate* about boys, young men and education needs to be understood in the broad context of gendered age, employment and educational politics of recent years, including the impact of the 1988 Education Reform Act and other legal and policy changes. These have entailed a shift from the language of equal opportunities to that of school effectiveness, standards and performance (Weiner *et al.*, 1996). Meanwhile the extent to which these changes have fundamentally affected the production of boys' and young men's *material practices* in and around schools remains in doubt (Jackson, 1996).

CRIME

A second policy arena where troubled masculinities have been explored, and particularly so in relation to young men, has been crime. In some ways this particular debate connects with a long-term historical debate around the fear of the mob, the underclass, the lumpenproletariat (Pearson, 1983). In this sense, contemporary 'lawless masculinity' (Campbell, 1993) is just a new variation on an old theme. In other ways, the current association of men and crime connects with the previous discussion on education, or for some men a lack of education may be closely linked with the pursuit of crime. Either way the prime issue that has been recognized in recent years is that it is men, especially young men, who specialize in crime. In 1992, 92 per cent of recorded violent crime against the person and 97 per cent of recorded burglaries were by men (Coote, 1994). Similarly, within academic criminology, the association of men, masculinities and crime is now being firmly and explicitly recognized and analysed, following many years of silence (Allen, 1989; Messerschmidt, 1993; Newburn and Stanko, 1994; *Masculinity and Crime*, 1994). Anna Coote, Deputy Director of the Institute of Public Policy Research, has put it clearly and bluntly: 'The problem with crime is a problem with men' (Coote, 1993).

Jack Cordery and Antony Whitehead (1992) have spelt out the features of (young) men's specialization in crime in more detail:

> 84 per cent of all recorded crime is committed by men;
> 25 per cent of all men are convicted of an offence by the age of 25;
> Two-thirds of all male offenders are young men below 30;
> Most men offend in groups;
> Many offences are committed under the influence of alcohol;
> Offending careers often end when young men settle down.

Clearly, crime is not performed equally by all men or all young men. Known or recorded crimes are concentrated among those who are relatively disadvantaged – men with no jobs or lower-paid jobs, with less education and with poorer health. They are also heavily concentrated in and associated with specific geographical localities, such that those who most suffer the effects of young men's crime are neighbours or near neighbours rather than distinct class antagonists. Similarly, in the United Kingdom at least, even acknowledging that official statistics underreport racist crime (Gilroy, 1987), crimes of rapes, robbery and assault are predominantly intra-racial rather than inter-racial (Brake and Hale, 1992). These age, class and ethnic patterns in turn create problems for some men, and particularly some young men, not least in the violence and potential violence of other men.

Recent commentaries, particularly in the mass media, have tended to focus on particular aspects of the association of men and crime. Above all, they have emphasized crime outside the offender's *own* house; that is, they have played down domestic violence (largely men's violence to known women) and other domestic crime and played on the threat of crime in the street and elsewhere in public. This is very much part of the public construction of the 'fear of crime' debate, that has at different times highlighted burglary, mugging, street crime more generally, joy-riding, ram-raiding and car crime more generally. Meanwhile, and almost quite separately, there has developed a more specialist professional debate about the kind of intervention that is appropriate with *adult* men in relation to violence to known women and sex offending. Group programmes for such men, whether in the community or in prison, appear to be gaining increasing attention (see Lees and Lloyd, 1994; Chapter 6, this volume). Here the focus is, however, defined as individual violence, not men (young, young adult, adult or older) and crime in some more general way.

At times the focus of debate in the public domain has been elaborated through more precise lenses. For example, the recent expansion of drug-trading and use has come to be understood as the major impetus behind crime carried out by drug-users, that is, in addition to the illegality of drug-trading itself and, in some cases, related organized crime. The increased concern with the association of crime, drugs and young men spans policy, policing and media discourses.

According to Keith Hellawell, Chief Constable of West Yorkshire, drug-taking and stealing to feed the habit is now an integral part of youth culture: there is now an unofficial tariff – a domestic iron would buy a reefer of cannabis; a new video recorder would buy two rocks of crack cocaine (Brindle, 1996: 2). There are signs that this association is increasingly affecting the younger people of 11, 12, 13 and 14 (Health Advisory Service, 1996). This shift in discourse to encompass a group younger still – of boys rather than young men – brings in a whole host of additional issues.

Special concern is reserved for younger or very young boys who commit crime, especially violent crime. The most publicized case of recent years of this type has been the murder in 1993 of Jamie Bulger by Jon Venables and Robert Thompson. Whereas much of the media presented the two killers as evil monsters, an alternative account is that they represent a brutal and horrifyingly extreme response to established ways of producing boys (see Jackson, 1995). More recently, considerable publicity has been given to the problem of young repeat offenders who cannot effectively be detained. In November 1995, the case of a Durham boy of 14, who had been arrested or reported to the police 72 times for offences ranging from house-breaking to car thefts, was made known. The boy was too young to be placed in youth custody and was blatantly contemptuous of police and others' attempts to control him (Randall, 1995).

Periodically, the young men and crime debate is intertwined with or overlaid by that around race, and specifically the behaviour of young black, particularly Afro-Caribbean, men. This has been the case with the very public debate in the press, on radio and television about the state of street crime in London. In July 1995 Sir Paul Condon, Chief Constable of the Metropolitan Police, made a speech suggesting that 80 per cent of muggers in some parts of London were black, as opposed to white or Asian. This led to public feuding between him and *The Voice*, the black tabloid with the largest circulation; Condon claimed that the paper's less than accurate reporting had fuelled discontent, including a riot outside Brixton Police Station in December 1995, following the death of a young black man, Wayne Douglas, in police custody (Beckett, 1996). In February 1996 *The Voice* produced a 'Men in Crisis' special issue, including details of 47 alleged deaths in police custody since 1969, of police harassment (black people are five times more likely to be stopped), internal police racism, and general distrust between black Londoners and the police.

The whole debate around race, crime and young men, particularly young black men, has now been subjected to considerable critical analysis (see Pringle, 1995: 84–5). Black people are more at risk of attack than white people, and official statistics continue to underreport racist attacks (Gilroy, 1987). Some commentators (for example, Cashmore and McLaughlin, 1991) argue that the police have been active in constructing through the media the notion of black criminality, and particularly the black (young male) mugger. What is usually missing from this debate in mainstream media and politics is an awareness of the specific intersections of race, class, age and gender in different localities. While official statistics, at least, do report relatively high levels of crime from young Afro-Caribbean men in some localities, such figures have to be placed in a broader context of racialized, gendered, aged and class power relations. This includes the specific forms of interaction that may develop between predominantly white young policemen and some young black men (Jefferson, 1991).

Interestingly, the focus on the public domain crime as against private domain crime is itself paralleled in legal constructions of men. For example, Richard Collier (1995) has expertly demonstrated how the explicit construction of 'dangerous masculinities' in law is itself premised on the implicit construction of the 'good father', the 'family man' and indeed heterosexuality itself (see pp. 23–4).

As with all these policy arenas, what we have here is a complex interaction of material conditions, in this case the occurrence of crime, and media, legal and policy representations of those conditions. Younger men do steal more cars than do older men; and at the same time, these material conditions figure unevenly and sometimes almost randomly in the construction of men, younger or older men in policy, legal and media debates, and hence in the construction of public consciousness of men more generally. Similarly, such social/political discourses themselves differ according to particular state welfare regimes and forms of policy development (Edwards and Duncan, forthcoming).

The debate on young men and crime, like that on boys and education, can be cast within a number of different political and ideological frameworks. As with debates on the causes, even origins, of violence and aggression, the full range of explanations, from biological or sociobiological determinism to social and psychological constructionism, are available. The taken-for-grantedness of biological explanations of young men's crime is difficult to shift, whether this is couched in terms of 'youthful high spirits', 'hormonal change', 'territorial imperatives', or simply the male 'propensity to violence'.

Although the threat of young men, and especially in groups and gangs and mobs is not new (Pearson, 1983), the struggle of commentators to make sense of this threat has become more intense. Often the preferred account involves a combination of biological and social factors – of, say, 'youthful high spirits' and the effects of social deprivation, unemployment and low educational attainment. This emphasis on deprivation as the cause of crime – that is, young men's crime – is particularly favoured by Labour Party spokespersons. It allows a critique without too much attention to the tricky problem of gender and gendered power. A slightly different emphasis in some accounts, regardless of whether they are feminist, anti-feminist, left or right, is to focus on the problem in terms of faulty socialization. Anna Coote summarizes this view, which explains young men's crime in terms of the lack of satisfactory 'rites of passage' in the following way:

> What is now being observed is that the old routes by which boys learned to be men have been severed and new routes have not yet been found. Not only are more women going out to work, but eight out of ten new jobs created between now and the turn of the century are expected to be women's jobs. The roles and expectations of daughters, wives and mothers have changed profoundly. So have the prospects for sons, husbands and fathers. But while women have *added* the role of wage-earner to their traditional role of home-maker and carer, men have so far simply *lost* their traditional breadwinning role. Young men grow up fearing there will be no jobs for them, and lacking (in Albert Cohen's words) the means of realising their aspirations to become men.
>
> In communities where there are no jobs for men or women, the girls still have their rites of passage: they can claim adult status by becoming mothers. Even if they do not, they can share in that possibility: they have, if they wish, an idea of what they can become. This may be far from ideal: poorly educated teenagers, themselves trapped in dependency, are not best placed to give their children a start in life. But they have to grow up fast – in a way they would not if they spent their time thieving, joy riding or selling drugs. Most young mothers make a good job of parenting, considering the odds stacked against them. When they fail to marry the fathers of their children, they may be making a realistic assessment of the available options. The boys who get them pregnant may appear to them to have very little else to offer.
>
> The young men must find other ways of growing up.
>
> (Coote, 1994: 2–3)

While few commentators would argue for a purely biological approach, many wish to supply a naturalistic sub-theme to this progression of boys to young men to adult men via the route of crime.

In other words, the problem is not located with boys and young men as such, either biologically or socially, but with how they become men, how they progress to that adult status. While this can be a way of moving beyond a merely biological or merely social-economic construction of young men's crime, it still tends to be a way of playing down gender, and absorbing of the particular forms of gendered power of boys and men into the natural gloss of growing up. The men and crime debate is in its early days; it does name gender, but often in such a way as to recast the problem within other pre-existing and non-gendered models and discourses.

WORK

The debates on boys and education, and on young men and crime intersect with debates on work, employment and unemployment. However, in some ways the debate on troubled masculinities in relation to work, employment and unemployment has been far less developed than might have been expected. Indeed, as will be seen, it is arguable if this constitutes a significant policy arena, or at least an explicit policy arena, in relation to men at all. Work, and particularly paid and employed work, has been established as a central life interest of many men, and especially those who are or have been in employment or expect to be in the future (Tolson, 1977; Collinson and Hearn, 1996b). Men's and young men's identities have often been formed through the predominance of certain kinds of jobs and occupations, and indeed for a minority of men through professional and managerial work (Collinson and Hearn, 1996a). The broad contours of change around men and work are well known: the loss of men's employment in the primary and heavy manufacturing sectors, and the associated cultural change in communities and regions; the transformation of manufacturing from direct manual/batch work to automated production lines to computerized and robotic systems; the associated redefinition of much manufacturing as 'light' rather than 'heavy', and as equally accessible to women's employment; the introduction of information technology; the expansion of tertiary and quaternary employment; and the increasing move to flexible and casualized work in the post-Fordist economy and corporation. While these changes have most clearly affected working-class men, there are also parallel changes in the lives of at least some middle-class men, in terms of their own casualization and redundancy through the effects of increasing

marketization (Brown, 1995). Over the last fourteen years, an estimated 90 per cent of new jobs were part-time and low paid (Achilles
Heel Editorial, 1996). All of these changes are of course gendered
and indeed racialized. In particular, in recent years there has been
a major relative expansion of women's employment, especially
women's part-time employment, so that 46 per cent of women's
employment is part-time (Dickens, 1995). More than 20 per cent
of men now have women domestic partners who earn more than
the man concerned (Cohen, 1996).

All of these changes are relevant to the changing situation of men
and young men. They have been extensively analysed in the academic and research literature. The landmark work here is the
appropriately named *Brothers* by Cynthia Cockburn (1983), in
which she describes the impact of the new technology on the newspaper industry, and in particular men's definitions of themselves as
masculine workers – 'brothers'. As unemployment increased in the
1980s, other studies turned to the effects of unemployment on men's
behaviour and identity.

While unemployment may mean that men spend more time at
home, this does not necessarily mean that men become more
domestic or domesticated in their orientation. Men continue to
do less than their fair share of housework (Morris, 1990; Jowell
et al., 1992). Loss of job is likely to involve loss of status, which
may be accompanied by frustration, financial problems, domestic
difficulties, and sometimes a greater assertion of a form of 'masculinity' through crime and violence. Men's unemployment may thus
have disproportionately negative effects on women partners (Hunt,
1980; McKee and Bell, 1985, 1986; Morris, 1985), and may reinforce rather than change men. There have also been detailed studies
of the interconnections of employment, redundancy, unemployment, community relations and personal identity for men in the
South Wales (steel) (Bytheway, 1987), Hartlepool (manufacturing)
(Morris, 1987) and South Yorkshire (mining) communities
(Waddington *et al.*, 1991; also see this volume, Chapters 9 and 11).
Some recent studies suggest that there are the beginnings of some
realignment of domestic work but here again men tend to be selective in their choice of tasks, and to avoid childcare, especially
early childcare (Morris, 1990; Wheelock, 1990; Brannen and
Moss, 1991). It is now widely accepted that change in work, employment and unemployment can have profound effects upon men, both
young and old.

Furthermore, differential patterns of employment and unemployment have been especially important for the differential experiences of young men in terms of racialization. Some of the highest rates of unemployment occur among young black men and these rates are themselves highly variable by locality. Furthermore, intervention by government has failed to shift this situation. As Herman Ouseley (1996), Chairman (*sic*) of the Commission for Racial Equality, notes: 'Much higher percentages of whites coming from training schemes get into jobs: irrespective of how long they stay there and of the modern apprenticeships that came out [in 1995] to make sure that training led to jobs, only 2 per cent went to ethnic minorities within that year' (p. 69). This points to the clear need for, at the very least, fair shares in training and employment, as well as more positive and focused state intervention.

References to change in the structure of work are prominent in discourses of troubled masculinities; the frequent assumption is that changes in work patterns for men cause or underlie other changes in the way men are. Men's relationship to paid work is seen as central in terms of its loss or potential loss; the possible marginalization of such men; the loss and transformation of work skills; men's relationship to women partners in work, especially those with higher pay or work status; and more generally, men's possibly uncertain identity with these changes. However, what are less clear are, however, the implications of such change for political debate and policy development.

Some new right and men's rights activists may propose a return of women to the domestic sphere, and so 'solve' the problem in that way. Others from the right, most notably Charles Murray (1990) and his British adherents locate the problem with those men who are marginalized from employment and comprise a persistent 'underclass'. Thus for such commentators, work is important when it is absent. This threat is seen as further complicated by the conjunction of unemployment, fragmented family forms and various constructions of cultural malaise. In contrast, even progressive commentators are remarkably reticent in addressing the policy arena of men and work directly. Perhaps, like the dominant ideology of men in many organizations, the labour market is seen as autonomous or relatively autonomous (Cockburn, 1990). Work, employment and unemployment often remain taken-for-granted social structures, all the more so within (troubled) discourses of troubled masculinities. The deep structure of work and employment, subject as it is to global economic forces, is often considered to be beyond the realm of social policy and even beyond the control of the government and the state. In contrast, discourses of troubled masculinities tend to be centred very much on these policy arenas that are constructed as part of state activity, state intervention and indeed state social policy. In this sense, discourses of troubled masculinities frequently construct 'masculinity' and 'men' as relatively ephemeral to the central formation of taken-for-granted capitalism, whether or not that particular economic system is supported or critiqued. In this way, patriarchal relations are generally left implicit.

There is, however, one aspect of the policy debates around men and work that may be in the process of development and that may not conform to the broad pattern described above. This concerns the growing realization that those men in long-term employment, and particularly high-status employment, may be subject to increasing demands and pressures on their time. Work schedules and time schedules remain deeply gendered. As Colette Fagan has recently commented,

> [m]en provide employers with flexibility through extensive involvement in long, unsocial, variable working hours. Not only do they (British men) have much longer paid work than women but they work far longer than men in most of the members of the European Union. Meanwhile British women also work unsocial and variable hours, providing employers with flexiblilty through part-time rather than long hours of work. . . . Women, and especially mothers, continue to bear the major responsibilities for domestic, and particularly childcare work, limiting their ability to take up paid work. Significantly, (m)others with young children are actually more likely to work unsocial hours . . . than are women without children under age sixteen . . . , and . . . fathers with children under age sixteen tend to work even longer hours – and more unsocial hours particularly overtime at weekends.
>
> (Fagan, 1996: 100–1)

There is a growing policy debate in the European Union on time-use and the case for maximum working hours in employment legislation. In November 1993 a European Directive on Working Time was approved, calling for minimum daily rest periods, a maximum working week of 48 hours, a maximum average daily working time of 11 hours, and providing for minimum periods of annual leave, and some restrictions on night working and shift working (Dickens, 1995). The then UK government's opposition to this progressive initiative is indeed a further attempt to obscure the social relations of men and work. Even though this is a cause for major concern, it is well worth noting that women in full-time work in fact work longer hours in paid employment, so that the issue of time-use is likely to be even more acute for them, and especially so with their added domestic responsibilities (see Bryson *et al.*, 1994). Breaking down the distinctions between 'full-time' and 'part-time', reducing the time men spend in paid work, and rethinking the relationship of work and time for men are all important policy issues.

THE FAMILY

The policy focus on the family has taken a wide variety of forms. They have variously centred on 'boys', 'sons', 'parenting', 'fathers and mothers', lone or otherwise. Most commentaries on boys and young men in the family have paralleled the earlier debate on boys and education. The family focus has been concerned with the disruption or breakdown or simple ineffectiveness of the parenting of boys in their becoming young men, then men. The most explicit text which addresses this issue is Angela Phillips (1993), *The Trouble with Boys, Parenting the Men of the Future*. This engages in some detail with how boys learn to become young men, particularly in the context of a changing society both nationally and familially. It bemoans the pressures on boys that go to make for unsatisfactory forms of manhood, and concludes by the need to bring boys and men back into families in a more egalitarian way.

However, the major theme in recent years has been the social position of lone mothers parenting sons and young men, and the associated relation of fathers, absent to lesser or greater degrees. Conservative criticisms, or rather attacks, on lone mothers have been both moral and financial; they have also been about the effectiveness of such mothers in bringing up sons into appropriate young men. Much of this debate has glossed over the research that is available on the positive effects of living away from conflict between a man and woman parent, and the benefits of separation, especially after the initial trauma (Heatherington, 1992). Other research has shown that the periodic scares about the effects of lesbian parenting and lesbian mothers are unfounded (Rights of Women, 1984).

Anna Coote and Jane Franklin summarize the moral panic about lone mothers succinctly:

> There are different ways of interpreting social change. But one version of events is threatening to overshadow the rest with a pall of moral panic and nostalgia. It tells us that civilization is collapsing – witness the rising rates of crime and divorce. It warns that we must shore up the old social structures and restore their fast-eroding features: discipline, order, certainty and authority.
>
> This view insists on a causal link between crime and the increase in non-traditional families. The roots of change in family structure are traced to four interconnected factors: Beveridge's welfare state model of the post-war years, corrupted by permissive Sixties liberalism, triggered an excess of female emancipation in the Seventies which was whipped into a lather of selfish individualism by the Eighties' free market boom, to produce that arch demon of the Nineties: the lone mother.[1]
>
> (Coote and Franklin, 1995: 1)

The central point of connection here is between family forms, especially lone mother families, and the production of boys, young men and men. The accusation from the right is that not only are such family forms morally problematic and financially expensive but also that they fail to produce appropriate sons and future fathers, as well as of course failing to reproduce husbands. At times, this is seen as the fault of the women concerned, becoming either too independent or too dependent on the state; at other times, it is the men who are blamed because of their 'flight from commitment', or their own excessive independence or indeed dependence on the state. Clearly, an important part of this policy debate has been the attempt to link lone mothers and young men's criminality. To put this simply, which seems an appropriate way to put a simple argument – lone mother families are accused of producing sons and young male criminals rather than husbands or (future) fathers. And so the cycle is assumed to go on as such would-be fathers fail to respond in the next generation. Although a 1993 NOP survey found that two out of three people did not accept this link (*Sunday Times*, 1993), the notion remains powerful in government and in political party circles. It is the family dimension of the threat of the mob.

What is particularly interesting is that the logics of government policy on the family, and men's place within it, have often been quite inconsistent. This is partly because of confusion around whether it is the 'family' or 'marriage' that is to be the focus of policy. The 1995 Family Homes and Matrimonial Act failed to give protection from men's violence to co-habiting women. The 1996 Family Law Act has reformed the divorce law in notoriously inconsistent ways, including the abolition of fault, the introduction of longer delays and conciliations, and pension-sharing. The Children Act of 1989 emphasized the importance of *'parenting'*, of both mothers and fathers, and the desirability of maintaining social and emotional ties with both parents, including fathers, after separation and divorce. While this reform of childcare and child protection was strongly influenced by civil service thinking, the transformation of child support was largely the product of governmental political direction. The subsequent Child Support Act of 1991 focused particularly on the financial responsibilities that had been neglected by fathers. While the Child Support Agency (CSA) has been primarily a means of transferring payments to mothers from the state to the pockets of fathers, its role has been complicated by a moral debate on the family and fatherhood. As Helen Wilkinson (1995) explained in November 1995, feckless fathers are also targets, with some moralists advocating an extension of the principles of the Child Support Act to punish men further. Others are eager to rein in liberal divorce laws.

The CSA superseded what was previously a fragmented and unequal system whereby fathers, and sometimes mothers, were, theoretically at least, given financial responsibilities after separation and divorce through the court system. However, over three-quarters of lone parents were previously not receiving financial support from the other parent, and 90 per cent were drawing social security benefits. As such, the CSA shifted these state operations from the legal to the administrative system, and, theoretically at least, moved those operations towards a more universalistic mode, in contrast to many other recent Conservative reforms. The House of Commons Social Security Committee pronounced in 1991 the introduction of the CSA as the biggest social change in that field in forty years. The original Act was not well thought out. While it was inspired by a moral panic around a relatively small group of young, 'irresponsible', feckless fathers, in practice it engaged with a much larger group of fathers, who saw themselves as much more responsible and not at all feckless.

The outcome of these measures is, not surprisingly, contested. It is strongly suggested that the main financial beneficiary has been the state, in that the absent parents, usually fathers, have in effect paid money that would otherwise have been paid by the state. The overall benefit to lone parents, usually lone mothers themselves, is not great (Millar, 1994). However, the extent of ideological movement can be appreciated by the fact that the second Child Support Act of 1995, which consolidated a number of amendments on the first Act, was given cross-party support for the broad principle in the Select Committee Report of February 1995. By 1996, 1.5 million cases had been dealt with.

Meanwhile, the last few years have also seen a growing debate on the positive benefits of fatherhood and indeed the need for positive models of fatherhood. The question of fatherhood, and particularly young fatherhood, is a recurring and synthesizing theme throughout these debates on the family and indeed other policy arenas. Fatherhood is assumed to be a possible fixed reference point within a world characterized by rapid change. The clear message from across a broad political spectrum is that families do need fathers. Despite the evidence from research on, say, lesbian mothers, families and parents (Rights of Women, 1984), it is now widely considered that:

> children need their fathers too – as much for emotional sustenance as for paying the bills. Men are caught in a different kind of trap, in which their traditional expectations conflict with life as they find it. They have a sense of failure if they cannot get work, and derive very little self-esteem from working unpaid at home. Those who are employed are exiled from their families, clocking up longer and longer hours to keep their place in the labour market.
>
> (Coote, 1995: 15)

The relationship, sometimes a paradoxical one, between the critique of 'feckless fathers' and the positive promotion of fatherhood is examined in the next chapter. Interestingly, this debate, like that on the family more generally, rarely addresses questions of sexuality or heterosexuality, and more rarely still in any kind of critical way.

Finally, in this section we may note that the debate on time-use which is developing in relation to men and work also bears on the re-appraisal of men and family life. This does not concern some abstract 'crisis of masculinity' or 'crisis of fatherhood' but rather how time is spent inside and outside families. Not only is this a matter of who does what kinds of work in the family, but also the quality of the contact between men and other members of families. Thus a recent study found that it was the amount of time young people spend with their families that is a key influence on how well they do at school and work, rather than whether they grow up in a family with both natural parents (*The Relationship* . . . , 1996). Interestingly, such 'nuclear families' now constitute less than 30 per cent of all households (Open University, 1988).

CONCLUDING COMMENTS

At the heart of these discourses of troubled masculinities is a concern about young men. With the exception of those debates that centre on men's health, young men are seen as the primary problem. Young men are seen as an uncertainty, a problem, by both women, particularly older women, and older men, across the political spectrum. What is the nature of this problem of young men?

Young men are defined as subordinate to older men within patriarchal relations, and are now seen to be questioning and challenging those relations by moving from being objects to becoming subjects. Thus concern about young men is partly about uncertainty around the place of young men in the family, and different kinds of family relations, whether as sons, brothers, husbands or fathers.

To put this rather differently, young men are seen as rejecting or potentially rejecting of patriarchy and, in particular, of patriarchal responsibility. They are seen as representing a particular form of male power – the fratriarchal as opposed to the patriarchal. Young men are seen to embody one version of male power – that which is uncontrollable and unpredictable, even unknown. This is in clear contrast to the male power of patriarchy:

Patriarchy traditionally meant the primacy of the father is kinship, and by extension an authoritarian and often antiquated yet paternalistic form of government, as well as the rule of the elders', the 'wise old men'.

Fratriarchy is a mode of male domination which is concerned with a quite different set of values from those of patriarchy. Although the *fratrist* can be expected to share all the assumptions about matters such as the origin of life in the father, together with the whole ideology which springs from this, he is preoccupied with matters other than paternity and parenting, raising children, providing for a wife and family, and acting as guardian of a moral code. Unlike patriarchy, fratriarchy is based simply on the self-interest of the association of men itself. It reflects the demands of a group of lads to have the freedom to do as they please, to have a good time. Its character is summed up in the phrase 'causing a bit of bovver'.

(Remy, 1990: 44–5; emphasis in original)

Thus, while the fratriarchy is most clearly seen in the performance of crime, its impact is also present in all other spheres of life – education, work, home life, sport and so on. It has also had a recent resurgence with the assertion of 'ladism' or 'new ladism'. These fratriarchal relations are particularly concerned with that dimension of male power that is founded in *the interpersonal power of the group of men* rather than, say, the power of the individual father or the power of the corporate body. Although, having said that, it is also important to recognize the links between individual power and corporate power, and between the power of rule and the power of force. Young men may of course have their own rules and may indeed re-affirm or break the rules of others, but they do not usually have access to control over the most important or powerful rules of society, such as the distribution of wealth, privilege and patronage. Their power is usually based on gendered force, influence, persuasion, status, use of space and the avoidance of domestic work – the personal, the interpersonal and the group rather than the rules of the corporate world. This is generally left to other, older men, with or without good health.

ACKNOWLEDGEMENT

I am grateful for discussions with David Jackson and Fiona Williams on the issues addressed in this chapter, and to Jeanette Edwards for comments on an earlier draft.

NOTE

1 Other invaluable commentaries have been provided by Laws (1994), Millar (1994) and Edwards and Duncan (forthcoming).

REFERENCES

Achilles Heel Editorial (1996) Working men, *Achilles Heel*, 20: 4.

Allen, Judith (1989) 'Men, crime and criminology: recasting the questions', *International Journal of Sociology of Law*, 17: 19–39.

—— (1991) 'Men, masculinity and criminology', *International Journal of the Sociology of Law*.

Anderson, Digby (1991) *The Unmentionable Face of Poverty*, London: Social Affairs Unit.

Arnot, Madeleine, David, Miriam and Weiner, Gaby (1996) *Educational Reforms and Gender Equality in Schools*, Manchester: Equal Opportunities Commission.

Beckett, Andy (1996) 'The voice in the wilderness', *The Sunday Review: Independent on Sunday* (February), pp. 4–7.

Bennett, Catherine (1996) 'The boys with the wrong stuff', *Guardian* (6 November).

Bleach, Kevin *et al.* (1996) *What Difference Does it Make? An Investigation of Factors Influencing the Motivation and Performance of Year 8 Boys in a West Midlands Comprehensive School*, Wolverhampton: Education Research Unit, University of Wolverhampton.

Brake, M. and Hale, C. (1992) *Public Order and Private Lives. The Politics of Law and Order*, London: Routledge.

Brannen, Julia and Moss, Peter (1991) *Managing Mothers*, London: Unwin Hyman.

Brindle, David (1996) 'Drugs fear for under-11s', *Guardian* (31 January), p. 2.

Brown, P. (1995) 'Cultural capital and social exclusion: some observations on recent trends in education, employment and the labour market', *Work, Employment and Society*, 9: 29–51.

Bryson, Lois, Bittman, Michael and Donath, Sue (1994) 'Men's welfare state, women's welfare state: tendencies to convergence in practice and theory?' in Diana Sainsbury (ed.) *Gendering Welfare States*, London: Sage, pp. 118–31.

Bytheway, Bill (1987) 'Redundancy and the older worker', in R.M. Lee (ed.) *Redundancies, Lay-off and Plant Closures*, London: Croom Helm, pp. 84–115.

Campbell, Beatrix (1993) *Goliath: Britain's Dangerous Places*, London: Methuen.

Cashmore, E. and McLaughlin, E. (eds) (1991) *Out of Order? Policing Black People*, London: Routledge.

Cockburn, Cynthia (1983) *Brothers*, London: Pluto.

—— (1990) 'Men's power in organizations: equal opportunities intervene', in Jeff Hearn and David Morgan (eds) *Men, Masculinities and Social Theory*, London: Unwin Hyman, pp. 72–89.

Cohen, D. (1996) 'It's a guy thing', *Guardian Weekend* (14 May), pp. 26–30.

Collier, Richard (1995) *Masculinity, Law and the Family*, London: Routledge.

Collinson, David L. and Hearn, Jeff (eds) (1996a) *Men as Managers, Managers as Men*, London: Sage.

—— (1996b) 'Men at work: multiple masculinities/multiple workplaces', in Mäirtín Mac an Ghaill (ed.) *Understanding Masculinities: Social Relations and Cultural Arenas*, Buckingham: Open University Press, pp. 61–76.

Coote, Anna (1993) 'The problem with crime is a problem with men', *The Independent* (16 February).

—— (1994) 'Introduction', in Anna Coote (ed.) *Families, Children and Crime*, London: Institute of Public Policy Research, pp. 1–13.

——(1995) 'The family: a battleground in fearful times', *The Independent* (30 October), p.15.

Coote, Anna and Franklin, Jane (1995) 'In place of moral panic', *IPPR In Progress* (Autumn): 1–2.

Cordery, Jack and Whitehead, Antony (1992) 'Boys don't cry: empathy, warmth, collusion and crime', in Paul Senior and David Woodhill (eds) *Gender, Crime and Probation Practice*, Sheffield: Sheffield City Polytechnic, PAVIC Publications.

Dench, Geoff (1994) *The Frog, the Prince and the Problem of Men*, London: Neanderthal Books.

Dennis, Norman and Erdos, George (1992) *Families without Fatherhood*, London: Institute of Economic Affairs.

—— (1993) *Rising Crime and the Dismembered Family*, London: Institute of Economic Affairs.

Dickens, Linda (1995) 'UK, part-time employees and the law – recent and potential developments', *Gender, Work and Organization*, 2(4): 207–15.

Edwards, Rosalind and Duncan, Simon (forthcoming) 'Lone mothers and economic activity', in Fiona Williams (ed.) *Social Policy: A Critical Reader*, Cambridge: Polity.

Fagan, Colette (1996) 'Gendered time schedules: paid work in Great Britain', *Social Politics*, 3(1): 72–106.

Gilroy, Paul (1987) *There Ain't No Black in the Union Jack*, London: Hutchinson.

Greenstein, Ben (1993) *The Fragile Male*, London: Boxtree.

Hacker, Andrew (1991) *Two Nations*, New York: Basic Books.

Harman, Harriet (1993a) *The Century Gap*, London: Vermillion.

—— (1993b) 'Women surge past men to cross the century gap', *Guardian* (4 June).

Health Advisory Service (1996) *The Substance of Young Needs*, London: HMSO.

Hearn, Jeff (1996) 'Is masculinity dead? a critique of the concept of masculinity/masculinities', in Mairtin Mac an Ghaill (ed.) *Understanding*

Masculinities: Social Relations and Cultural Arenas, Buckingham: Open University Press, pp. 207–17.

Heatherington, Mavis (1992) *Coping with Marital Transition*, Monographs of the Society for Research in Child Development.

Hofkin, Diane (1995) 'Why teenage boys think success is sad', *Times Educational Supplement* (18 August).

Hunt, Pauline (1980) *Gender and Class Consciousness*, London: Macmillan.

Jackson, David (1995) 'Breaking out of the binary trap: boys' underachievement, schooling and gender relations', unpublished ms., Nottingham for ESRC, Seminar on the Educational Underachievement of Boys, the Institute of Education (January 1997).

Jefferson, Tony (1991) 'Discrimination, disadvantage and police work', in E. Cashmore and E. McLaughlin (eds) *Out of Order? Policing Black People*, London: Routledge, pp. 166–88.

Jowell, Roger, Brook, L., Prior G. and Taylor B. (eds) (1992) *British Social Attitudes: the 9th Report*, Aldershot: Dartmouth.

Judd, Judith (1996) 'Girls sweep past boys in exam race', *The Independent* (22 April), p. 1.

Laws, Sophie (1994) 'Un-valued families', *Trouble & Strife*, 28: 5–11.

Lees, John and Lloyd, Trefor (1994) *Working with Men who Batter Their Partners*, London: WWM/The B Team.

McKee, Linda and Bell, Colin (1985) 'Marital and family relations in times of male unemployment', in Bryan Roberts, Ruth Finnegan and Duncan Gallie (eds) *New Approaches to Economic Life*, Manchester: Manchester University Press.

—— (1986) 'His unemployment: her problem. The domestic and marital consequences of male unemployment', in Sheila Allen, Kate Purcell, Alan Waton and Stephen Wood (eds) *The Experience of Unemployment*, London: Macmillan.

Masculinity and Crime (1994), Conference Report, Uxbridge: Brunel University.

Messerschmidt, James (1993) *Masculinities and Crime*, Lanham, MD: Rowman and Littlefield.

Millar, Jane (1994) 'State, family and personal responsibility: the changing balance for lone mothers in the United Kingdom', *Feminist Review* 48: 24–39.

Morris, Estelle (1996) *Boys Will Be Boys: Closing the Gender Gap*, London: Labour Party.

Morris, Lydia (1985) 'Renegotiation of the domestic division of labour in the context of male redundancy', in Bryan Roberts, Ruth Finnegan and Duncan Gallie (eds) *New Approaches to Economic Life*, Manchester: Manchester University Press.

—— (1987) 'Constraints on gender: the family wage, social security and the labour markets: reflections on research in Hartlepool', *Work, Employment & Society*, 1(1): 85–106.

—— (1990) *The Workings of the Household*, Cambridge: Polity.

Murray, Charles (1990) *The Emerging British Underclass*, London: Institute for Economic Affairs.

Newburn, Tim and Stanko, Elizabeth (eds) (1994) *Just Boys Doing Business: Men, Masculinities and Crime*, London: Routledge.

Open University (1988) *Family, Gender and Welfare*, Milton Keynes: Open University Press.

Ouseley, Herman (1996) 'Keeping men mainstream', in Trefor Lloyd and Tristan Wood (eds) *What Next for Men?* London: Working with Men, pp. 65–76.

Pearson, Geoffrey (1983) *Hooligan: A History of Respectable Fears*, London: Macmillan.

Phillips, Angela (1993) *The Trouble with Boys, Parenting the Men of the Future*, London: Pandora.

Pratt, Simon (1996) 'Could do better', *Achilles Heel*, 20: 20–1.

Pringle, Keith (1995) *Men, Masculinities and Social Welfare*, London: UCL Press.

Randall, Colin (1995) 'Police powerless to stop gang leader, 14', *Daily Telegraph* (3 November), p. 7.

The Relationship Between Family Life and Young People's Lifestyles (1996) Findings, Social Policy Research 95, York: Joseph Rowntree Foundation.

Remy, John (1990) 'Patriarchy and fratriarchy as forms of androcracy', in Jeff Hearn and David Morgan (eds) *Men, Masculinities and Social Theory*, London: Unwin Hyman, pp. 43–54.

Rights of Women (1984) *Lesbian Mothers on Trial*, London: Row.

Salisbury, Jonathan and Jackson, David (1996) *Challenging Macho Values: Practical Ways of Working with Adolescent Boys*, London: Falmer.

Sarre, Sophie (1996) *A Place for Fathers: Fathers and Social Policy in the Post-war period*, London: Discussion Paper WSP/125, London School of Economics and Political Science.

Sunday Times (1993) (14 November).

Tolson, Andrew (1977) *The Limits of Masculinity*, London: Tavistock.

Waddington, David, Cricher, Charles and Wykes, Maggie (1991) *Split at the Seams? Community, Continuity and Change after the 1984 Coal Dispute*, Milton Keynes: Open University Press.

Weiner, Gaby, Arnot, Madelaine and David, Miriam (1996) 'Is the future female? Female success, male disadvantage and changing gender patterns in education', in A.H. Halsey, P. Brown and H.Lauder (eds) *Education, Economy and Society*, Oxford: Oxford University Press.

Wheelock, J. (1990) *Husbands at Home*, London: Routledge.

Wilkinson, Helen (1995) 'Fundamentally wrong on families', *The Independent* (3 November), p. 21.

Chapter 3

Troubled masculinities in social policy discourses
Fatherhood

Fiona Williams

The previous chapter looked at masculinities in relation to the problematization of young men. A second area on which troubled and troubling discourses of masculinities have settled is the debate and concern over fatherhood. Fatherhood is said to be in crisis (Knijn, 1995). The social, economic and cultural conditions which sustained traditional meanings of fatherhood – particularly those attached to male breadwinning, moral authority and undisputed paternity – have been subject to challenge and change, especially over the last decade. This process has generated, and been generated by, a variety of discourses about the family, divorce, lone motherhood and children, crime, education, unemployment and sexuality, which have in common an attempt to question or assess the nature and role of fatherhood. In some ways, the shifting of ideas and practices around this aspect of masculinity is not new. It is possible to track the historical construction of fatherhood over the last 100 years and to understand this contemporary debate as part of the attempt to 'modernize fatherhood', to 'reconstitute paternal masculinity' (see Collier, 1995, 1996) and to anchor troubling masculinities by fixing them to men's rights and responsibilities within families. At the same time, the significance given in current social, political and policy discourse to men's role as *fathers*, rather than as workers, citizens, husbands/partners or soldiers, *is* new. To some extent, fatherhood has become the lens through which these other roles (with the possible exception of soldiering) are now signified.

The aim of this chapter is to set out the dimensions of this process of the signification of men as fathers and to chart the contemporary discursive positions which have helped produce this signification. Some of the discourses around fatherhood have been more central than others to policy-making; some are prescriptive and others analytical. Although it is possible to differentiate positions in the debate on fatherhood as 'traditional' or 'progressive' or 'anti-feminist' or 'pro-feminist', such distinctions are too simple, for what is interesting is the way some of these positions overlap, drawing upon shared discourses of masculinity and normality in relation to family life. However, and in spite of this, for heuristic purposes I also classify these concerns with fatherhood into two camps. The first set of positions is characterized by a concern with the *absence* of the father, especially in an economic and moral sense, whilst the second set problematizes the *distance* of the father in his emotional and caring capacity.

THE CHANGING CONDITIONS OF FATHERHOOD

The problematization of the nature of fatherhood is, as I have suggested, new. This newness represents the very contingent terms in which the concept has been constructed over the past century. The symbolic, and in some areas, actual, separation of the public and private spheres in the nineteenth century gave motherhood a new practical and ideological importance within the private sphere, deemed to be separate from paid work, natural but requiring control and supervision.[1] It was constructed as a state of activity and involvement.

Fatherhood, in contrast, was reconstituted as a state of being, contingent upon other conditions or states of activity. Central to these conditions was, over this century, a man's breadwinning capacity. The economic power derived from this gave him responsibilities to provide for and protect his wife and children but it also legitimated his legal and informal rights of control over his wife and children, his patriarchal authority, his position as chief arbiter and decision-maker. Added to these economic, moral and legal dimensions was a fourth, more long-standing, dimension – the biological. Marriage ensured a man's undisputed paternity of his children, and it ensured his children's legitimacy. Historically, it was marriage rather than paternity which determined the economic, legal and social rights and responsibilities which constituted fatherhood (Collier, 1995: 185). These conditions, through which a modern notion of fatherhood became constructed, have in policy, law and popular culture, been deemed to be *natural*; that is, to be part of being a man. Going out to work, providing for a family, having power, authority and control over a wife and children, establishing undisputed paternity have, culturally speaking, been seen as essential and defining characteristics of manhood and, as such, central to the construction of twentieth-century masculinities. Fatherhood, in its turn, has been seen as the natural state of being, seen to flow from these rights, duties and desires, even though the images of fatherhood have themselves changed – from paterfamilias to family man – and are diversely constituted within different class, ethnic, sexual and religious groups.

Within the context of the British welfare state which, relative to other welfare states, has developed as a strong male breadwinner regime (Lewis, 1992), social policies for men have prioritized their role as workers, citizens and soldiers or ex-soldiers, rather than directly as fathers. This contrasts with social policies for women, which have been framed in terms of their roles as mothers and wives rather than as workers or citizens. It is within this context that the active prescription of 'good mothering' in the domestic sphere was spelt out in relation to the welfare of children, particularly through maternalist health and welfare measures in the first two decades of the century, and later through the influence of child-care psychology. On the other hand, men's role as fathers was deemed to follow largely from their engagement with the discipline of paid work in the public sphere, and, until recently, prescriptions for paternal activity were vague and general rather than specific. This parental/sexual division of labour and the surveillance of mothering (the designation of 'good' or 'fit' and 'bad' or 'unfit' mothers) was to have consequences, as we shall see below, for women taking on the custody of children following separation and divorce in the 1970s and 1980s.

What is also interesting, in contrasting the greater visibility of motherhood with fatherhood in social policy in Britain, is the differing constitution of social rights in this century attached to motherhood and fatherhood. For women, the winning and granting of social rights (family allowances, health provision and so on) have flowed from their carrying out what are deemed to be *natural female responsibilities* (as wives and mothers). For men, however, responsibilities – for example to provide for families – have been predicated upon the existence of what came to be deemed to be *natural male rights* – to earn a wage, to exercise control over wives and children. Indeed, as Richard Collier argues, the history of legal intervention in men's economic responsibility for their families demonstrates the belief that it is necessary to furnish men with rights in order to expect them to carry out their responsibilities (Collier, 1995: 209). The tendency for women, on the other hand, is that they have claimed or been granted rights by virtue of pre-existing responsibilities and obligations. In other words, it is possible to discern a gendering of (male) rights and (female) responsibilities in the modern history of parenting.[2] The contradiction for fatherhood is that it is deemed to be both an essential component of masculinity (a natural extension of breadwinning and male authority) yet, at the same time, unnatural to men (in that it will only be exercised through the granting of male rights). The main point here is that what is new about the current concern over fatherhood is that it has begun to question (if only sometimes then to defend) the taken-for-grantedness and assumed naturalness of fatherhood.

However, it is important to say that the above depiction of this particular form of paternal masculinity, resting, as it does, on 'the economic and familial order of gender hierarchy and compulsory heterosexuality' (Collier, 1995: 176), has represented a universal ideal rather than a diverse reality. To begin with, over this century the breadwinner ideal was not accessible for many poorer, working-class families where women had to work to supplement a low male wage or were even an equal or main wage earner. Similarly, wars, men's high mortality rates and the vagaries of migration and racist immigration controls meant that lone parents, female breadwinners and reconstituted families were never that uncommon. The symbolic representation of fathers as protectors and providers was also challenged by campaigns such as those for temperance (and thereby an end to men's violence and profligacy) in the nineteenth century and, from the 1960s, campaigns against domestic violence.

Just as importantly, every part of this ideal of paternity has been challenged by social and economic changes. To begin with, the decline of the industrial base and increasing male unemployment have undermined the capacity of many men to act as breadwinners; men's economic power has also, to some extent, been dented by their wives' earning power; claims for women's autonomy, especially through lone motherhood, cohabitation, separation, divorce and same-sex relationships and parenting, along with moves towards the democratization of child–parent relations have challenged men's assumptions about their natural authority over women and children. The naming of domestic violence and child sexual abuse has also overshadowed the representation of fathers as protectors. Finally, reproductive technologies have made possible the separation of sexuality not only from reproduction, but also from paternity (although to date they have often been used to reinforce paternity). Fathers no longer need attend the conception of their child. All these different changes have challenged the economic, legal, moral and biological conditions of fatherhood and the masculinities which they feed and upon which they depend. Furthermore, new cultural representations of fathers as active, involved and equal partners in the business of childcare, whether married or unmarried, have forced reconfigurations of the more traditional image of the semi-detached, present-but-distant, breadwinning family man for whom marriage granted rights and responsibilities. It is this destabilizing of the taken-for-granted notions of paternal masculinity which is at the heart of the debate over the 'crisis' in fatherhood, to which we now turn.[3]

DEBATES OVER FATHERHOOD

Not only is the question 'what are fathers for?' a new one, but what is also interesting is the number of different perspectives being brought to bear on the question and the difficulties of classifying them in traditional political terms. In some cases the question represents a cause or symptom of another perceived social problem, or constellation of problems: for example, the emergence of an 'underclass', or the increase in divorce, single and never-married mothers. For others, the question 'what are fathers for?' signifies a shift from prescribed and fixed gender roles; it opens up opportunities for new forms of familial relations based upon diverse, individually negotiated and fluid identities. I take the view here, drawing on Collier's (1995, 1996) analysis, that the question represents a new discursive terrain upon which the reconstruction of the 'modern man' is being contested. At the heart of this struggle is an attempt to redefine men's relationship with women and children in the family, drawing in different ways upon discourses of responsibility, sexuality, authority, equality, care and support. Many of these redefinitions presuppose a particular relationship to paid work and a particular investment in heterosexuality, although some attempt to recast these too.

Key contributors to this debate are enormously diverse, and mapping the debate in terms of existing political ideologies (left, right, feminist and so on) poses difficulties. Dividing the groups or policies into 'traditional' and 'progressive' camps according to their view of gender relations would not account for the ways in which discourses of male and female equality and shared parenting have been pulled into the debate to bolster a traditionalist perspective on men.

Similarly no one feminist position alone exists in relation to issues of fatherhood and masculinity, and more importantly, views on women's autonomy, the context in which it can be supported, and how far it already exists, vary among those who claim to promote such autonomy.

Another form of categorization used by Trudie Knijn is to distinguish between different explanations for a crisis in fatherhood (Knijn, 1995: 11–17). She distinguishes between *feminist* explanations – which problematize male power in the family and demand greater equality in the sexual division of labour in the household – and a *structuralist* one which identifies the transition to a post-industrial economy as one which has stripped many men of their capacity to fulfil their central fatherhood role, that of male provider. A third explanation – a *cultural* one focusing on changing lifestyles – is associated with 'new school' sociologists (Giddens, 1991). Knijn's categorization is useful but carries the danger of over-emphasizing the differences between these explanations and over-looking the ways in which they overlap.

What is equally interesting to examine is the interlacing effect of discourses on men, masculinities and fatherhood. Different positions travel and traverse the same and different networks – the view from the train can be different according to where you sit. With these observations in mind I have used a distinction which is, first, highly specific to the debate itself and, second, represents two of the main recent historical paths which have cut their way through to this new terrain. On the one side, there has developed a concern, or a panic, about the *absent father*. On the other side, there have been calls for a reconstruction of paternal masculinity in terms of greater involvement with childcare and greater sharing of parental roles. In this case the problem is with the *distant father*. The distinction made is therefore around the discourses of absence and distance. However, to some extent, as we shall see, each discourse leaks into the other.

THE PROBLEM OF ABSENCE

The problematizations of absent fathers that we look at here are those articulated by New Right US sociologist and commentator Charles Murray, ethical socialist sociologists, Norman Dennis and George Erdos, the Child Support Act 1991, and the organizations representing divorced and separated men, such as Families Need Fathers and Dads After Divorce. The problematization of absence points to the significance of a father's presence in the family. In addition, the problematization of absence in the following accounts is premised upon the separation of good fathers from bad fathers – or the 'safe' from the dangerous (Collier, 1995: chapter 6). In this way, it mirrors the promotion, control and supervision of motherhood in the earlier part of this century which similarly depended upon the classification of good/fit and bad/unfit mothers, and was, as such dichotomies often are, underscored by the bigotry of class and racial superiority. The absent or errant father in this scenario represents the bad, and the present father, the good. Charles Murray's essay on the 'underclass' starts by quoting Henry Mayhew's writing on the 'undeserving poor' in the 1850s and compares this with his own contemporary experience:

> In the small Iowa town where I lived, I was taught by my middle-class parents that there were two kinds of poor people. One class of poor people was never called 'poor'. I came to understand that they simply lived with low incomes, as my own parents had done when they were young. Then there was another set of poor people. Just a handful of them. These poor people didn't lack money. They were defined by their behaviour. Their houses were littered and unkempt. The men in the family were unable to hold a job for more than a few weeks at a time. Drunkenness was common. The children grew up ill-schooled and ill-behaved and contributed a disproportionate share of the local juvenile delinquents.
>
> (Murray, 1990: 1)

In this way Murray begins to identify bad fathers as those without jobs and drunk (therefore unable to provide a wage or discipline) and their children as disorderly and delinquent. Further on in the same essay he discusses the importance of fathers as role models:

> It turns out that the clichés about role models are true. . . . Little boys don't naturally grow up to be responsible fathers and

husbands. They don't naturally grow up knowing how to get up every morning at the same time and go to work. . . . And most emphatically of all, little boys do not reach adolescence naturally wanting to refrain from sex, just as little girls don't become adolescents naturally wanting to refrain from having babies . . . boys and girls grow into responsible parents and neighbours and workers because they are imitating the adults around them.

(Ibid.: 10–11)

Murray combines naturalistic and essentialist discourses of masculinity, femininity and sexuality with psychological ideas of the importance of the father's presence as a role model, constraining and disciplining his sons into sexual and economic responsibility. So who constrains men's natural irresponsibility when they are grown up? The answer is work, wives and paternal responsibility, which also act as essential pillars to masculine identity:

> Just as work is more important than merely making a living, getting married and raising a family are more than a way to pass the time. *Supporting a family is a central means for a man to prove to himself that he is a 'mensch'.* Men who do not support families find other ways to prove that they are men, which tend to take various destructive forms. As many have commented through the centuries, young males are essentially barbarians for whom marriage – meaning not just the wedding vows, but the act of *taking responsibility for a wife and children* – is an indispensable civilising force.

(Ibid.: 22–3; my emphasis)

What Murray is saying is that a father's presence is important because not only does he socialize his male children, but three things – work, a wife and responsibility – civilize and socialize the father, too. This places women in a peculiarly ambiguous position which is not explained – for it would appear that they possess sufficient *savoir-faire* to act as a civilizing force for their husbands, but not, it seems, their sons, and yet they also possess so little that they need to submit to the authority of the man they have civilized. In this scenario men's presence in families denotes hierarchy, discipline, financial responsibility and heterosexual order.

I have quoted Murray at length because these discourses are picked up by others concerned with father absence. A.H. Halsey, Norman Dennis, George Erdos and Jon Davies all come from an ethical socialist tradition and provide analyses not dissimilar from Murray's. They have also been published by the right-wing think-tank, the Institute of Economic Affairs (for example, Dennis and Erdos, 1992; Davies, 1993). They identify a link between the growth of fatherless families and the growth of crime: men have been made redundant both through economic restructuring and by women's independent lifestyles. This has broken up the working-class communities and the families within them, along with the values of hard work, respectability and co-operation. These have been further undermined by the promotion of a marketized individualism which has reached beyond the public world to the private world of social and sexual relationships. Jon Davies calls this 'an ethos of Privacy and Appetitive Individualism' which promotes 'an endless variety of sexual and procreative relationships which lack both internal stability and a clear articulation within society in general' (Davies, 1993: 99). Here again, the discourses of work, working-class respectability, male authority and female dependency and an ordered and restrained heterosexuality are welded on to ethical socialist values of co-operation in family and community relations. Social order and an authoritative paternal masculinity are threatened by male unemployment, female independence and sexual and moral irresponsibility and relativism.

These ideas from the Old Left and New Right have influenced government ministers and policy-makers. Conservative Cabinet ministers, John Redwood and Peter Lilley, have both publicly demonized errant fathers and lone mothers. For example, John Redwood suggested, after a visit to a housing estate in Cardiff in July 1993 where he had been shocked to find high numbers of lone mothers, that benefits should be withheld from mothers until the errant father were to be found (cited in Collier, 1995: 227). Interestingly, Redwood also appealed for the return of absent fathers so that they could provide 'love and support' to their families, drawing upon more recent discourses of fathers as involved, loving and supportive. However, the targeting of absent fathers as economic providers has found its most tangible expression in the passing of the 1991 Child Support Act. As explained in the previous chapter, this Act gave powers to the Child Support Agency (from 1993) to locate errant/absent biological fathers and make them liable for the maintenance of their children. Practically, the Act calculates to shift the cost of maintenance of children away from the state and on to fathers. At the same time the discursive context of the Act was an appeal by the Conservative government to family values and self-sufficiency which had been given extra urgency by the moral panic they and others generated around lone mothers and absent fathers.

The Child Support Act represents two shifts in the problematic of fatherhood. The first is to attempt to turn absent fathers into responsible fathers, although this notion of responsibility is limited to his economic contribution. In this way, it moves away from a legal concern with fathers' rights over their wives and children to a concern with fathers exercising their responsibilities towards their children. Collier (1995) describes this as a shift from father-rights to father-absence. At the same time it also casts the net of responsibility far more widely to pull in *unmarried* as well as married fathers. This signification of the responsibilities of unmarried fathers has also been accompanied by shifting boundaries in claims by unmarried men to fathers' rights, for example, having rights in the decision whether to terminate a pregnancy. This has further had an effect in displacing the old good/bad dichotomy of men in which married men were safe and constrained and unmarried men were dangerous and free, and replacing it with a new dichotomy of the (good) family man and the (bad) absent father.

However, whereas the Child Support Act has limited itself to an older idea of straightforward economic responsibility, the 1989 Children Act appeals to newer discourses about the constituents of fatherhood. One could say the Child Support Act deals in the discourses of bad fathers, whilst the Children Act buys into the discourses of good fathers. One of the key concepts underpinning the Children Act is that of *parental* responsibility, rather than *paternal* responsibility. One of its key aims is to minimize conflict in the post-separation and divorce process, to encourage the involvement of both parents in the care of their children after divorce or separation, and, through this, to encourage the best interests for the child's welfare. There are two key assumptions underlying the Act: first, that children are best cared for by both parents; and second, that contemporary parenting is a universally shared and complementary activity between mothers and fathers. Together these assumptions draw on an old discourse of the superiority of the nuclear, heterosexual family (broken-but-still-together) along with a new image of the role of men within that family – not only as a (detached-but-present) breadwinner but as a key pillar in a 'symmetrical' family set-up, loving, compassionate, supportive and involved.[4] The Act does not spell out what it means by the 'involvement' of parents; more specifically, it does not spell out what it means by the involvement of either mothers or fathers. The term 'parent' provides a gender-neutrality to mothers' and fathers' roles and also presents an image of already-existing equality in gendered familial relations. Although this image might be preferable to that of 'paterfamilias' and subservient wife, it is in danger of obscuring existing inequalities in the domestic sphere in terms of income, time and division of labour.[5] In effect, this blurs the distinction between gender parental equality as a *given* and gender parental equality as a *goal*. This blurring between the actual and the desired surfaces in many of the positions argued in the debate on fatherhood; it is central to the next group we look at.

An influential voice in the debate on absent fathers has come from absent fathers themselves.[6] A number of fathers' rights organizations have been formed over the last decade – for example, Dads After Divorce, Families Need Fathers – with the aim of restoring what is perceived to be the erosion of men's legal rights, particularly in relation to child custody following divorce. Unlike earlier men's organizations and networks represented, for example, by the magazine *Achilles Heel* and the *Men's Anti-Sexist Newsletter* (*M.A.N.*), and the academic development of critical studies on men and masculinities which are explicitly pro-feminist, these groups identify feminism and women's autonomy as one of the causes of family breakdown and the separation of fathers from their children. But more than that, it is the support for women's autonomy in *family law* which has become the focus of campaigns by these fathers and rights groups. So, for example, the Campaign for Justice on Divorce, Families Need Fathers and Dads After Divorce have all focused on changing the way in which they perceive the balance to have been tilted in favour of women in custody cases. Custody after divorce (now settled by a residence order) is generally granted to mothers on the basis that continuity of care is in the best interests of the child. Given the conventional division of childcare responsibilities in families this usually means that women are acknowledged by the court as the resident parent. (There are exceptions, of course; known lesbianism has sometimes been used to deny custody to mothers.) This general situation has been presented by fathers' rights groups as, on the one hand, anomalous, out-of-date and out of accord with equal rights for men and women.

But it has also been presented as undermining men's authority within the family.

In this way, these organizations have sought to mobilize two quite different discourses about fathers: one which appeals to a notion of gender equality, and a second which appeals to a notion of patriarchal authority. The first is further elaborated in terms of claims to the mutual emotional investment men and their children have in each other which is broken on divorce. One would not want to deny this pain of separation for either party, but, at the same time, these claims are built upon a notion of men's equal involvement in the care of their children and one might want to question the actuality and reality of this. Research by Charlie Lewis (Lewis, 1995) comparing fathering in the 1950s and 1980s suggests that it is easy to overestimate the changes that have occurred in men's involvement with their children. Whereas many men *perceive* their commitment and involvement to be greater than that of their own fathers, parental accounts of fatherhood from the 1950s bear considerable similarities with those gathered in the 1980s. (A similar disparity between mothers and fathers' perceptions of paternal involvement in childcare has been noted in other studies – see Ferri and Smith, 1996, discussed later.) The second point of the argument – that father's authority has been displaced – and that this displacement is compounded by other social and economic changes is explained by Roger Whitcomb, Chairman of the self-named UK Men's Movement[7] in these terms: 'Our problem is not a crisis of masculinity, but that the anti-male ethos of feminism has infiltrated the law courts and popular culture to such an extent that men have been reduced to divorceable sperm donors and disposable cheque-signing machines' (Cohen, 1996: 30).

In terms of the influence of these arguments upon policy, it is possible to see some aspects of the Children Act's gender-neutrality and acknowledgement for the role of the non-resident divorced parent (usually the father) as an appeasement of this position (Piper, 1995: 17). However, these fathers' organizations were far more influential in discrediting the operations of the Child Support Agency (CSA) between 1993 and 1995. The Child Support Agency, as has already been detailed, was premised upon the objective of finding errant fathers. However, in its scope it was universal – all fathers not living with the mothers of their children became potential targets. This scope meant that white middle-class, 'respectable' working-class ex-family men or reconstituted family men were tarred with the same brush as the absent fathers of the (sometimes racialized) 'underclass', and it also brought them, for the first time, within the span of the DSS (Collier, 1994). The CSA's narrow emphasis upon the father's contribution as a financial one offended the father-rights organizations' attempt to reconstruct their paternal masculinity in both emotional and authoritative terms.[8]

The backlash against the Child Support Agency revealed the classist assumptions underlying images of errant fathers. In the United States, more so than in the United Kingdom, these assumptions about so-called 'deadbeat dads' have also been far more explicitly racialized. One response to this from part of the African-American community was the organization of the Million Man March Day of Atonement in Washington, DC on 16 October 1995. The call for the march was initiated by Louis Farrakhan, the leader of the black Nation of Islam organization. It aimed to mobilize (and was successful in so doing) black men to demonstrate their concern with increasing racism, deteriorating social and environmental conditions and the urgent need for a transformative and progressive leadership in such a context (Organizing Committee, 1995: iv). The theme of the march was upon the need for black men to express atonement, reconciliation and responsibility within the context of black family and community life. This was expressed by the Organizing Committee's Mission Statement in the following terms:

> Our priority call to Black men to stand up and assume this new and expanded sense of responsibility is based on the realization that the strength and resourcefulness of the family and the liberation of the people require it; that some of the most acute problems facing the Black community within are those posed by Black males who have not stood up; that the caring and responsible father in the home; the responsible and future-focused male youth; security in and of the community; the quality of male/female relations, and the family's capacity to avoid poverty and push the lives of its members forward all depend on Black men's standing up . . . and that unless and until Black men *stand up*, Black men and women cannot *stand together* and accomplish the awesome task before us.
>
> (Organizing Committee, 1995: 2–3)

The organization of the march (male-led, male-dominated), and the responses to it, can be read on many different levels (which there is not space here to develop): for its exclusion of women from the march;[9] for its implicit homophobia;[10] for its overlaps with victim-blaming notions of the underclass; for its assertion of self-help along with a commitment to justice and equal rights for men and women. However, what it also represents is an attempt to recon-struct and restore dignity to black households through the assertion of a breadwinning, responsible, hard-working masculinity. On the one hand, men and women (and children) are identified as joined together for the fight against racism (and in this sense, unlike defen-sive white men's organizations in Britain where men's interests are pitted against women's) but, on the other hand, racism is held responsible for having destabilized the hierarchical heterosexual order within the black family. In these terms, the restoration of a stable, hierarchical if complementary, heterosexual family order is seen as essential for self-preservation and the united fight against racism.

A final point to make about these discourses of the absent father is that whilst many draw on these newer representations of the caring, supportive father, this caring is definitively confined to the care and support of *children* and, to some extent, wives. At no point does this image of the caring father extend to the care of old or frail parents or relatives, nor are any demands being made in terms of sons' rights to care for their own ageing parents or parents-in-law. This suggests that the discourse of care which under-pins this new form of paternal masculinity locates itself more closely to a notion of care as moral authority and control than to care as a form of practical and emotional tending.[11] In this sense, shared parenting is underpinned by a relatively unconstructed sexual division of labour but one in which the subjective emotional investment of a father's *identity* may well be as near or as equal to that of a mother's investment, but in which the objective costs of time and labour involved in this investment weigh far more heavily on the mother.

This section has looked at the construction of the problem of the absent father and responses to this. It has identified a number of different perspectives which draw from and contribute to attempts to reconstitute a new paternal masculinity. These perspectives are heavily reliant but in different ways on old discourses of father-hood – as economic provider and figure of authority within a hier-archical, heterosexual order. But they also draw on new classist and sometimes racist discourses of good and bad fathers, and on resistance to these, as well as new notions of involved, loving and supportive fatherhood.

THE PROBLEM OF DISTANCE

The second way in which fatherhood has been problematized is in terms of the lack of involvement and practical commitment to shared parenting by fathers, along with an attempt, first, to provide an understanding of the reasons for this, and second, in some cases, to work towards strategies to change the situation. These reasons range from the lack of structural and attitudinal support for fathering to men's responses to the rupture in the power relations between men and women, or the limits of expressive forms of masculinity available to men. Various groups can be identified representing these arguments: practitioners involved in active fathering projects; differently placed feminists (Campbell, 1993; Hewitt, 1996; Coward, 1996); left-wing think-tanks – especially the Institute for Public Policy Research (IPPR) – sociological accounts of the nature of social relationships in late modernity (Giddens, 1991; Beck, 1995); the pro-feminist men's movement and critical studies of men and masculinity (Connell, 1987, 1995a; Hearn, 1983, 1984, 1987, 1992; Morgan, 1992; McMahon, 1993; see also Chapters 1 and 2, this volume); the mythopoetic men's movement (Bly, 1990); psychoanalysts (Samuels, 1993, 1995); and studies of gay and lesbian parenting (Weeks *et al.*, 1996). I concentrate here mainly on the different feminist, practitioner and psychoanalytic perspectives. With the exception of the mythopoetic men's movement, most groups represented here would probably see their attempts to reconstruct (or account for the reconstruction of) fatherhood as a positive and progressive response to claims for women's autonomy, and unlike some of the groups in the previous section, they do not envisage a return to traditional gender roles. However, the mythopoetic men, best represented by Robert Bly, whose book, *Iron John: A Book about Men* (Bly, 1990), which sold in great numbers in the United States, advocates male-bonding rituals as a way for men to retrieve their lost – and strong – masculinity. At the root of these lost masculinities is the pain of the memory of fathers who remained too distant for their sons to get close to and to bond with.

In Britain, Wild Dance, a mixed-gender organization, has run male-bonding groups bearing similarities to the Bly approach. Its founder, Richard Olivier, explains its rationale thus:

My problems were that I blamed my father for not being around me and that I had difficulty dealing with his fame [his father was Sir Laurence Olivier]. . . . The group gives me the space to develop emotional vocabulary and look afresh at my identity as a man. It offers a forum for men to dispense with goals and just sit in the pain, sit in the process . . . we are . . . in the middle of a huge cultural shift for which there are no easy solutions.

(Cohen, 1996: 30)

Although it reckons with the cultural shift and acknowledges the need to bring fathers and (especially) sons closer together, this position embraces social change. At the same time, however, Bly, in particular, also identifies women's independence as undermining the strength of true masculinity and is essentialist in its approach to both masculinity and femininity (for a full critique, see Samuels, 1993: 184–94).

What, then, is more interesting is to examine those perspectives which seek to reconstitute paternal masculinity in line with women's greater autonomy. For some groups – especially practitioners involved in developing supportive parenting groups and those concerned with public policy – the real problem lies in the lack of policy, political, legal, practical and attitudinal support for fathers wanting to become active parents. In some areas, fathers' support centres have been set up, such as *A Dad's Place* in Newcastle upon Tyne. This is, as its briefing paper describes, 'a voluntary project that enables men to enjoy and take a pride in their role as fathers . . . the project promotes active fathering by creating a range of opportunities for men and their children. The project recognises that fathers play an important role in children's successful development' (Knight and Duckett, 1996).

Such centres are in line with the recommendations in an IPPR pamphlet entitled 'Men and their Children: Proposals for Public Policy' (Burgess and Ruxton, 1996). This argues that the cultural representations of fatherhood are often negative and discouraging – for example, focusing upon child sexual abuse, errant fathers or rendering men's caring capacities as deviant or invisible – and are at odds with the dominant view of the majority of parents who would like to see more active involvement by fathers. In addition, major social institutions – such as education, employment, the law – do not recognize fathers' potential needs for support and rights to care. Apart from the Children Act, they argue, government policy has been largely rhetorical on the question of encouraging active fathering; for example, the UK government opted out of the European Union directive on parental leave, and has framed its moral panic around absent fathers, through the Child Support Act, in traditionalist family terms. In contrast, the IPPR propose a policy for fathers which would: widen cultural images of father-hood; improve education and support for fathers; adopt a chil-dren's rights perspective; develop a positive legal framework which encourages men to be involved with their children; reduce conflict between parents post-separation; and maintain contact between children and their parents (Burgess and Ruxton, 1996: vi).

These principles would be put into effect through education for boys and would-be fathers; encouraging health, welfare and child-care professionals to direct their advice and support services to fathers as well as mothers, and encouraging employers to foster father-friendly employment policies such as parental leave, career-breaks, job-shares and so on. A Fathers Resource Centre would identify fathers' needs and would work towards shifting public atti-tudes to fathers. The rights and responsibilities of married fathers should be extended to unmarried fathers, both in terms of these fathers' rights to a declaration of parentage and to contact with their children except in difficult cases such as rape. This is argued for both in terms of encouraging fathers to be involved and also in terms of children's rights to identity. Children's rights are also the basis for strengthening policies to encourage non-resident parents (mainly fathers) to maintain contact after divorce or separation.[12] Non-custodial penalties are recommended for wilful child support defaulters along with a reframing of child support in terms of the costs attached to maintaining a child, as well as a recognition of the costs to the non-resident parent of keeping in contact.

It is possible to identify two sets of influences in these recommen-dations. In some ways they appear to put flesh on earlier demands dating back to the 1980s from feminists and from anti-sexist men's groups which aimed to break down the sexual division of labour in the home as well as in access to paid employment. On the other hand, the extension of fathers' rights and the focus on parenting over and above the separate interests of men and women reflects the thinking in the 1989 Children Act discussed earlier. In terms of the first influence, it is interesting to track the shifts in analysis.

So, for example, Susie Orbach and Luise Eichenbaum argued in 1983 for shared parenting, shared jobs and shorter hours for both parents (Orbach and Eichenbaum, 1983). Many of the practical demands from this time focused upon a re-assessment of the relationship between paid work and domestic work for both men and women, and envisaged the transformation being effected through changed working conditions – a shorter and more flexible working day, parental leave and public provision of day nurseries, after-school and holiday facilities under carers' control. As Anne Phillips wrote: 'We have to adapt work to fit in with the rest of life and particularly adapt it to fit with children' (Phillips 1983: 5).

This scenario envisaged creating the material conditions in which opportunities would exist for men and women to care equally. It rested upon the capacity of men and women to have leverage to make demands in the work place and upon claims of the state, and it supposed that, given the right conditions, men would take up, under the encouragement of women, the opportunities to care. However, by the 1990s, it was clear that few of these goals had been achieved. Although women have entered paid employment in greater numbers, no major reassessment of either the relationship between paid work and domestic work or of a more equitable gender division of time and labour has taken place. One explanation for this is in terms of the changed conditions for negotiation of these objectives – there has been a weakening of trade-union power; a restructuring of paid work, resulting in higher male unemployment and increased part-time employment for women; and cutbacks in public expenditure with particular consequences for the decline in affordable day-care facilities for children and older people; along with much longer working hours for the employed.

At the same time, however, part of the explanation also lies in men's apparent resistance to sharing domestic and childcare responsibilities in the home. So, for example, in 1995 women in full-time employment spent, on average, eight hours more a week on housework, cooking and shopping compared with men in full-time work. The presence of dependent children reduces the amount of free time a week by about 20 per cent for women but only by 10 per cent for men. Even comparing men and women who work part-time, women still spend twice as much time as men in doing the shopping, cooking and housework. Whereas men may do household tasks such as repairs, these, in general took up less than a quarter of the time for all forms of domestic and care work (HMSO, *Social Trends*, 1996: 216) These figures, of course, generalize men's and women's activities. More detailed research by Elsa Ferri and Kate Smith (1996) suggests that, in so far as men are taking up domestic and childcare responsibilities, then these are when their female partners are in paid work: the greater mothers' hours in paid work, the greater men's involvement in domestic and childcare responsibilities. At the same time, women tended to take responsibility for more time-intensive activities (such as caring for a sick child).

Against popular ideas of the middle-class 'new man' this research found a marked *inverse* relationship between social class (measured by occupation) and equal parental responsibility for childcare. Interviews with mothers and fathers found that shared childcare was more common among semi-skilled and unskilled workers than professional and managerial workers, in spite of the fact that middle-class parents are more likely to express more egalitarian attitudes (Ferri and Smith, 1996: 27–8). Whilst part of the explanation might lie in professional and managerial men's longer working hours, there were still marked class differences when among professional and managerial men working under fifty hours a week. On the other hand, where fathers were unemployed and mothers working, the sharing of care was not significantly different from dual-employed families. In other words, unemployment does not result in a major role reversal of domestic and childcare responsibilities (1996: 26).

These research findings present something of a contradiction – on the one hand, fathers appear to be resisting an equal sharing of domestic commitments, except in some situations where their partner has equal earning power, yet on the other hand, they also appear to be claiming greater involvement in their children's lives. Burgess and Ruxton, for example, rest their demands upon evidence of a groundswell of popular opinion in favour of men's greater involvement with their children (1996: 3, footnote 12). How this contradiction – between the nature of men's resistance and the nature of men's demands – is explained marks the key differences in approaches to retrieving the distant father.

The IPPR approach, which has been supported by high-profile British feminists such as Patricia Hewitt, Rosalind Coward and Anna Coote, has been central to the debate about distant fathers in the mid-1990s, yet it differs markedly from earlier feminist approaches referred to above and, indeed, from other current feminist approaches, which are discussed later. First, the analytical context in which the demands in the 1980s were argued was one in which the *unequal relations of power between men and women* – at home and at work – were central. The aim was to change those policies which underpinned gender inequality especially in relation to the unequal division of labour in the home and unequal access to paid work and income. In the 1996 IPPR document, the analytical context has changed. Here it is *men's loss of power* and/or rights (rather than men's submission of privilege or women's lack of power and/or rights) which is the key issue. Fathers are not only losing opportunities to be the breadwinner, it is argued, but also losing out on opportunities for involvement with their children. They have, as fathers and as workers, become marginalized, de-skilled and excluded. In these terms, policies are proposed which *compensate* men – in terms of practical support and legal and moral recognition – in terms of their role as fathers.

Second, in the 1980s, whilst policies were demanded which could create the material conditions which made male caring more possible, there was also an emphasis upon men (and women) as the *agents* of this change – both individually in the home, and collectively in trade unions and other organizations. In the IPPR pamphlet, the responsibility for change is taken off fathers and put on to social institutions – education, welfare professionals, judges, policy-makers, employers: British fathers have been discouraged from playing a full and rewarding role in the intimate lives of their families (ibid.: 4). Fathers are presented not as resistant to active involvement by their own actions, but held back by structures and attitudes.

> Within families, fathers have become increasingly marginalized: long hours working limits many; family breakdown alienates others. Today mothers are the 'preferred parent' among teenagers of all families . . . fathers' private lives remain largely hidden, and in the media, fathers are often negatively represented.
>
> (Burgess and Ruxton, 1996: v)

Words such as 'invisible', 'hidden' and 'marginalized' convey an oppression of fathers.

Two further aspects which mark a shift away from a notion of women as subordinate in gendered power relations and of men as responsible for change are first, the idea that women, too, are responsible for men's lack of involvement. For Burgess and Ruxton this has happened in two main ways. They suggest that 'recent debates on family work . . . have been mainly conducted in a feminist voice' and that this has meant that caring for children has been portrayed as onerous and burdensome, rather than as pleasurable. In addition, attempts to involve men have not been framed in terms of the emotional gains to men of involvement with their children, but in terms of justice for women in the household. Both of these, they argue, have been counterproductive in appealing to men's interests. This approach could be read as a positive acknowledgement of women's power and pleasure in the household division of labour (rather than understanding it as dreary and oppressive). At the same time, the approach conveys the idea that women's exercise of power should *not* be disruptive to men's interests. And whilst it acknowledges the arena where women have power, it does not set this against other arenas where they still exercise – in comparison to men – less power, for example, employment or work-related benefits such as pensions.

This negative impact of women's power in childcare arrangements is taken further by other feminist writers. For example, Ros Coward identifies feminism in general and women in particular as carrying some of the blame for the failure of men to be more involved in caring. Of the first she writes: 'Some time ago feminists stopped talking about getting men to care and share more and started wondering . . . exactly what, in the 90s, is a father for?' (Coward, 1996). She suggests that a positive view of fathering has been taboo in feminist debates as it undermines the role of single parents. She also suggests that women fail to surrender care to the fathers of their children: 'Women may have been working but few have given up their central role with the child and fully delegated primary care of their children to their fathers' (ibid., 1996). Patricia Hewitt, too, has talked about the need for women to move over and give men space and support to care for their children (Hewitt, 1996). On the one hand, this approach provides a positive view of women's lives which acknowledges their power and pleasures rather than seeing them as victims of inequality and oppression, yet this notion of women's power as the cause of men's resistance fails to square with the gender differentials in time spent on household and caring work quoted above, nor on similar statistics on other forms of care, particularly of older or disabled people.

A further change can be seen in the nature of the demands. The demands of the 1980s were seen to involve both men and women, separately and together, campaigning in women's groups, anti-sexist men's groups, in trade unions, in single-issue campaigns, for policies around the collective and shared care for children. In fact, over the last decade, demands for changes in policies to make shared care more feasible, such as work-place nurseries or job-shares have tended to come from organized women, though often with organized men's support. The IPPR pamphlet setting out a policy for fatherhood has also been spearheaded by women. Where organizations of men have been most active around father-hood is among the fathers' rights groups discussed in the previous section. These make little reference to the need for nurseries or crèches, but are framed almost entirely in terms of the legal rights of fathers. The IPPR pamphlet also makes little reference to the dismal state of pre-school provision for children in Britain.[13] However, it does focus about one-third of its proposals on the extension of legal rights to fathers – especially unmarried fathers.

In this way it is possible to see the position represented by Coward, Hewitt and the IPPR pamphlet as drawing upon dis-courses in which men are encouraged to take up responsibilities through the inducements of further rights rather than on the basis of a commitment to gender equality. The loss of power or pri-vilege in one area (breadwinning, authority) is seen to require com-pensation by the extension of rights in another. One could also speculate whether the men who lose and win in this scenario are the same men. The decline of industrialized industries has mainly affected the economic rights of working-class men. The claim for and exercise of legal rights to parentage and custody after divorce and the resistance to maintenance levies has come from men's orga-nizations led by the middle-class. Indeed, the feelings of exclusion, loss and marginality from fatherhood have been most keenly articu-lated by both middle-class and working-class men on the point of separation and divorce – and understandably so. However, whether one should generalize these particular feelings of pain and loss to a generalized feeling of loss felt by *all* fathers in *all* situations is again questionable. It is at the point of separation that the loss of privi-leges attached to being 'a family man' are most clearly outlined in law.[14] The law, in usually acknowledging mothers as the resident parent, is in part reflecting the greater practical investment that women have made in caring for their children. Just as it is mistaken to generalize the feelings of one group of men at a particular moment in their lives, so too is it misplaced to generalize mothers' greater access to custody to a view that the balance of power between mothers and fathers everywhere is tilted in women's favour, and needs to be readjusted.

What the 1980s feminism and the IPPR pamphlet do share, however, is a view that the capacity to care for children is not determined by biology. Care combines practical skills and emotional commitments which are open to all, regardless of gender. This means that, aside from birth and lactation, there need not be a separate and distinctive role for parents of either sex. It implies that the advantages that stem from having two parents are not that a child has male and female adult figures, but that there are, potentially, two socially approved sources of income and time and two pairs of hands, eyes, ears and two hearts. Nevertheless, arguments for the reconstruction and validation of fatherhood are often caught between moving towards a notion of parenting accessible to both men and women and an idea of the distinctive and separate role that fathers and mothers – through their gender – provide. For example, Ros Coward talks about an active and affectionate father bringing homosociability to sons and offering daughters sources of identification other than motherhood (Coward, 1996). What Coward does not make clear is that these are the symbolic characteristics that fathers bring to family life within a segregated system of the gender division of labour. The whole debate about fatherhood is riven with slippages between the *actual,* the *potential* and the *essential.* For example, women's *potential* for equality through their greater involvement in paid work and greater autonomy is assumed in many of the positions we have looked at to represent *actually existing* equality or even advantage, or, in traditionalist discourse, it is seen to be a repudiation of a natural or essential position for women. On the other hand, Coward's position, quoted above, defends the *potential* for fatherhood in terms of an *actually existing* position that fathers currently occupy, one that has been naturalized as an essential aspect of masculinity. Similarly, in other arguments, men's desire for greater recognition of their involvement with their children is taken to be evidence of their *actual*, practical involvement in childcare.[15]

A contrasting feminist perspective on the crisis of fatherhood is provided by Beatrix Campbell (Campbell, 1993, 1996). She locates the public recognition of a perceived social problem around single mothers and absent fathers within, on the one hand, structural economic changes and, on the other, men's and women's different responses to the disruptions these changes have brought:

> Fathers – and masculinities – have emerged as new political problems in the 90s both because of global restructuring and because feminism put them under greater scrutiny.
>
> We are all participating in a new historic settlement between genders and generations.
>
> (Campbell, 1996: 11)

Whereas underclass theorists blame mothers, especially single mothers, Campbell identifies masculinity and masculinist responses to unemployment and poverty as the root of the problem:

> If the New Right ventured into the estates and saw the streets captured by thin, pale boys, it did not see the menacing response by men to the abolition of work, nor the street megalomania of boys trying to be men; in short, it did not see a *masculine* response to an economic crisis – it saw instead the failure of the *mothers* to manage men.
>
> (Campbell, 1993: 303)

In her book *Goliath* (Campbell, 1993), she also documents the way in which women have responded to economic crisis. This is largely through collective and individual strategies of survival and solidarity. For men, particularly young men, their responses – which in extreme forms are manifested in petty crime, brutal control over urban spaces, and doing drugs – represent an attempt to re-assert in different ways the power and privileges attached to men and masculinity:

> in pauperised places where men have no escape from the space they share with women and children (the home and the neighbourhood) masculinity is still defended as difference and domination. This is the legacy that the history of mainstream masculinity has given to men.
>
> (Campbell, 1996: 11)

For Campbell, the problem is not that men have *lost* their identities, but is in the ways they have chosen to *assert* them. The particular response she documents and dissects is the rash of riots in Britain in the summer of 1991 across municipal suburbs in Cardiff, Oxford and Tyneside by, in the main, young white men resulting in the random destruction of parts of those communities. Similarly, for Campbell, the problem is not an *absence* of role models but a superabundance of cultural and global representations of macho propaganda – 'they were soaked in globally transmitted images and ideologies of butch and brutal solutions to life's difficulties' (Campbell, 1993: 323).

In more general terms, this masculine response has also, in Campbell's analysis, prevented working-class and middle-class men from being able to offer women and children what they really want – co-operation. To support this, Campbell cites the fact that women, even when their male partners are unemployed, do more than three-quarters of the domestic work and childcare. Among both the poor and the prosperous, when men and women share the same time and space, something is still more important to men than co-operation – their masculinity (Campbell, 1996: 11). In working-class communities Campbell acknowledges the point made by Dennis and Erdos on the decline of what has been termed 'respectability', but emphasizes the way it has given rise to different consequences for women and men. For women, it has enabled them to break out of the constraints of domestication and dependence and to cross the divide between the public and private spaces. For men, however, it has removed the political, personal, cultural and institutional rationales for their co-operation with women. This has left women with the responsibility of challenging men to work with them rather than against them in these new conditions. For Campbell, strategies to overcome this impasse should aim to support women and to challenge men and violent forms of masculinity (Campbell, 1993: 253). Although she does not spell what this might mean, it represents a different focus from that of the IPPR, which emphasizes support aimed at men and compensation for their losses along with an encouragement to women to surrender their power in the home.

Both sets of arguments rely, however, on unitary and generalized conceptions of women and men, and although Campbell makes it clear that her analysis is about working-class women and men, it also depends upon fixed differences between men's and women's behaviours. In these terms, it is difficult to assess the validity of either argument, for what we need to know is the different ways in which men construct and negotiate their masculinities as well as the common and differentiated responses they have to different social, economic and personal condtions. For example, Bob

Connell's work presents a complex understanding of the processes through which different masculinities are expressed and experienced (Connell, 1995a, 1995b). Among the concepts Connell develops to examine different forms of masculinity are those of the *patriarchal dividend* and *hegemonic masculinity*. The patriarchal dividend represents the advantages that accrue to men by virtue of generally higher wages and better promotion prospects compared with women. Hegemonic masculinity is the dominant and culturally authoritative form of masculinity in any given gender order (namely, society). However, other forms of masculinity are generated at the same time – for example, a *subordinated* masculinity may be the product and process of gay men's culture; a *marginalized* masculinity may co-exist with the hegemonic for minority ethnic men, whilst men who accept and benefit from but do not necessarily defend the patriarchal dividend may operate a form of *complicit* masculinity. From his life history research upon men who have lost out on the patriarchal dividend – in this case, men who are long-term unemployed – Connell shows that they neither buy fully into hegemonic ideologies or practices nor fully buy out of them; for example, contemptuous misogyny may coexist with an admiration of women's strength and survival techniques; fatherhood may be both feared and desired (Connell, 1995b).

This brief reference to an understanding of multiple masculinities and the contradictory and complex responses they generate when men lose out on the patriarchal dividend may indicate how to cut through the excessively optimistic scenario of masculinities presented by the IPPR and the deeply pessimistic one given by Campbell, as well as, of course, some of the traditionalist notions of fathers discussed earlier in the chapter. A set of interviews conducted for the *Guardian* newspaper provides case studies which illustrate how both these scenarios exist. The interviews included as respondents two married miners made redundant from the same colliery in Nottinghamshire. The first has a daughter and a wife who has become the sole breadwinner whilst he has become a full-time 'housewife' – a role in which he is both effective and contented. What undermines his ease with his role is public attitudes: 'It's only when I see myself through other people's eyes, like when a travelling salesman rings the doorbell and I answer it in my apron and duster that I feel embarrassed that he'll think I'm not a proper man' (Cohen, 1996: 26).

This situation would clearly be improved by the sort of supportive framework suggested by the IPPR, and discussed earlier. On the other hand, this would be unlikely to help the situation faced by this man's ex-colleague and his wife and two children. Their situation far better fits the analysis offered by Campbell, where, when the chips are down, men's overriding concern is with their loss of masculinity rather than co-operation with their wives. This second man says:

> Until I was made redundant, I put the bread on the table and I made the decisions. Now she does. It's bad enough that I've lost my job, but I've lost my authority as head of the family as well.
> His wife's response is:
> It's not just a job he needs, it's retraining in how to be a man. He can't understand that men are no longer the head of the household, that decisions need to be made jointly. And he can't express how he feels about it. When I ask him what's wrong he says: Nothing. Nothing. Then he takes out his frustration and anger on me and the kids.

> (Cohen, 1996: 26)

A final perspective on this problem of the 'distant' father is provided by the work of psychoanalyst Andrew Samuels (1993, 1995). The significance of Samuels' work in the debate under discussion is that, whilst he is concerned with a project of involving fathers more in the care of their children, he does not unhook this project from the issue of gender equality, nor does he seek to compensate men for their losses in the public sphere with gains in the private sphere. This is because he sees current social and economic changes as undermining the fixity of men's *identities* more than their *power*. He does not fall into the trap of misreading a desire by men for greater emotional involvement with their children with a reality of more equality between men and women in the household:

> The huge change in Western consciousness concerning men does not mean that men and women have identical agendas; I have become suspicious of simplistic calls for partnership between the sexes. Men will not give up their power that easily. But the notion of a partnership between the sexes in pursuit of social justice remains an ideal at which to aim.

> (Samuels, 1995: 515)

More significantly, though, Samuels argues that in so far as there are lessons to be learned about how to carry out non-fixed gender parenting roles then we should look to the experiences of those families who transgress the conventionally accepted family form – namely, lone parents/mothers and same-sex parents. In this way, Samuels turns upside down the conventional placing of transgressive families as, in traditionalist family discourse, problematic and pathological and, in much progressive discourse, as diverse family forms to be acknowledged and tolerated. Instead, he sees these forms of parenting as carrying within them the seeds of non-gendered parenting identity and practice and, thereby, offering fathers, in particular, insight into the possibilities of a more fluid parent identity. The sorts of policies which flow from this analysis are ones which provide lone parents with support, resources and approval as well as the opportunity for others to learn from their experiences.

The different positions on the distant father draw in different ways upon the discourses of gender equality, masculinities, children's rights, gendered parenting practices, men's and women's agency and the role of social policy and law. Whilst many are explicitly feminist, they nevertheless occupy different positions on gender relations. Some seek to redress a perceived loss of power for men as a step towards shared gender roles; others are more concerned to challenge those expressions of masculinity which distance men from shared caring and which serve to bolster men's remaining areas of power and privilege. In policy terms this leads some to support an extension of both men's rights as well as their responsibilities in relation to the care of children, whereas others emphasize the continuing need for vigilance, restraint and resistance to male power and privilege and yet others to look to the possibilities for support to enable women and men to share care in non-gender-specific ways. Common to all is a call for socialized forms of provision to support mothers and fathers to care, although policies involving cash transfers and affordable day care are noticeably lower down on the agenda in campaigns in the 1990s. Implicit in these different approaches are also varying degrees of acknowledgement of the nature of changing family forms. For some, the emphasis is clearly upon the dual-earner, two-parent heterosexual family as the object of social support, whereas others are more keen to emphasize non-conventional family forms, not simply as deserving of social support, but as signifying the transformatory potential of new forms of non-hierarchical, cross-gendered forms of parenting. In this way, there are differing positions within these discourses of distance between those who would seek to reconstruct father-hood through shifting and recontextualizing masculine identities, and those who would deconstruct fatherhood in order to disconnect the points at which paternal masculine identities fuse with expressions of hierarchy and power.

CONCLUSION

More generally, a number of points can be drawn out of this discussion on the fatherhood debate. To begin with, social and economic changes have challenged the economic, legal, moral, cultural and biological conditions of fatherhood. The debates around this have, on the one hand, expanded the discursive space to include an area previously closeted in the taken-for-granted quarters of domestic privacy. On the other hand, much of the room in this contested space is currently occupied by those who would seek to retain, but reconstitute in new ways, a hierarchical, heterosexual gender order.

In order to examine this issue, the chapter utilized a distinction in the discourse between those focusing on absence (in the economic and moral sense) and those focusing upon distance (in the emotional and caring sense). This distinction allowed for a setting out of some of the key components of fatherhood – the economic, the legal, the moral, the authoritative, the sexual, the biological, the emotional and the practical. In mapping the various contributions to the debate, this distinction also demonstrated the difficulty of identifying clear political lines of attachment, either in terms of 'old' politics of left and right, or 'new' politics of social movements, particularly feminism. In addition, although positions were identified in terms of a concern with absence or distance, some overlapped – such as the concern on both sides with the extension of fathers' rights – and some fell on the cusp – such as the Children Act. Indeed, the differing discourses of the Child Support Act, with its emphasis on fathers' responsibilities, and the Children Act, whose legal consequences have emphasized fathers' rights, find reflection in different feminist positions.

In order to assess this shift in emphasis in some feminisms, from women's rights to equality and men's responsibilities in equality struggles to men's rights in relation to their children and women's responsibilities to facilitate those rights, I suggested that it was necessary to examine and make sense of, first, the dissonance between men's *emotional investment* and their *practical involvement* in and with their children and, second, the idea that men's loss of rights and privileges in the public sphere require compensation through enhanced rights in the private sphere. One possible consequence of this shift is that it repositions mothers within a new form of relations of domination – one based no longer on the husband in marriage, but on the rights and responsibilities of the biological father of her child.

At the same time, we need to question how far many of these discourses rely upon fixed and separate notions of male and female parenting roles as well as upon unitary notions of male and female identities. Some of the arguments for shared parenting are based on implicit assumptions of the different and gender-based contributions of mothers and fathers which serve to obscure the manner in which that difference, in practice, sustains inequalities in the sexual division of childcare, especially when measured in terms of time and space. They also serve to reinforce the marginalization of those family forms which are not based upon gendered parenting. Furthermore, such assumptions ignore different expressions of masculine identities and the differential structuring of interests that fathers have in sustaining or abandoning old and new forms of power and privilege. Differences of class, 'race' and ethnicity, sexuality, age, generation and disability position men differently in relation to masculinities and the heterosexual gender order, in general, and fatherhood, in particular. Making fatherhood a public issue has revealed the layered and criss-cross nature of public discourses, the gendering of rights and responsibilities and new interpretations of gender equality; it also provides the space for the articulation of these more challenging ideas about the relationship between identities and power.

ACKNOWLEDGEMENTS

This chapter has benefited greatly from comments from, and discussion with, Jeff Hearn and Ruth Hubbard. For information on specific points I would also like to thank Gail Lewis and Carol Smart.

NOTES

1 The separation of public and private spheres should not be overstated – see Hearn (1992).

2 This point has been made in different ways by Smart (1991) and Svenhuijsen (1992).

3 By 'crisis', I mean a point of contestation and change, rather than catastrophe (see Moran, 1988).

4 This notion of the symmetrical family has a relatively long history emerging out of the sociological work of Young and Willmott in the 1950s and 1960s and spelt out in the 1970s (Young and Willmott, 1957, 1973).

5 Carol Smart has argued that there is, in effect, a hierarchical ordering within the moral and legal discourse of care in custody cases. She distinguishes between the form of care that in many cases mothers provide, and see themselves as providing ('caring for'), and that provided by men ('caring about'). However, in legal discourse, mothers' claims to have cared for their children could often find no legitimate mode of expression, or recognition, whereas fathers' claims to 'care about' their children are accommodated into a rights discourse. By contrast, mothers rarely used a notion of rights to express their feelings of identity to their children (Smart, 1991).

6 Not only were these groups influential in discrediting the Child Support Agency, they actually influenced some subsequent policy changes including an increase in the level of income of the absent parents to be ignored in the assessment of maintenance contributions, the phasing in of increased maintenance payments (for a full account, see Clarke *et al.*, 1996). This is in contrast to the limited influence of organizations of lone mothers.

7 The term 'men's movement' has become increasingly problematic in recent years. In the 1970s and 1980s it generally referred, in the UK at least, to anti-sexist (pro-feminist) groups and networks; in the late 1980s and early 1990s it came to be used, particularly in the US, to refer to mythopoetic groups and networks; and now there is a very small UK organization calling itself the 'UK Men's Movement', which adopts a men's rights position (see Hearn, 1993).

8 It may also be that the pressure placed on the Child Support Agency to meet performance targets meant that the fathers they followed up first were those who were already paying some maintenance because they were accessible, unlike entirely absent fathers.

9 Not all black organizations went along with this; for example, the African-American Agenda 2000 put out a leaflet which said, 'no march, movement or agenda that defines manhood in the narrowest of terms and seeks to make women lesser partners in their quest for equality can be considered to be a positive step. Therefore we cannot support this march' (E. Hammonds, 'In Response to the Million Man March' leaflet, Massachusetts Institute of Technology).

10 The Nation of Islam (NOI) Organization has a reputation for its fundamentalist, traditionalist religious views about women and sexuality as well as a virulent anti-Semitism. Whilst some African-American

groups boycotted the march, others went along to it with a view that the march had touched a nerve among Black communities. So, for example, the Black Gay and Lesbian Leadership Forum joined the march despite NOI's hostility to them. A post-march commentary, by James Hanna-ham, an African-American gay activist writing in the *Village Voice*, 31 October 1995, summed up the complex significance of the march:

> The crowd got impatient for the arrival of impresario Minister Louis Farrakhan, or as we called her, Miss Louise-Farrah Khan . . . she went off for two and a half hours, straying far and wide with feeble attempts to reprise earlier themes. She spent at least a half hour on a close reading of the word 'atonement' unpacking that sucker like a Gucci handbag. . . . We had to hand it to her though. White America perceives Farrah Khan as dangerous. . . . Sure, Louise is a lunatic and we don't trust her as far as we could throw her. Neverthe-less, she managed to pull off a much-needed (if only precursory) step in the self-determination of black American men.
>
> (Hannaham 1995: 39–40)

11 This is borne out by the research of Ferri and Smith on parenting roles where men claimed greater involvement in teaching children good beha-viour than in 'generally being with and looking after children' and 'looking after children when they are ill' (Ferri and Smith, 1996: 23–4). They also point out that this aspect of childcare is less time-intensive than the other aspects.

12 This close connection of children's rights with fathers' rights can also be seen in other areas of policy; for example, the Human Fertilization and Embryology Act (1990), which requires licensed clinics to consider the welfare of any child who may be born as a result of the treatment (including the need of that child for a father) (s. 13(5)).

13 This is in contrast to the recommendations from the research by Elsa Ferri and Kate Smith, which includes expansion of affordable day-care provision along with family-friendly employment practices and parenthood education (Ferri and Smith, 1996).

14 Ulrich Beck and Elisabeth Beck-Gernsheim suggest that it is upon divorce that men are confronted by the consequences of an inequality with which they had, up until that point, lived quite happily:

> Becoming a father is not difficult, but being a divorced father cer-tainly is. At the moment when it is too late, the family personified by the child becomes the centre of all hope and concrete effort; the child is offered time and attention in a manner which during the marriage was out of the question.
>
> (Beck and Beck-Gernsheim, 1995: 154)

15 Carol Smart refers to a similar distinction in her work on child custody (see note 5 above). 'There is, moreover, a tendency to defeat these tentative moral claims by reference to the fact that men are perfectly capable of caring for as if this *projected activity* should carry the same moral weight as *actual activity*' (1991: 494).

REFERENCES

Beck, U. (1995) *Risk Society*, London: Sage.

Beck, U. and Beck-Gernsheim, E. (1995) *The Normal Chaos of Love*, Cambridge: Polity Press.

Bly, R. (1990) *Iron John: A Book about Men*, Shaftesbury, Dorset: Element Books.

Burgess, A. and Ruxton, S. (1996) *Men and their Children: Proposals for Public Policy*, London: IPPR.

Campbell, B. (1993) *Goliath: Britain's Dangerous Places*, London: Methuen.

—— (1996) 'Good riddance to the patriarch', *Guardian* (15 April).

Clarke, K., Glendinning, C. and Craig, G. (1996) *Small Change: The Impact of the Child Support Act on Lone Mothers and Children*, London: Family Policy Studies Centre.

Cohen, D. (1996) 'It's a guy thing', *Guardian Weekend* (14 May), pp.26–30.

Collier, R. (1994) '"Detached fathers" and "family men": representations of masculinity in the campaign against the Child Support Act, 1991', Paper presented to the *British Sociological Association Conference*, Sexualities in Social Context, University of Central Lancashire, March 1994.

—— (1995) *Masculinity, Law and the Family*, London: Routledge.

—— (1996) 'Coming together? Post-heterosexuality, masculine crisis and the New Men's Movement', *Feminist Legal Studies*, 4(1): 3–48.

Connell, R.W. (1987) *Gender and Power: Society, the Person and Sexual Politics*, Cambridge: Polity Press.

—— (1995a) *Masculinities*, Cambridge: Polity Press.

—— (1995b) 'New directions: gender theory, masculinity research, gender politics', English version of 'Neue Richtungen fur Geschlechter theorie, Mannlichkeitsforschung und Geschlechterpolitik', in L. Christof Armbruster, Ursula Muller and Marlene Stein-Hilbers (eds) *Neue Horizonte? Sozialwissenschaftliche Forschung uber Geschlechter und Geschlecht verhaltnisse*, Opladen: Lesker & Budrich, pp. 61–83.

Coward, R. (1996) 'Make the father figure', *Guardian* (12 April).

Davies, J. (1993) 'From household to family to individualism', in J. Davies, B. Bergen and A. Carson (eds) *The Family: Is it Just Another Lifestyle Choice?* London: IEA Health and Welfare Unit.

Dennis, N. and Erdos, G. (1992) *Families without Fatherhood*, London: IEA Health and Welfare Unit.

Ferri, E. and Smith, K. (1996) *Parenting in the 1990s*, York: Joseph Roundtree Foundation.

Giddens, A. (1991) *Modernity and Self-identity*, Cambridge: Polity Press.

—— (1992) *The Transformation of Intimacy: Sexuality, Love and Eroticism in Modern Societies*, Cambridge: Polity Press in association with Basil Blackwell.

Hearn, J. (1983) *Birth and Afterbirth: A Materialist Account*, London: Achilles Heel.

—— (1984) 'Childbirth, men and the problem of fatherhood', *Radical Community Medicine*, 15 (Spring): 9–19.

—— (1987) *The Gender of Oppression: Men, Masculinity and the Critique of Marxism*, Brighton: Wheatsheaf.

—— (1992) *Men in the Public Eye*, London: Routledge.

—— (1993) 'The politics of essentialism and the analysis of the men's movement(s)', in *Feminism and Psychology* 3(3): 405–9.

Hewitt, P. (1996) 'Women moving over', Talk given at IPPR Conference, Men and Their Children (30 April).

HMSO (1996) *Social Trends*, London: HMSO Publications.

Knight, B. and Duckett, R. (1996) 'A Dad's place', Information supplied for IPPR Conference, Men and Their Children (30 April).

Knijn, T. (1995) 'Towards post-paternalism? Social and theoretical changes in fatherhood', in M. Van Dongen, G. Frinking and M. Jacobs (eds) *Changing Fatherhood, A Multidisciplinary Perspective*, Amsterdam: Thesis Publishers.

Lamb, M. (1995) 'Paternal influences in child development', in M. Van Dongen, G. Frinking and M. Jacobs (eds) *Changing Fatherhood, A Multidisciplinary Perspective*, Amsterdam: Thesis Publishers.

Lewis, C. (1986) *Becoming a Father*, Milton Keynes: Open University Press.

—— (1995) 'Men's aspirations concerning childcare: the extent to which they are realized', in M. Van Dougen, G. Frinking and M. Jacobs (eds) *Changing Fatherhood, A Multidisciplinary Perspective*, Amsterdam: Thesis Publishers.

Lewis, J. (1992) 'Gender and the development of welfare regimes', *Journal of European Social Policy*, 12(3): 159–73.

McMahon, A. (1993) 'Male readings of feminist theory: the psychologization of sexual politics in the masculinity literature', *Theory and Society*, 22(5): 675–96.

Moran, M. (1988) 'Review article: crises of the welfare state', *British Journal of Political Science*, 18: 391–414.

Morgan, D. (1992) *Discovering Men*, London: Routledge.

Murray, C. (1990) *The Emerging British Underclass*, London: IEA Health and Welfare Unit.

Orbach, S. and Eichenbaum, L. (1983) *What Do Women Want?* Glasgow: Fontana.

Organizing Committee, Washington, D.C. (1995) *The Million Man March Day of Absence. Mission Statement*, Los Angeles: University of Sankove Press; Chicago: Third World Press; Chicago: FCN Publishing Co.

Phillips, A. (1983) *Hidden Hands: Women and Economic Policies*, London: Pluto Press.

Piper, C. (1995) 'Marketing the Children Act 1989: the invisibility of mothers and fathers', Paper presented to the Social Policy Association Annual Conference, (18 July), Sheffield Hallam University.

Samuels, A. (1993) *The Political Psyche*, London: Routledge.

—— (1995) 'The good-enough father of whatever sex', *Feminism and Psychology*, 5(4): 511–30.

Smart, C. (1991) 'The legal and moral ordering of child custody', *Journal of Law and Society*, 18(4): 485–500.

Svenhuijsen, S. (1992) 'The gendered juridification of parenthood', *Social and Legal Studies*, 1(1): 71–83.

Van Dongen, M., Frinking, G. and Jacobs, M.(eds) *Changing Fatherhood: A Multidisciplinary Perspective*, Amsterdam: Thesis Publishers.

Weeks, J., Donovan, C. and Heaphy, B. (1996) *Families of Choice: Patterns of Non-heterosexual Relationships. A Literature Review*, London: South Bank University, School of Education, Politics and Social Sciences: Research Paper 2.

Young, M. and Willmott, P. (1957) *Family and Kinship in East London*, London: Routledge & Kegan Paul.

—— (1973) *The Symmetrical Family*, London: Routledge & Kegan Paul.

Part II
Women and men on men and welfare

Chapter 4

Are men good for the welfare of women and children?

Ann Oakley and Alan S. Rigby

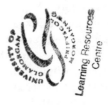

> But our concern is with the mothers and children. How are they maintained? The answer is, of course, broadly speaking by their husbands and fathers.
>
> (Rathbone, 1927: 14)

> He was never bloody here when I wanted him here, and when he was here he was – well, when I needed him most he was drunk, stoned out of his blooming mind.
>
> (Woman in Social Support and Pregnancy Outcome study)

Conventional accounts of welfare ignore gender relations. Ungendered individuals populate both welfare inputs and outputs, and the places where welfare is enacted – the 'home', the 'family', 'the state' and 'work' – appear as homogenized stages for casts of ungendered players sharing essentially the same scripts. The key concepts and ideas attract by their blandness – by the spectacle they conjure up of a conflict-free existence. Whether we look at the history of the development of the welfare state (Lowe, 1994), at how sociologists have defined the functions of the family (Elliot, 1986), or at the way in which epidemiologists have traditionally studied the social patterning of health and illness (Tuckett, 1976), we see the same tendency to assume that the differences between men and women are not part of power relations.

THEORIZING 'THE TURK COMPLEX'

The social reformer and feminist, Eleanor Rathbone, was fortunate in having a father who believed in her (Stocks, 1949). It was Rathbone's inquiry into the circumstances of widows in Liverpool in

1913 which impressed on her the need to liberate women from their fragile dependence on male providers. Their lives were poor, dreary and marked by constant hard domestic labour in services to the community of quite as much value as those of 'a dock labourer, or a plumber, or a soldier' (Stocks, 1949: 62–3). Rathbone argued that the case for the 'family wage' ignored the different sizes of different families, and the position of single men and women, but most importantly it swallowed up mothers' needs to be able to provide for their children in an insultingly specious view of wives as luxuries on a par with beer and cigarettes to be afforded by men, most of whom suffered from an urge to dominate and deny women's rights – otherwise known as 'the Turk complex' (Rathbone, 1924).

Rathbone annoyed the Miners' Federation by pointing out that although producing coal was dangerous, producing human beings was some four times more so (Rathbone, 1927: 43). But although her defence of working-class mothers was absolute, she, like other founders of the welfare state, took certain key aspects of the traditional division of labour within the family for granted. Men often handed over a 'preposterously small proportion' of their wages to their wives, but they deserved a 'quiet corner' away from housework and childcare for a pipe or a read or 'a talk on politics or football with a friend'. Because of this, many women were disappointed to find their notions of companionship in marriage reduced to separate spheres, with hardly a link between the two. The separation could cross-cut class lines: even in middle-class homes the best food had to go to the men because they were the breadwinners. Significantly, Rathbone noted that failed male providers were none the less capable of indulging in 'orgies of parental fondness' (Rathbone, 1927: 42–4). Good men were good for women and children, but bad men had their good sides, and were better than none.

In most conceptions of welfare, the presence of a man in the family is presumed to benefit both women and children. The assumption of male beneficence is manifested in many different ways, from the condemnation of single-parent (meaning lone-mother) households as bad for children, to the prescription of normality in family life as being essentially *about* the presence of a man (Institute of Economic Affairs, 1992), and the observation that families without men are generally worse off materially than those with men (Coote *et al.*, 1990). The *consequences* of patriarchy – women's inferior labour-market position, their economic vulnerability – are conflated with the *personal* help that may or may not be given to women and children by men. This conflation is common in the attitudes of health, welfare and education professionals who tend to view families without men as deviations from a moral norm (Edwards and Popay, 1995; Mayall and Foster, 1989), despite the fact that statistically such families are increasingly likely. Thus, for example, normal childbearing is now considered to involve the father's presence, and some health workers refuse to accept deliveries unless the father's presence is guaranteed: 'I just make sure I get them there any way I can. I'd castrate them if necessary' (Seel, 1994: 16). This moral imperative conflicts with a good deal of ambiguity, if not uncertainty, about what it is that fathers are expected to do at childbirth and whether women really find it helpful (Barbour, 1990).

As Hanmer *et al.* (1992) observe, one of the main ways in which the Turk complex has been, and is, maintained in the welfare field is through the valuing of non-gendered constructions and accounts of welfare above those highlighting the unequal experiences of men and women. The 'social division of welfare' means a 'sexual division of welfare' (Oakley, 1987; Rose, 1981). Neither the welfare state, nor welfare services, nor the informal provision of welfare within the family and community can be understood in terms of an ungendered scenario. So far as welfare within the family goes, we now understand that women not only do housework and bring up children, they also perform 'people work' (Stacey, 1982), care work (Graham, 1983), child work (Hearn, 1983), solidary work (Lynch, 1989) and emotional work (Hochschild, 1983). We also understand that violence against women is a neglected public health issue, and the most endemic form of violence against women is their abuse by intimate male partners (Kornblit, 1994).

Theorizing the Turk complex means understanding not only the role of gender in welfare but the position and function of the state as the biggest patriarch of them all (Walby, 1990). The state appropriates women's labour by depending on it for servicing the capitalist system. The patriarchalism of the state expresses itself partly in relation to concepts and practices of family life, and partly by upholding in social policy a notion of 'the family' as the happy and comfortable place we all live in, despite the fact that many of us either do not, or we experience it differently. The 'pro-family' politics of the 1990s are as much a resistance to women's rights as the Turk complex of the 1920s (Oakley, 1994). We need to see behind the screen of 'The Family' in order to ask important questions about what this cultural and material arrangement does to the personal welfare of those who live in it. Families are better for men's mental health than for women's; prime among the conditions of ordinary life that depress women is the condition of ordinary family life (Dennerstein and Farish, 1993). For both women and children, the risk of being exposed to violence is greater in the home than anywhere else (French, 1993; Romito, 1993). While fathers are capable of 'orgies of parental fondness', there is no evidence that children deprived of fathers do worse because of this than other children. They are, on the other hand, very likely to do worse because of the economic dependence of women that remains uncorrected, despite the staunch efforts of Eleanor Rathbone and many other social reformers before and since her time.

MEN AND THE WELFARE OF WOMEN AND CHILDREN: SOME EMPIRICAL QUESTIONS

This chapter interrogates data collected from a sample of women and children living in four areas of England in 1986–94 with a set of specific questions about the role of men in women's and children's welfare. The principal question is: do the women and children who live with men have better or worse health and welfare outcomes, and, if so, can any such differences be attributed to the presence or absence of men in the household? To put it bluntly, do men make a positive contribution to the welfare of women and children?

THE SAMPLE

The Social Support and Pregnancy Outcome (SSPO) study was originally designed as a randomized, controlled trial of a research, midwife-provided, social support intervention in 'high risk' pregnancy. The hypothesis tested was that providing extra social support in pregnancy would improve the health of women and their babies. A total of 509 women took part in the original study, which was based at two centres in the South of England and two in the Midlands, and carried out between 1985 and 1989. Because of an interest in the class-related phenomenon of low birth-weight, only women with a history of low birth-weight ($<2,500\,g$)

delivery were asked to take part in the study. The original period of data collection spanned 18 months in families' lives beginning in early pregnancy, and included information from medical records, qualitative, tape-recorded home interviews, and postal questionnaires. The home interviews were offered to the half of the sample allocated to receive the social support intervention: 92 per cent of the 255 women in this group completed all three of the planned home interviews. The postal questionnaires were carried out at six weeks, one year and seven years after birth, with response rates of 94 per cent, 78 per cent and 67 per cent respectively.

The findings of the analysis of the SSPO study as a controlled trial of a social support intervention have been extensively published (see, for example, Oakley *et al.*, 1990; Oakley, 1992a and 1992b). Briefly, providing social support as a research intervention was associated with significantly better health for both women and their children. The follow-up questionnaire undertaken when the children were 7 years old confirmed the continuing benefits to intervention group families of the social support provided before the children were born (Oakley *et al.*, 1996).

The SSPO women were on average 28 years old at recruitment to the study; 90 per cent had living children. In addition to the index child born during the study, 28 per cent had had further children by the time of the seven-year questionnaire. Because of the selection criterion used (a history of having had a low birth-weight baby), most of the women were socially disadvantaged; 73 per cent were working class in terms of either their partners' or their own present or past occupation; and 40 per cent smoked in pregnancy[1] (see Graham, 1987).

In this chapter, we explore five particular sub-sets of data collected in the SSPO study which throw some light on the question, 'Are men good for the welfare of women and children?' These sets of data relate to (1) health and welfare outcomes in households with and without men; (2) the allocation of material resources in the household; (3) men's contribution to the division of labour; (4) men's role in providing emotional and social support; and (5) the relationship between men and stress in women's lives. The tables below show percentages based on the number of women answering particular questions. The base figures at the three time points are 467 (six weeks), 362 (one year) and 241 (seven years); the data from the home interviews with the women offered the pregnancy support intervention are derived from a sub-sample of 248.

HOUSEHOLDS WITH AND WITHOUT MEN:
HEALTH AND WELFARE OUTCOMES

Most women (around 90 per cent) have children either in marriage or within a cohabiting relationship with the father of their child. However, one in five mothers are caring for children in one-parent households. Single mothers tend to be younger and poorer than separated and divorced mothers (Coote *et al.*, 1990). But formal marital status is increasingly a poor guide to actual living circumstances (Cunningham-Burley, 1986). Married couples may be living apart, and non-married women may be living with part-ners in long-lasting relationships. At the time of the first postnatal questionnaire, 93 per cent of the SSPO study women were living with the baby's father. This had declined to 83 per cent when the children were a year old. Information about partner status was not asked for at the seven-year time point, but 27 per cent of the women reported a change in their living arrangements, and 17 per cent were not living with the child's father at this point.

Some idea of the flux that attended some partner relationships is given by one young mother, Sheena Briffit*:

INTERVIEWER   Have you had any important decisions to make since you've been pregnant?

SHEENA BRIFFIT   Yes, I have really, because, like, me boyfriend is living with his mum, and when I had the double bed about a couple of months ago, he said, 'I'll move in with you' . . . well, his mum and dad are out of work . . . which they always have been and they are quite dependent on his money which I can understand . . . but I need his help . . .

INTERVIEWER   So is the flat in your name?

SHEENA BRIFFIT   Yes, it's in my name and he sleeps here every night in case anything happens . . . but he is moving in in the holidays which I am a bit wary about . . . because last time he promised me and it never happened, but this time I said if it does happen that he doesn't move in with me I'm finishing with him. I say, 'you either want me or your mum.'

Sheena thinks her boyfriend will move in with her despite the fact that 'his mum's always going on at him, saying it's too soon and you're too young for responsibility. So I just said to him well,

_____
* All names are pseudonyms.

Table 4.1 Social characteristics of households with and without men†[2]

	Living with husband %	Living with partner %	Neither %
Woman left school before 16	20	32	43
Woman aged under 25	17	45	46
Woman not in paid work in pregnancy	64	74	86
Husband/partner not in paid work	16	33	56
Family income under £85 per week	13	33	93
Woman has no access to a car	21	47	56
Not owning or buying home	33	71	86

Note:
† Data from 6-week questionnaire

you weren't too young to make love to me and you aren't too young to stand up to these responsibilities.'

There were considerable social differences between women living with their husbands, living with a partner and living alone, as shown in Table 4.1. The proportions of women who left school before 16, were aged under 25, had paid work during pregnancy, unemployed partners, low family income, no access to a car and were not home-owners were higher in the group who lived with a partner than in the group who lived with husbands, and higher still in the group of women who lived with neither. Being married may therefore be a proxy for higher social status, either because socially advantaged women are more likely to get married and/or because being married may confer material and social advantages.

These data fit what is known about the position of lone mothers, who are one of the most disadvantaged groups in Britain. For example, 65 per cent of lone mothers live in rented accommodation, while 76 per cent of mothers in two-parent households live in owner-occupied housing (OPCS, 1994). Whereas lone-mother families represent 18 per cent of all families in Britain, they make up two-thirds (68 per cent) of those on income support (Department of Social Security, 1993). Lone-mother families and two-parent families headed by an unemployed parent face the greatest

Table 4.2 Children's health by family status

	Father living with mother %	Father not living with mother %
Birth-weight (mean gm)	2,896.7	2,968.1
No health problems at 6 wks	82	83
Very healthy at 1 yr	64	56
Very healthy at 7 yrs	61	50
No long-term illness at 7 yrs	88	67
Mother happy with child's development at 7 yrs	75	60

risk of debt of all population groups in Britain (Berthoud and Kempson, 1992).

It is interesting that the differences by marital status shown in Table 4.1 did not hold for some other important indicators of social support, including the amount of contact with relatives and the number of friends the women reported having. There were no differences here between the three groups of women.

Table 4.2 shows some of the data on health outcomes for the children collected at the three time-points by whether or not there was a man in the household. Generally, the health of children in households with men is better than that of those in households without. However, the figures show little difference at birth and shortly after. By 7 years, only 67 per cent of children whose fathers are not living with their mothers are reported to have no long-term illness or health problem, compared with 88 per cent of those in father-present households.

Table 4.3 presents similar data for the women. On most of the variables shown in the table, women without partners appear to do worse than those with partners. The differences are greatest for depression at 1 year. With respect to the control variable, women living with partners may have more control because their households are better resourced. But they are dependent on their partners' comings and goings, and on the way *they* do things:

INTERVIEWER   Do you feel that you're under any stress at the moment?

LORRAINE MARTIN   Yes, the house. It's just the worry of it, you know, but I know that when he gets home everything will be

Table 4.3 Women's health by family status

	Father living with mother %	Father not living with mother %
Good physical health:		
at 6 wks	93	93
at 1 yr	89	83
at 7 yrs	92	85
Not depressed:		
in hospital after birth	56	48
at 6 wks	89	82
at 1 yr	53	33
at 7 yrs	93	85
Felt in control of life:		
at 6 wks	67	56
at 1 yr	84	16
at 7 yrs	7	28
Confident as mother:		
at 6 wks	99	96
at 1 yr	92	94
at 7 yrs	72	74

alright, it's just not knowing when he's coming home, it's just worrying, because I do worry about everything like that, I mean he is the sort that would say, oh, wait until the reminder comes in, and then he'll wait another couple of weeks before it gets paid, whereas me, as soon as it arrives I go and pay it there and then.

INTERVIEWER   So you know it's paid?

LORRAINE MARTIN   Yeah, that's right.

Another way to express the data in Tables 4.2 and 4.3 is in terms of the odds of women and children living with men having good health compared to the health of those of women and children living without men. Table 4.4 shows these odds ratios adjusted for class and previous health problems. Women who live with men are 10 per cent less likely than those who live without men to report good health for their children and to say that their own psychological health is good at six weeks. At all other time-points and in relation to women's physical health, the chances of good health are higher in

Table 4.4 Association between household status and women's and children's health outcomes*

	Father living with mother OR** (95% CI)
Children's health:	
at 6 wks	0.9 (0.2–4.2)
at 1 yr	1.2 (0.5–3.2)
at 7 yrs	2.1 (0.9–4.4)
Mothers' physical health:	
at 6 wks	1.2 (0.6–2.6)
at 1 yr	1.7 (0.5–5.6)
at 7 yrs	1.2 (0.5–2.7)
Mothers' psychological health:***	
at 6 wks	0.9 (0.3–2.4)
at 1 yr	2.4 (0.8–7.3)
at 7 yrs	1.8 (0.7–4.5)

Notes:
* All odds ratios adjusted for social class and previous health problems; odds ratios for women's health also adjusted for life events
** Odds ratio is set at 1.0 for father-absent households
*** Composite variable including mothers' answers to questions about levels of stress, unhappiness, anxiety, satisfaction and control

father-present households. However, it is notable that the confidence intervals here all include one, which means that our findings are compatible with the real differences being in the direction of men's presence either lowering or promoting health.

MATERIAL RESOURCES

One of the ways in which men may positively benefit women and children's health is through the material resources provided by the second or sole income associated with their generally more financially advantaged position in the labour market. This, of course, assumes that men *are* employed, which is not necessarily the case. At six weeks, 19 per cent of partners of the SSPO study women were unemployed.[3] Table 4.5 shows some key material resources in father-present and father-absent households. It is evident that father-present and father-absent households are different, not only in terms of income, but with respect to other resources

Table 4.5 Material resources by family status

	Father living with mother %	Father not living with mother %
Household income:*		
below poverty level†	35	96
above poverty level	65	4
Housing:* rented	37	86
owner-occupier	63	14
Crowded housing:*		
yes	21	29
no	79	71
Household amenities*‡		
poor	18	48
good	82	52
Use of car:*		
yes	55	22
no	45	78
Enough money to provide for child::**		
yes	57	22
no	43	88
Worried about money:**		
yes	18	10
no	82	90

*   Information taken from 6 wk questionnaire
**   Information taken from 1 yr questionnaire
***   Information taken from 7 yr questionnaire
†   Household income was classified as above or below poverty level by taking broad household income groups reported by women and judging these against the then (1987) prevailing poverty standard of less than 140 per cent of supplementary benefit level.
‡   A household amenity 'score' was constructed on the basis of women's answers to questions about own/shared kitchen, bathroom, toilet and bedroom, running hot water, washing machine, telephone, central heating and paid domestic help.

which have an important impact on the work of parenthood, including quality of housing and household amenities and access to transport.

Within father-present households, material resources are not necessarily allocated equally between mothers and fathers. Indeed, the tendency for women *within families* to be materially disadvantaged compared to men is a finding that emerges from a considerable number of diverse research studies (see Brannen and Wilson, 1987; Morris, 1990). So far as financial resources are concerned, 'control', 'management' and 'budgeting' are different and normally gender-differentiated functions. Most power rests with the controller of the domestic income, who is usually also the person who earns the most, namely, the man (Morris, 1984; Pahl, 1983). The weaker power position of the non-earning or lower-earning partner is a key feature of most types of household finance management.

In addition to the questions asked in the postal surveys, the women who were interviewed at home in pregnancy as part of the social support intervention were asked for some additional information on material resources and their intra-household allocation. These data on intra-household resource allocation and management generally confirm the findings of other studies (see Morris, 1990).

More than half the SSPO study women who provided data in home interviews said that they made no financial contribution to the household income because they were not in paid work. About a quarter said they contributed less than a quarter of the total amount; about one in seven contributed between a quarter and a half. Forty-three per cent reported being given a fixed amount of money for the housekeeping, and a majority of these (55 per cent) said their housekeeping money was not enough. Table 4.6 shows who paid for particular items of expenditure. Women were most likely to pay for food and for their own and their children's clothes. Partners were most likely to pay for the major routine and non-routine expenses, including bills other than food, the rent/mortgage, insurance and holidays and other 'luxuries'. Between one in five and a third of all the expenditure categories were shared by both partners (which means that most were not). The highest dependence on state benefit was for children's clothes (33 per cent) and the rent/mortgage (23 per cent).

DIVISIONS OF LABOUR

The data on the division of labour come from a series of questions about to what extent partners 'helped' with household and child-care tasks at four time-points (pregnancy, six weeks, 1 and 7 years), whether they were considered generally helpful, and the extent to which they were interested in the child.

Table 4.6 Who pays for what?*

	Woman	Partner	Both	State benefit	Other
	%	%	%	%	%
Food	30	31	24	15	<1
Rent/mortgage	10	47	18	23	2
Household bills	13	49	21	16	1
Incidental household expenses	15	40	29	15	1
Children's clothes	20	19	27	33	2
Woman's clothes	27	31	29	12	0
Holidays/luxuries	11	53	31	2	3
School fees/trips	15	36	34	13	2
Insurance	11	53	28	7	1
Other major outgoings	15	48	24	13	<1

Note:
*Information taken from the first home interview during pregnancy with the intervention group women (N=248)

Framing questions about male domestic participation in terms of 'helping' assumes that the primary responsibility for taking care of the home and children rests with women. Empirical data show this to be the case in most households (Brannen and Moss, 1988; Gregson and Lowe, 1994; Luxton, 1980; Oakley, 1974). In couple households, 75 per cent of women are mainly responsible for domestic work; even where men and women are employed full-time, women are mainly responsible in 67 per cent of households (Jowell *et al.*, 1991). Against this backdrop of unequal responsibility, even a man reported to be 'very helpful' is unlikely to be assuming a significant share of his partner's domestic workload. Tables 4.7 and 4.8 show the percentages of men who were described by their partners as helping either 'rarely' or 'never' with a set of core domestic and childcare tasks.

Three main conclusions can be drawn from these tables. The first is that the *absolute* level of help from men is rather low: between one in ten and three out of four men 'never' or 'rarely' help with the tasks listed in the tables. The lowest figure is for playing with the child at 1 year; the highest is for fetching 7-year-olds from school. Second, there is a clear tendency for men to become less helpful as children get older, both in relation to looking after

Table 4.7 Percentage of men helping 'rarely' or 'never' with domestic
tasks during pregnancy and when children are 6 weeks, 1 year
and 7 years old

	In pregnancy %	At 6 wks %	At 1 yr %	At 7 yrs %
Cooking	40	39	51	61
Housework	29	29	46	47
Shopping	18	18	31	36
Childcare (other children)	9	9	16	18

Table 4.8 Percentage of men helping 'rarely' or 'never' with childcare
tasks

	At 6 wks %	At 1 yr %	At 7 yrs %
Changed nappies	51	50	–
Got up at night	57	62	–
Took child out on own	–	61	41
Played with child	–	8	19
Took child to school	–	–	70
Fetched child from school	–	–	73
Look after child when ill	–	–*	58

Note:
*Question not asked at 1 year

them and in relation to housework, cooking and shopping. The
8 per cent of men who 'never' or 'rarely' play with the baby at
1 year becomes 19 per cent who 'never' or 'rarely' play with their
7-year-olds. While 40 per cent 'never' or 'rarely' help with cooking
in pregnancy, this figure has become 61 per cent when the children
are 7. The corresponding figures for housework at 29 per cent and
47 per cent, and for shopping 18 per cent and 36 per cent. Third,
there is a clear hierarchy of male preferences. Men are most likely
to help with childcare and least likely to help with cooking. The
order of priority is the same at each of the four time-points: childcare followed by shopping followed by housework followed by
cooking.[4]

SOCIAL AND EMOTIONAL SUPPORT

What women say about men's helpfulness can be interpreted both as a description of the amount they do in the home and as a reflection of how the women feel about both it and them. The merging of these issues in male–female relationships was clear in much of the interview data, including the early pregnancy interview with Marilyn Palmer during one of her home interviews:

INTERVIEWER   Now what about Derek, how much support and help does he give you?

MARILYN PALMER   Not a great deal, really. It seems as if he thinks this is my bit . . . like last night . . . I said 'I want to give Rosie a bath', so I filled the baby bath, she does occasionally have a baby bath still in here when I can't be bothered to bath her with me, and it was quite full because it has to be to bath her, and he just walked into the kitchen and walked out again. And I says, 'Well, aren't you going to carry the bath for me, because I can't carry it in' – and he just expected me to carry this big bath full of water. . . . I get fed up with asking him to do things like that for me.

INTERVIEWER   What about being able to talk to him? Do you sit down in the evenings and talk about anything and everything?

MARILYN PALMER   Well we talk, yes, but not about the pregnancy.

INTERVIEWER   You don't actually tell him how you are feeling?

MARILYN PALMER   No I don't. He doesn't understand . . . and I don't think he knows what he should do . . . so I just don't bother.

At the last home interview shortly before the new baby was born, an exchange between the research midwife doing the interviewing and Marilyn Palmer demonstrated the shared understandings women may have about men's roles in the household:

INTERVIEWER   What is Derek like when you aren't pregnant?

MARILYN PALMER   Well, he is a bit thoughtless. I mean, if you are ever ill, he wouldn't ask you how you are, or, do you want me to get you anything? You have to muddle through on your own . . . whereas when he's ill, I suppose it's the same with every other man . . .

INTERVIEWER   We all run round after them! And if they have a cold, they're dying, sort of thing . . . but we have to be on our knees before anybody comes to bring you a cup of tea in bed, sort of thing. Yes. [Returns to interview schedule.] How is your sex life, then?

MARILYN PALMER   Well, what was it last time? [Laughs.]

Each of the postal questionnaires asked the women whether a list of people (partners, mothers, fathers, mothers-in-law, fathers-in-law, sisters, brothers, other relatives, friends, neighbours, workmates, doctors and health visitors) were helpful or not. At each of the four time-points men were more likely than anyone else to be described as particularly or quite helpful: 87 per cent at six weeks, 85 per cent at 1 year and 87 per cent at 7 years. A subsidiary question asked women to name the most helpful person: 65 per cent at six weeks, 55 per cent at 1 year and 44 per cent at 7 years named their partners.

Thus, the proportions of women describing their partners as generally helpful were higher than the figures in Tables 4.7 and 4.8 would suggest. In fact, cross-tabulating answers to the two questions about whether partners were helpful and who was the most helpful person showed that at six weeks 15 per cent of the women who said their partners were not helpful actually described them as the *most helpful* people. Such figures may reflect the very low levels of support available to some women, in the light of which any contribution from male partners, however paltry, must be welcome. But descriptions of men as the most helpful people around also importantly embody an ideological view about marriage being an intrinsically supportive relationship (Brannen and Moss, 1988, 1991). The contribution men make in terms of domestic labour and support has to be seen in the context of other social support resources mothers are able to draw on to help them in bringing up children. Female relatives, particularly mothers, are especially important here. Unlike help from partners, that provided by women's mothers is a more stable resource over time (Oakley *et al.*, 1994a; Oakley and Rajan, 1991).

In a previous analysis of some of the same data (Oakley *et al.*, 1994a), we showed that *qualitative* indices of support (whether people are felt to be helpful) are more closely related to women and children's health outcomes than *quantitative* ones (whether women live with partners, have close contact with relatives, and so on). These generally stronger associations were particularly the case for women's psychological health outcomes: the feeling of

Table 4.9 Partners' levels of interest from pregnancy to 7 years

	Pregnancy %	6 wks %	1 yr %	7 yrs %
A lot	44	72	57	55
Enough	33	20	27	26
Not enough/none	23	8	16	16

being supported was linked with increased emotional well-being. One dimension of partner support relates to the extent of partner's psychological involvement with the child. A total of 68 per cent of the women reported that their partners had been with them during the births of their babies (22 per cent had someone other than the partner with them). Table 4.9 shows levels of partners' interest in the child from pregnancy through to 7 years. Whatever the women interpreted 'interest' to mean, this is apparently, like men's helpfulness in the home, a declining resource over time.

THE STRESS OF LIVING WITH MEN

Our data show that being married to or living with a man is not co-terminous with being helped or supported by him. Some men may be highly involved with their children and may provide high levels of help and support to their partners, but others may not. Women are also involved in *giving* support to men (Delphy and Leonard, 1992). Living with a man means being exposed to events affecting him and his life. Table 4.10 shows the incidence of life events involving partners at the different time points. Life events involving partners were not the most frequently mentioned life events, but three of these in particular – problems with partner's work, changing jobs and becoming unemployed were among the ten most frequently mentioned life events at six weeks and one year, and two of these (work problems and unemployment) were among the ten most frequently mentioned at seven years.

   Most types of life event are negatively related to women's psychological and physical health and to the physical health of children at six weeks, 1 year and 7 years. These relationships hold independently of class and previous health problems. Grouping the life events, women were asked about into five categories (family, work, health, finance and partner), we found that at six weeks the category

Table 4.10 Life events involving partners

	During pregnancy* %	Over 1st yr** %	During last yr*** %
Got engaged/married	5	4	3
Got separated/divorced	4	5	6
Partner began new relationship	3	3	4
Partner changed jobs	15	20	14
Partner had problems at work	16	20	22
Problems in relationship with partner	14	17	2

Notes:
*   Information given at 6 wks
**   Information given at 1 yr
*** Information given at 7 yrs

of life events most strongly related to mothers' psychological health was that associated with partners. Women who had problems with their partner were 3.2 times more likely to have poor rather than good psychological health (95 per cent CI: 1.6–6.6), and those who reported problems with their partner's work were 3.6 times more likely to be in poor psychological health (95 per cent CI: 1.8–7.1). At 1 year, both psychological and physical health were most strongly related to financial problems; women who reported these were three times more likely to have poor psychological and five times more likely to have poor physical health (95 per cent CI: 2.1–5.5 and 2.0–13.3). However, women reporting problems in their relationships with partners were 6.3 times more likely to have poor psychological health (95 per cent CI: 3.1–12.7) and 3.3 times more likely to have poor physical health (95 per cent CI: 1.6–7.0). At six weeks, financial problems doubled the chances of poor physical health in babies (95 per cent CI: 1.1–4.0) and at 1 year, problems with partners, finance and family health problems reported by mothers significantly increased the chances of their saying that their children were in poor health.

At 7 years the category of life events most strongly related to the mothers' psychological health was that related to problems with their partners; women who reported problems with their partners were 5.7 times more likely to have poor rather than good psychological health for themselves (95 per cent CI: 2.3–14.3). Also associated with poor psychological health at 7 years were financial problems. Women reporting these were 4.5 times more likely to have poor rather than good psychological health (95 per cent CI: 2.3–8.7). Other important predictors of poor psychological health at 7 years included problems at work (both for themselves and their partners) and problems with their housing.

In contrast, becoming engaged or married was associated with better psychological health for the women (OR = 0.5, 95 per cent CI: 0.3–1.1) as was a divorce/separation. At 7 years, the category of life events most strongly related to the women's physical health was also that related to their partners. Women reporting these were twice as likely to report their physical health as poor (95 per cent CI: 1.3–4.9). Other predictors of poor physical health at 7 years included financial problems and unusual expenses. At 7 years, separation or divorce from their partners quadrupled the chances of the women reporting poor health for their children (95 per cent CI: 1.1–13.2). Becoming engaged or married was also associated with adverse health outcomes for their children (OR = 1.3, 95 per cent CI: 0.3–5.7). These latter two findings are in contrast to those for mothers: here an engagement/marriage or divorce/separation was associated with better rather than worse health outcomes. Finally, problems at work (for both the women and their partners) also significantly increased the chances of the women saying that their children were in poor health.

Two of the most consistent factors associated with adverse health outcomes of the women and children are those relating to their partners and their partner's work. Figures 4.1a to 4.1c show these associations graphically (plotted as odds ratios and 95 per cent confidence intervals) at six weeks, 1 year and 7 years. Three conclusions in particular emerge from these graphs. First, the associations between partner-related events and health outcomes are stronger for women's psychological health (all odds ratios are significantly above 1.0, Figure 4.1a). Second, the main associations with the women's physical health (Figure 4.1b) are those relating to the partner *directly*. Third, the women seem to act as a buffer between adverse partner-related events and their children's health. These odds ratios tend to lie around 1.0 or just below (Figure 4.1c) rather than well above 1.0 (as in Figure 4.1a), which indicates some kind of protective effect operating from the mothers to their children.

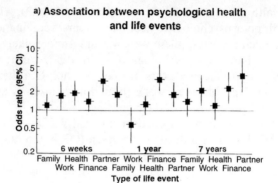

a) Association between psychological health and life events

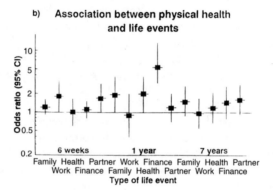

b)   Association between physical health and life events

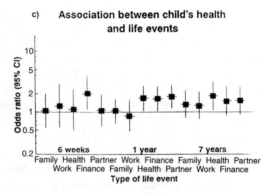

c)   Association between child's health and life events

Figure 4.1 Relationship between life events and health outcomes at 6 weeks, 1 year and 7 years. Reproduced by kind permission of Oxford University Press from *European Journal of Public Health* (1994) 4.

There were numerous examples in the interviews of women talking about how issues in their partners' lives had affected them, including in this interview with Andrea Maxton:

INTERVIEWER   Since I've seen you, has anything particularly difficult or unpleasant happened to you?

ANDREA MAXTON   My husband has been in and out of work.

INTERVIEWER   Oh, no, really – he's self-employed, isn't he?

ANDREA MAXTON   That's right, yes, so things just aren't going smoothly at the moment . . . the building industry is just getting worse, and less and less is happening, and there are more and more people, you know, joining, the work's just not there.

INTERVIEWER   It's difficult, isn't it, you don't really know where you are . . . and with you going to give up work as well?

ANDREA MAXTON   Yes, I don't know what to do.

INTERVIEWER   You must see that as quite a big worry . . . or are you used to it?

ANDREA MAXTON   You get used to it to a certain extent. Obviously if I do give up work then we shall have to be a lot more careful when he is earning.

In the six-weeks and 1-year questionnaires, the women were asked whether the birth of the child had made a difference to their relationships with their partners. At six weeks 42 per cent said that it had, and half of these said it had brought problems. At 1 year, of the 45 per cent who reported the child making a difference to the relationship, over a third judged that it had brought problems. There were no questions designed specifically to measure the quality of the emotional relationship with the partner, but in answer to a question in the 7-year questionnaire about how they were getting on with their partners, 54 per cent said 'Very well', 25 per cent said 'Well', 15 per cent said 'Okay' and 6 per cent said 'Badly'.

THE LOVE OF UNTRAINED WOMEN

It was William Beveridge who in 1932 considered that there were at least two important unanswered questions about women and the family. One was whether children might not be better looked after by experts than subjected to the love of untrained women. The other question was whether the economic independence of wives and mothers was really compatible with family life (Beveridge, 1932). Data of the kind drawn on in this chapter suggest a third question – one about the compatibility of traditional family life with the maximization of women's and children's welfare.

In several respects, it is clear that men's presence in the home is not automatically a gain for women, and thus for those for whom women care. The vulnerability of women and children to stresses in men's lives demonstrated above is one sign of the equivocal value of men to the welfare of women and children. As Delphy and Leonard (1992: 226) note, 'The work which wives do for their husbands' occupations, for men's leisure activities, and for their emotional and sexual well-being, gets completely lost sight of because it is so varied, so personalized and so intimate.' The levels of men's participation in domestic tasks quantified in this chapter are not impressive; neither is the extent to which they provide significant psychological and social support for their partners. In this respect, our data echo the findings of others. For example, Hartmann (1981) compared households with children and mothers but no husbands with those containing husbands using time-budget studies, and showed that husbands represent a net drain on women's time. The domestic division of labour between men and women is at its sharpest when children are young: it is among families with pre-school children that fathers make the smallest contribution to childcare and housework (Piachaud, 1984), and although there is some evidence that men do more in the home than they used to, this increase is from a low baseline (Gershuny and Jones, 1987). Even in the 'most liberated, young, two-job household', the husband averages only 15 per cent of routine domestic work (Gershuny, 1982). Middle-class families may be marked by as much gender segregation (Edgell, 1980) as working-class families traditionally exhibit (Dennis et al., 1956). Where waged domestic labour is annexed to support the child-rearing function, this role is one largely assumed and managed by women in order to help them rather than both parents equally (Gregson and Lowe, 1994).

While the data from the SSPO study drawn on in this chapter support and expand similar findings from other studies, a novel aspect of the SSPO data is its longitudinal nature. This demonstrates that the positive contribution men make in terms of domestic work, childcare and psychological and social support is a declining resource over time. The contraction of this resource also occurs in a context in which fathers are less likely to be present in the households of women and children as children get older.

Some disbenefits of traditional father-present households can easily be demonstrated. In view of the established importance of social support to health, including the health of mothers and young children (Oakley, 1993), it would be surprising if the *failure* of men in some households to provide this did not have some impact on the health of their partners and children. But other essential questions about the role of men are more difficult to answer. Women living on their own with children are discriminated against as a group, both through inadequate state support for motherhood and because of women's disadvantaged labour market position. This makes it difficult to quantify the contribution men make to women's and children's welfare. The advantages that men appear to offer may be mainly in the form of protection from the deficits of a system loaded against lone-mother families.

In other words, so long as men and women are treated differently, it is impossible to tell what difference men really make. This caveat makes it difficult to know how to interpret the findings of studies which suggest that lone mothers do worse than mothers in two-parent families – for example, in reporting higher rates of physical illness and psychological distress than women living with male partners (Huppert and Weinstein, 1991). The analysis described above suggests that some of these differences disappear when the impact of other social and health factors is controlled. Similarly, careful analyses of the data on the impact of fathers on children's development indicate that it is mainly the poorer material circumstances of children brought up in lone-mother families which adversely affects their development, rather than the absence of the father *per se* (Richards and Dyson, 1982).

A notable feature of the findings reported on in this chapter is the role women appear to play in buffering the impact on *children's* health of negative events associated with the presence of fathers. So far as we know, this has not been reported before. It suggests that, while children benefit materially from the presence of their fathers, this benefit in part depends on the ability of their mothers to protect them from some of the disbenefits associated with living in a nuclear family.

A reasonable conclusion from this would be that it is primarily patriarchy that is bad for women and children's health. This fact is disguised by the rhetoric of heterosexual love and protection which encourages women to see men as their saviours, and to 'excuse behaviour in our men that we would never permit ourselves or pardon in others of our kind' (Johnson, 1978: 30). None the less, there is evidence, including from the study described in this chapter, that women themselves are often aware of the ambivalence of their relations with men: the co-existence of affection, support and a shared life with the exploitation of women's work and caring to prop up both the economy of family life and the world outside the home.

NOTES

1 Graham (1987) points out that cigarette smoking among women is increasingly a marker of poverty.
2 We are grateful to Jo Garcia for her analysis of the SSPO study data here.
3 The question about partners' employment was not asked at the later time-points.
4 Women who lived with, and without, men reported similar weekly house-work hours at 7 years; 42 per cent of both groups said they spent more than 20 hours on housework each week. The average was 20.5 hours for those living with men and 19.7 for those living without men.

REFERENCES

Barbour, R.S. (1990) 'Fathers: the emergence of a new consumer group', in J. Garcia, R. Kilpatrick and M. Richards (eds) *The Politics of Maternity Care*, Oxford: Clarendon Press.
Berthoud, R. and Kempson, E. (1992) *Credit and Debt: The PSI Report*. London: Policy Studies Institute.
Beveridge, W. (1932) *Changes in Family Life*.
Brannen, J. and Moss, P. (1988) *New Mothers at Work*, London: Unwin Hyman.
—— (1991) *Managing Mothers*, London: Unwin Hyman.
Brannen, J. and Wilson, G. (1987) *Give and Take in Families*, London: Unwin Hyman.
Coote, A., Harman, H. and Hewitt, P. (1990) *The Family Way*, London: Institute for Public Policy Research.
Cunningham-Burley, S. (1986) *Marital Status and Pregnancy Outcome*, Glasgow, MRC Medical Sociology Unit.
Delphy, C. and Leonard, D. (1992) *Familiar Exploitation*, Cambridge: Polity Press.
Dennerstein, L. and Farish, D. (1993) 'Mental health, work and gender', in *Women, Health and Work, Proceedings of an International Congress*. Barcelona, Spain.

Dennis, N., Henriques, F. and Slaughter, C. (1956) *Coal is Our Life*, London: Eyre & Spottiswoode.

Department of Social Security (1993) *Households Below Average Income: A Statistical Analysis 1979–1990/1*, London: HMSO.

Edgell, S. (1980) *Middle Class Couples*, London: Allen & Unwin.

Edwards, J. (1994) 'Parenting skills and gardening: views of community health and social service providers about the needs of their "clients"', *Journal of Social Policy*, 24(2): 237–59.

Elliot, F.R. (1986) *The Family: Change or continuity?* London: Macmillan.

French, M. (1993) *The War Against Women*, Harmondsworth: Penguin.

Gershuny, J.L. (1982) *Household Work Strategies*. Presented at International Sociological Association Conference, Mexico City (August).

Gershuny, J.L. and Jones, S. (1987) 'The changing work/leisure balance in Britain 1961–84', *Sociological Review Monograph*, 33: 9–50.

Graham, H. (1983) 'Caring: a labour of love', in J. Finch and D. Groves (eds) *A Labour of Love*, London: Routledge & Kegan Paul.

—— (1987) 'Women's smoking and family health', *Social Science and Medicine*, 25: 47–56.

Gregson, N. and Lowe, M. (1994) *Servicing the Middle Classes*, London: Routledge.

Hanmer, J., Hearn, J. and Bruce, E. (1992) *Gender and the Management of Personal Welfare*, Bradford: University of Bradford Research Unit on Violence, Abuse and Gender Relations.

Hartmann, H. (1981) 'The family as the local of gender, class and political struggle', *Signs*, 6: 366–94.

Hearn, J. (1983) *Birth and Afterbirth: A Materialist Account*. London: Achilles Heel.

Hochschild, A. (1983) *The Managed Heart: The Commercialization of Human Feeling*, Berkeley, CA: University of California Press.

Huppert, F.A. and Weinstein, A.G. (1991) 'Qualitative differences in psychiatric symptoms between high risk groups assessed on a screening test', *Social Psychiatry and Psychiatric Epidemiology*, 26: 252–8.

Institute of Economic Affairs (1992) *Families Without Fatherhood*, London: Institute of Economic Affairs.

Johnson, J. (1978) *Bad Connections*, London: Virago.

Jowell, R., Brook, L., Taylor, B. and Prior, G. (1991) *British Social Attitudes – the 8th Report*, London: Social and Community Planning Research.

Kornblit, A.L. (1994) 'Domestic violence – an emerging health issue', *Social Science and Medicine*, 39(9): 1181–8.

Lowe, R. (1994) 'Lessons from the past: the rise and fall of the classic welfare state in Britain 1945-76', in A. Oakley and S. Williams (eds) *The Politics of the Welfare State*, London: UCL Press.

Luxton, M. (1980) *More than a Labour of Love*, Toronto: Women's Press.

Lynch, K. (1989) 'Solidary labour: its nature and marginalisation', *Sociological Review*, 37(1): 1–14.

Mayall, B. and Foster, M-C. (1989) *Child Health Care*, London: Heinemann.

Morris, L.D. (1984) 'Redundancy and patterns of household finance', *Sociological Review*, 32: 492–593.

Morris, L. (1990) *The Workings of the Household*, Cambridge: Polity Press.

Oakley, A. (1974) *The Sociology of Housework*, London: Martin Robertson.

—— (1987) *Social Welfare and the Position of Women*. London: Thomas Coram Research Unit.

—— (1992a) *Social Support and Motherhood: The Natural History of a Research Project*, Oxford: Basil Blackwell.

—— (1992b) 'Social support in pregnancy: methodology and findings of a 1-year follow-up study', *Journal of Reproductive and Infant Psychology*, 10: 219–31.

—— (1993) *Social Support and Maternity and Child Health Care: A Guide to Good Quality Practice for NHS Purchasers*, Salford: Public Health Research and Resource Centre, Purchasing Guide 1.

—— (1994) 'Family values and the politics of "the" family: a view from the battleground', Keynote address to the Annual Social Services Conference, Harrogate (November).

Oakley, A., Hickey D. and Rigby, A.S. (1994a) 'Love or money? Social support, class inequality and the health of women and children', *European Journal of Public Health*, 4: 265–73.

Oakley, A. and Rajan, L. (1991) 'Social class and social support: the same or different?' *Sociology*, 25(1): 31–59.

Oakley, A., Rajan, L. and Grant, A. (1990) 'Social support and pregnancy outcome: report of a randomised trial', *British Journal of Obstetrics and Gynaecology*, 97: 155–62.

Oakley, A., Rigby, A.S. and Hickey D. (1994b) 'Life stress, support and class inequality: explaining the health of women and children', *European Journal of Public Health* 4: 81–91.

Oakley, A., Hickey, D., Rajan, L. and Rigby, A.S. (1996) 'Social support in pregnancy: does it have long-term effects?' *Journal of Reproductive and Infant Psychology*, 14: 7–22.

Office of Population Censuses and Surveys (1994) *General Household Survey*, London: HMSO.

Pahl, J. (1983) 'The allocation of money and the structuring of inequality within marriage', *Sociological Review*, 31: 237–62.

Piachaud, D. (1984) *Round about 50 Hours a Week: The Time Costs of Children*, London: Child Poverty Action Group.

Rathbone, E.F. (1924) *The Disinherited Family: A Plea for the Endowment of the Family*, London: Edward Arnold.

—— (1927) *The Ethics and Economics of Family Endowment*, London: The Epworth Press.

Richards, M.P.M. and Dyson, M. (1982) *Separation, Divorce and the Development of Children: A Review*, Cambridge: Child Care and Development Group.

Romito, P. (1993) 'Work and health in mothers of young children: who cares?' in *Women, Health and Work: Proceedings of an International Congress*, Barcelona, Spain.

Rose, H. (1981) 'Re-reading Titmuss: the sexual division of welfare', *Journal of Social Policy*, 10(4): 477–502.

Seel, R. (1994) 'Men at the birth', *New Generation*, 13(4): 16–17.
Stacey, M. (1982) 'Masculine or Feminine Powers? Action in the Public Domain', Presented at International Sociological Association Conference, Mexico City (August).
Stocks, M.D. (1949) *Eleanor Rathbone: A Biography*, London: Victor Gollancz.
Tuckett, D. (ed.) (1976) *An Introduction to Medical Sociology*, London: Tavistock.
Walby, S. (1990) *Theorizing Patriarchy*, Oxford: Basil Blackwell.
Wingard, D.L. (1984) 'The sex differentials in morbidity, mortality and life style', in L. Breslow, J.E. Fielding and L.B. Lave (eds) *Annual Review of Public Health*, 5: 433–58. Palo Alto, CA: Annual Reviews.

Chapter 5

Out of control
Men, violence and family life

Jalna Hanmer

Violence against women is not diminishing in frequency or intensity even though violence from men to women began to be recognized as a major social problem over twenty years ago (Parliamentary Select Committee, 1975). The experiences of women, the frequency of abusive behaviour from men, and the responses of professionals are drawn upon to provide frameworks for policy and interventions (Dobash and Dobash, 1980; Hanmer and Saunders, 1984, 1993; Mooney, 1993; Mirlees-Black *et al.*, 1996). Over the past two decades considerable effort has gone into providing women and their children with effective assistance, although this remains for the most part patchy and partial.[1] Resistance to identifying violence against women as crime, as serious, as worthy of agency intervention have been examined in health, housing, social services and policing services (Binney *et al.*, 1091; Borkowski *et al.*, 1983; Edwards, 1989; Hague and Malos, 1993; Hague *et al.*, 1995; Hanmer, 1995; Hanmer and Saunders, 1993; Maynard, 1985). Resistance by informal contacts, and the actions taken by the women and men involved, have received less attention.[2]

This chapter examines social processes that sustain violence against women. The focus is on the different responses women and men experience from the many others who are part of the social context in which violence against women takes place. The analysis is derived from interviews held with sixty women living in refuges and in the community, with first languages of English, Punjabi and Urdu, and from agency personnel with whom they had contact.[3] Thirty women have personal or family origins from the Asian sub-continent, primarily Pakistan, but also Bangladesh and India. The remaining thirty women are not completely homogenous in terms of personal and family origins, but almost all are white and see their origins as within the area of interview.

Women's accounts of their lives provide information on how hierarchy and privilege is structured within families, how cultural boundaries apply to men and women, how individual women negotiate within and move beyond culturally and socially pro-scribed limits on their behaviour, and how individual men maintain their socially superior position without altering their behaviour. The analysis focuses on the areas of struggle between women, men, families and others, how these develop over time, and the strategies women and men adopt in order to achieve their desired outcomes. In these interviews women describe men's relationships with members of his family of origin, with her and the children, with his and her friends, with work colleagues, and with other women. As with women, men's strategies involve relationships with his family, her family, his, her and their children, his friends, her friends, other women and other men. Families, friends and acquaintances may actively or passively support, even encourage, or restrain men in their violence. Agencies too, participate in these processes.

Whatever the 'race', 'ethnicity' or 'culture', women experiencing violence have in common devastating relationships with men. All the women interviewed live in a web of relationships bound by family and culture in which expectations of correct behaviour for women and men differ substantially. When confronted with repeated violence, women describe how family members and others intervene in women's lives and how women attempt to use networks of family and friends to mitigate, if not resolve, problems with their men.[4] Women's accounts demonstrate that men from varied cultural and ethnic groups have in common cultural and family advantages that come from being male, from being sons, husbands and fathers.

These dynamics raise a number of key questions around differ-ence and commonality and, when considering violence, call into question the use of 'race' or 'ethnicity' and their associated 'cultures' as dominant markers of sameness and variation in experi-ence. There are many differences between the women interviewed in this study, but these cannot be placed neatly into the cate-gories 'race', 'ethnicity' or even 'culture', when focusing on violence and the responses of women, men, the larger family and other in-formal relationships and groups. Differences often thought of as

major, such as the type of marriage entered into by women and
men, do not produce fundamentally different gendered experiences
of violence.

Amongst the sixty women interviewed there are three types of
marriage characterized by two factors: who arranged the marriage
and kinship. Marriages arranged by families may be between those
related by kinship, in particular first cousins, or between those who
are not kin; or marriage may be arranged by the individual marriage partners. These differences are important to the lives of men
and women, but domination, control and violence towards
women and children occur whatever the preferred form of marriage
and, whatever the preferred form of marriage, families and others
attempt to mediate relationships characterized by violence. The
pattern of marriage within white British society, which is seen as
freely entered into by both parties and based solely on personal
choice, seems no more likely to produce marriages free of violence
than those arranged between either family members or strangers.
Women and men who live together without marriage also may
have relationships characterized by violence.

Others do act to restrain a husband and/or other family members
who may be abusing an individual woman. While these interventions may work for some women, these interviews are with
women for whom individual and family modes of intervention are
not effective. These ineffectual interventions suggest that, for men,
other cultural values can take precedence. The most basic factor
constituting the cultural framework that either fully or partially
legitimates home-based violence by men against women is that
the boundaries specifying correct behaviour for women are not
those that bind men to society and cultures, however diverse cultures may be in other ways. Men stand outside community and
family accountability as understood by and applied to women.

These differential values and boundaries are the subject of this
chapter. The accounts of women expose the advantages men experience as male, sons, husbands and fathers. The chapter describes
women's perceptions of the feelings men express about women
and children, how this affects women's feelings about themselves
and the relationship, and their subsequent responses. The intangible
and tangible benefits men gain from the abuse of women are
described. Women's experiences of the responses of others to the
violence, to women, children and men then follows. The acceptability of violence has shifting boundaries and men vary their strategies

when women begin to leave. Leaving is a process that can occur over a brief to a very long time period.

ADVANTAGES MEN EXPERIENCE AS MALE, SONS, HUSBANDS AND FATHERS

Men gain many advantages as males, sons, husbands/cohabitees and fathers, and these advantages are interrelated. A man's status as son is an aspect of his behaviour as husband and father. His status as husband is an aspect of his behaviour as father, and all three statuses are predicated on being male. Men's statuses are cumulative from son to husband to father. This is seen more clearly with men living in extended families as they have daily interaction with parents, siblings and other family members, than with men living in nuclear families where contact with the wider family is less frequent. The general principle of status interrelatedness, however, still applies. The cumulative statuses of men are reinforced by public policy and its implementation. For example, men retain considerable authority over women and children upon divorce or relationship break-up, through residence and contact orders and their threat, and through non-intervention by the criminal justice system in their continued violence to and harassment of women.

The advantages men gain from violence have been known for some time with both service provision to women and research demonstrating certain key elements (Hearn, 1995). However, these elements are usually described as forms of women's oppression, rather than personal and social benefits to men. In order to develop an analysis that incorporates the actions of others, it is necessary to bring the man on to centre stage. He is both a primary force in the construction of social life characterized by degradation, humiliation and personal harm, and the upholder of deeply held cultural values which make it very difficult to effectively intervene in his violence. Women describe major benefits gained by men through the use of violence.

VIOLENCE AND THE EXPRESSION OF FEELINGS

Men express many feelings through violence and their feelings may determine their actions. Men may enjoy inflicting violence. 'The more violence he did to me, the more happy he would be.' 'After he had hit me, he would say, "Sit here in front of me, if I see any tears in your eyes then see what happens." Then he would say, "Laugh and talk to me".' This form of behaviour may also involve children. In a long session of violence, 'he slapped her [the child] and she became unconscious. He said [to the wife/mother], "You hit her; if you hit her you'll save yourself."' And he continued to abuse her until she did. Knowledge of this type of personal behaviour is well documented in the study of war and political regimes in which torture and genocide are part of the social process, but it is yet to be incorporated into family studies.

A more frequently met pattern of emotional response is to hold women responsible for the men's feelings. 'If I were to say to him like a couple of days after he'd hit me, my head's still hurting me, he'd say, "It will fucking hurt in a minute. What have I told you, don't keep starting. You always start me off. You're the one who fucking always winds me up. It's all your fault."' Women may respond by accepting responsibility for his feelings: 'And in the end I got to believing it was my fault.' Once in a domestic situation of recurring violence, women seek explanations for the abuse they suffer and self-blame is a widespread initial, if not long-term, way of understanding his behaviour.

A further development is to re-interpret his violence as caring for her. One form this takes is to re-create the man as baby. His baby self becomes the love object:

He is happy with me; he does love me; he doesn't want no one else to get my feelings. He is like a baby to me because I've seen him upset and I know the way he feels and he's come to me for help. I know he does need me and he's nobody else to turn to.

Another way to interpret violence as caring is to perceive threats and fear of death as proof of the strength of the man's positive feelings.

He is so jealous I've even been accused of knocking about with his own dad! That's how jealous he is, but he's really caring with it as well. There is no way on earth he wants anyone else to have me, no way. That because he cares. If I ever left him he'd literally kill me.

When women interpret violence in this way, then leaving him can feel like a betrayal. 'Now I feel as though I've let him down.' Emotional conflict may delay or inhibit women leaving. Women may leave temporarily as the conflict of feeling generated by leaving becomes too intense for them to remain away. Women can experience deep conflict, for example, one woman did not want to lose her highly controlling husband, but she had to ensure that her eldest child who had reached the mandatory school age could be taken to school, otherwise she feared the children would be taken from her by social services. Women who permanently leave violent men move beyond taking responsibility for the feelings of men. Women who permanently leave recognize the feelings of men in relation to violence as negative. It may take women some time before they begin to re-interpret the expression of his feelings in this way.

When men demonstrate an obvious lack of interest in the abused woman through relationships with other women or demonstrate a lack of concern for their children, women more easily recognize the feelings of men in relation to violence as negative. Men from Asian origins may have white women as sexual partners while being married to women brought into England as wives. This causes great unhappiness to women who said, for example, that their husband would take the white girlfriend out in the car, but never themselves, or that they brought their white girlfriend into the home, expecting the wife to cook and serve as if the other woman occupied her place within the marriage. White women, too, were expected to put up with other women, 'he used to make me leave the house at the weekends so he could bring his girlfriend to stay.' These patterns of behaviour went along with jealousy so that 'If I were walking anywhere I had to look straight ahead'. Or women could be commanded to keep their heads down, 'I weren't allowed to look this way or that way'. Men saw themselves as in control of their own lives and as having the right to have extramarital or other cohabitant relationships at the same time. One man explained to the woman he was abusing why he behaved as he did in this way, 'I'm my own boss'.

Pregnancy and having children can result in strong negative feelings for some men, with violence beginning at this point. This too can be an aspect of sexuality. For example, 'He said, "You're not a woman, you're finished." He said to me, "After bearing a child, the woman is no longer a woman."' The strength of negative feelings generated in men with pregnancy and childbirth may be expressed as wish for the child's death. 'When pregnant, he hated me, he hated her. He said, "I hope you lose it, I hope it dies."' This child was seriously ill in hospital and when pressed to come and see her, he sent a message saying, 'No, I hope she fucking drops dead'.

While men gain status as fathers as well as sons and husbands, not all men want women to have children, or to have a particular child. Women can undergo abortion in order to meet the demands of the man with whom they live. Once children are born, men may use violence and threats as ways to get rid of them, particularly when a child is the result of an earlier relationship. A man may begin a relationship by expressing interest in a woman's existing children, but once he is taken into the woman's household his behaviour can become abusive. Woman may decide to send a child to its natural father or allow the child to be taken into the care of the local authority as a way of maintaining marital harmony. The anguish and contradictory feelings then experienced by women may lead to repeated attempts to leave men who are both stepfathers to children from her previous relationship, and biological fathers of subsequent children borne by the woman.

SERVITUDE AND FINANCIAL EXPLOITATION

Women's domestic labour is essential for maintaining family life and is an important aspect of their existence as wives. The movement from 'normal' demands to excessive is a matter of degree. One Asian woman in an extended family said, 'They didn't think anything of me. They didn't think "she is part of the household also", but like a servant all day cleaning, washing clothes, doing everyone's ironing, putting it away. All day doing the work.'

Women from all cultural groups have their money taken from them. This begins with dowry or wages and moves on to child benefit and other state welfare entitlements. The man may give her no money, and all household bills including food for her and the children must come from her income, whether wages or welfare. Both white and Asian women can be forced to leave home because of lack of food for themselves and their children. When women do not know that the state will provide a minimum to ensure life, as with some recently arrived Asian women, they may leave home, regarding themselves lucky for not having died through starvation as a result of the extended family ceasing to feed them.

CULTURAL VALUES, BOUNDARIES AND SOCIAL PROCESSES: RESPONSES TO VIOLENCE AGAINST WOMEN AND CHILDREN

Other family members, friends and acquaintances respond to these types of behaviour from men to women and children in contradictory ways. The responses of others are frequently characterized by alternating behaviours as support moves between her and him. Thus a son may be told to stop hitting his wife when directly observed, to which he may nor may not respond, while his parents may demand that she apologize for upsetting him when she has been badly beaten on another occasion, but it has not been seen by them. Interventions may be ambiguous and erratic, as family members are pulled this way and that by competing and contradictory values, views and feelings.

One way this ambiguity can be expressed is when a family member assists a woman to leave and later, which can be within days, informs the husband of where she is. Once out of danger the more profound value of maintaining men's access to their wives predominates. Another is that directly observed violence can generate an immediate intervention to that specific situation. In the heat of the moment the wider issues of why this is happening and what the appropriate response of the wife should be to ensure her husband does not beat her are not of immediate relevance. While directly viewed violent attacks are more likely to result in raising the more general issue of appropriate behaviour between women and men in family life, unseen but verbally recounted attacks may also have this impact on other members of a woman's family and friends. On occasion in-laws may intervene as well as her family of origin. However, non-intervention in violence from husbands to wives may occur when it is directly seen as well as when unseen. One white woman said, 'Friends came around and saw from the beginning. He smacked me in front of them, saying, "Oh shut up, you're getting on my nerves." They got up and walked out saying they can't get involved.'

She may be told to accede to his demands whatever these may be. No demand may be too excessive so, for example, one Asian woman was told by her in-laws to agree to his second marriage to a white woman and to her joining the household. To refuse was to bring violence upon herself, understandable in the eyes of other family members. Further, her refusal to obey provided a justification for not intervening. Family members may tire of intervening with the man, particularly when the more general aim of maintaining the man's access to his wife is predominant. Another Asian woman said, 'It was getting that when he hit me, my dad didn't even do anything about it.' This woman was expected to obey her husband as a way of obtaining marital harmony.

Women described how men's violence against children is responded to in the same ways by others. As discussed earlier pregnancy and/or the birth of children can trigger violence, and can also escalate and extend violence from men in all cultural groups. For example, a young white woman found that with late pregnancy her problem turned from arguments to violent attacks. After the birth of her daughter he also began to assault the child. He would come home, wake the infant to say 'hello', and when she began to cry he would smack her to make her go to sleep. Because her family and in-laws did not live with them, they did not see the assaults on the infant and therefore could remain unaware. Although they knew about the assaults on the woman, no one asked about the child. Unawareness is not innocent, it contains a social value, that of non-intervention. His superior status as son, husband and father not only makes knowledge of his abuse unwelcome, it serves as a protective force or shield.

The relative lack of value of females may be directly expressed. For example, one Asian young woman from Pakistan, who married into an Asian family in Britain, found that her abuse moved from verbal to physical with the birth of her daughter. The family would intervene by removing the daughter when she was being directly assaulted and by remonstrating with her husband for assaulting the baby. The family explained the abuse of the baby as 'daughters are loans' and the continued abuse of the woman by 'once you have a girl, all the rest will be girls'.

CULTURAL VALUES, BOUNDARIES AND SOCIAL PROCESSES: RESPONSES TO VIOLENT MEN

The cultural boundaries of family and community accountability for men incorporate privileging male over female. Men as head of households have the role of maintaining family hierarchies and of ensuring that women and children recognize and respond to the authority vested in sons, husbands and fathers. Men can both protect social hierarchies within the extended family and be protected from criticism.

Sons may be expected to ensure the dominance of their mothers and fathers in relation to the daughter-in-law. For example one Asian woman was beaten because she verbally contradicted her mother-in-law. 'He said, "You can't say anything. Whatever my mother says, that is right. It's not that you are right, you are not right. You are wrong."' This also happens to other women. A white woman was beaten because her mother-in-law objected to her refusal to allow her grandson to have something from a shop. When this was relayed to her son, he 'came in and went bloody mad, hitting me and saying, "Don't fucking speak to him like that again and don't do this and don't do that."'

In turn men are to be protected from others finding out about their behaviour to their wives and children. When interventions from family members fail to be effective or non-intervention is the strategic response of others, self-interest may eventually surface. He may be told to treat her better because more problems may ensue if he does not; that is, serious injury or death, which would adversely affect the family as a whole. Families, and abused women too, may actively participate in protecting men; so, for example, if the police are looking for a man or wanting information that may lead to his arrest and prosecution no help is given. 'I said, "I'm not going to get him arrested."'

When women cannot be trusted to keep silent about violence, other family members, in both white and Asian families, may assist their violent male relative. Women may be kept within the home or under surveillance at all times when they leave the home or others call at the house. When external contacts are absolutely necessary, such as visits to the doctor, women will be accompanied. If a stay in hospital is necessary – for example, for childbirth – then the extended family may become particularly solicitous and kindly as well as warning the woman to say nothing about her husband and his behaviour. These strategies are effective and at the very least postpone outside intervention.

Women's independence may be restricted. 'I wasn't allowed to go up to town without one of his family. I had to go around to his sister's and say, "Oh, are you coming up to town?"' Alternatively, the restrictions on women's movements outside the home can be so extreme that women never leave the house without his accompanying her. These experiences of white women are not simple parallels with the situation of Asian women who are kept indoors within the extended family home, as the cultural justifications for this practice do not exist in the same way within white British society. Asian women, however, can be so tightly supervised that they are never allowed to speak to visitors to the home, including other family members, for fear they will disclose the abuse.

Gaining and maintaining control over women also involves using children. Men may abduct children if women leave or start civil law actions to gain contact with children in order to find out where she has gone or to have access to her so that the abuse can continue. This occurs even when men have seriously damaged the relationship with children or when they have never previously expressed any interest in the children. Both contact and residence orders can be made in favour of men who have violently abused both women and the children, although these may also be refused by family courts. The use of the civil courts in this way prolongs the emotional agony for women and children who are seeking to re-establish a life free from violence (Hester and Radford, 1996). Contact visits by men often mean leaving the children at their mother's or another relative's home. When his family express no or little interest in the children and he is not seeking contact as a way of trying to return to the marital home or to further attack her, his visits can become erratic and then cease.

Men obviously understand the boundaries that define their privilege and can be irate when these are challenged. A white women said:

> I had all his boot marks in my back. His sister went mad like and when he came from work she said, 'What are you playing at? Have you seen her back?' He told her to mind her own business and it was nothing to do with her. It was our problem and we'd sort it out. And then he went mad at me for showing her my back. I weren't allowed to talk about it. I weren't allowed to cry.

SHIFTING BOUNDARIES OF ACCEPTABLE VIOLENCE

Cultural values governing the boundaries of acceptable violence are not static. Gradations of violent behaviour may become acceptable or unacceptable to others as time passes. The cultural boundaries that are threatened with transgression remain intact if values shift to accommodate a wider range of behaviour from the husband/

father. Acceptance of violence to wives and children can increase over time, if family and the interventions of others to limit violence from the husband/father are not successful. Family dynamics also may shift in contradictory ways. For example, as violence increased for one Asian woman the extended family became more polarized. Over time both efforts to intervene with her husband on her behalf and positive responses to her decreased. Her husband's negative evaluation and behaviour towards her and the child became increasingly acceptable to all but one member of the family, another low-status woman who risked her personal security in helping this woman obtain effective assistance outside the family. This help was offered in secrecy and had to remain undisclosed to protect the quality of life of this second woman as she breached the cultural boundaries of hierarchy and privilege that governed this family's life.

There are other reasons why acceptance of violence to wives and children increases over time. Families may make little or no effort to intervene to protect their daughter and sister. A British-born Asian woman experienced a growing acceptance of violence and restrictions on her from her family once her husband had joined her from Pakistan. Married at 15 years of age in Pakistan, she returned to England a few months later and was allowed to work, to control her own money, to wear Western clothes, and to go out with friends and workmates. When her husband joined her several years later upon receiving his visa from British immigration, her life became progressively more restricted and ultimately she was not allowed to work, to have access to any money, to wear Western dress or to go out, and her family became progressively more tolerant of his abuse of her and her young daughter. This young woman was married to her mother's brother's son and not to her father's brother's son, although one was eligible. 'My mum didn't want to be proven that she's wrong [about insisting on this match] and my dad didn't want to prove to his relations that yes, he listened to his wife' (rather than pursue the culturally preferred patrilineal first-cousin marriage between the children of brothers).

If the values of others do not shift towards greater toleration of violence and the further enmeshing of women in the relationship, then the cultural boundaries of hierarchy and privilege may be transgressed and the husband/father deprived of his wife and child. This requires the woman to want to end the relationship and often for at least one other to support and to help her, although if agency staff are obstructive leaving can be delayed (Hanmer, 1995). Then actions around children in the civil courts may permit male-dominated family hierarchy and male privilege to be restored. Through residence and contact orders the hierarchical order between the ex-husband and the ex-wife and children can be re-established. This is a very commonplace outcome (Hester and Radford, 1996).

For example, one white woman with a child by her boyfriend feared leaving as he always threatened he would take the child. Even though he had children by his wife, with whom he still lived, and other girlfriends, when she turned to the police for help she was told she could not take the child from the home nor, although in her name only, would the police remove him from the premises. The local social services disagreed with this interpretation of the law and told her she could leave with her child. After leaving he assaulted those who helped her and criminally damaged several family properties. After arrest by the police, no further action was taken in relation to these crimes. The DSS gave the boyfriend the refuge address, although the policy is to not do this, and the court welfare officer supported contact even though he continued to be violent on access. While it may seem strange that this woman feared leaving because he would take the child, her fears were not that unreasonable given this outcome.

Statutory agencies may also force women to make a choice between their husband and their children. With the birth of a child violence creates new conflicts of values. Women may be required by others to transgress either the boundaries of being a wife or of being a mother. Women may respond by giving up one or more children in order to prioritize the man, or alternatively providing for their children can lead women to transgress the boundaries of family and marriage hierarchies. Amongst the sixty women the forced choice, with and without agency involvement, between their children and their husband/father/boyfriend often led to their permanently leaving violent men.

MEN'S STRATEGIES WHEN WOMEN LEAVE

After violent attacks or when women leave, men frequently utilize several strategies simultaneously in response. These include tears, apologies and expressions of a desire for the relationship to continue. 'When I left he comes down and says, "I'm really sorry, please come back." He would cry.' Men could enlist the help of others. 'He would get his sisters to phone me up.' As well as continuing violence, another strategy is threats to the woman's personal security and to that of her children, 'he would threaten to take the children off me'. These strategies might accompany or supplant trying to shift the blame, 'He would try to twist it so that he was justified to do what he did. If I hadn't made him jealous that night it wouldn't have happened.'

When the limits to his acceptable use of violence are reached, various strategies are used by men to reinstate themselves with family and friends. One way to deflect attention from having gone too far is for the husband/father to turn himself into a victim. This is accomplished through self-injury. For example, one white woman rushed to her in-laws on having been seriously assaulted by their son, 'I thought, they're going to see this time, what he had done.' His mother who previously refused to believe her son was assaulting his wife now accepted it and turned to help her. He took a drug overdose the same night and when he returned to the home of his mother and father he asked his wife, 'Don't you feel sorry for me?'

With persistent repeated violence men may refuse to let women leave. This is a serious problem as violence to women is likely to increase at the time she indicates an intention to end the relationship, or if she does leave without his knowledge and he finds her new home. But when women succeed in leaving, men often form another relationship and have further children continuing the pattern of violence and control. 'He's got a little daughter and apparently he's got fed up of her as well. She's left him a few times because I think he's got violent with her.'

While most women who leave violent men recount multiple ways men try to keep them from going, not all men seek to retain their wives. A small proportion are violent as a way of encouraging women to leave. 'He'd got his girlfriend in the family way, and he just wanted to get rid of me. He used to fetch her over when I was at my mum's, and take her into my bed.' Whether the aim is to retain or replace a woman, violence can be a strategy.

CONCLUSION

These sixty interviews demonstrate that in the last analysis, while there may be objections, the reality is that men can place their affections, loyalties, income and time elsewhere and still maintain their position as son, husband and father in the eyes of others. The reverse situation is not possible for a woman. She owes him affection, loyalty, income/money and time, expressed as both physical and emotional labour. Women who place their affections, loyalties, income and time elsewhere are inevitably defined by others as bad wives and mothers, against whom social sanctions must and will be introduced and enforced. Violence against women and their children demonstrates that these basic requirements of the good wife need not be reciprocated for a man to be seen as a good enough husband and father. Although not all women are equally affected, there is a clear double standard in operation that, regardless of their cultural group, impacts on women to the advantage of the men with whom they live.

In all cultural and ethnic groups husbands have cultural and family advantages that come both from being male and from being sons, husbands and fathers. This may partly explain why men are often so loath to give up the women and children they abuse. They lose the gendered social advantages gained by being a husband and father and have only those of being male and a son to fall back upon. When women establish themselves as single parents, men who are not immediately moving on to another woman become single and itinerant, a lowly social position especially as men age. To be head of a nuclear family, or married within an extended family, carries considerable power and status for the male in the wider community.

The maintenance of family hierarchy and male privilege within the family group conflict with interventions to control violence against women and children. Prioritizing men, their needs, wants and desires, means tolerating behaviours that would not be permitted from lower-status members of the family group, namely, women and children. Women share the values that sustain this basic social organization, as do other family members, friends, acquaintances and often formal agency personnel (Hanmer, 1995). The primary modes for handling the conflict that arises between the valuing of non-violent behaviour towards wives and children and the valuing of men in hierarchically organized family group relations are to not know or, if knowledge is inevitable, to view the matter as private. If knowledge is inescapable then the wife may be expected to control her husband through her behaviour, and/or to accede to his demands, or to view his behaviour as appropriate. The point of these strategies adopted by others outside the marital pair, is to avoid making a value judgement on his behaviour and to avoid the need to intervene, thus leaving intact values supporting gendered family hierarchies.

This is, however, a terrain of cultural conflict as the boundaries of family hierarchy and privilege are transgressed by others outside the marital or cohabiting pair and by the women themselves, frequently ambivalently and sometimes without question, and in ever-increasing numbers. These others include family members, friends, acquaintances and formal agency personnel. The view that women and children are not required to live in violent relationships appears to be gaining social support, but at the same time traditional family values are being increasingly promoted. The conflict of values observed among individuals within families is paralleled by wider social pronouncements on family values by government and other public figures in the 1990s, and by increasing governmental actions to restrict state benefits to one-parent, i.e. women-headed families (Harne and Radford, 1994).

Transgression can be experienced as being given back half a life or as a new beginning. Some women have the pleasure of face-to-face confrontations in which men cannot retaliate. One man saw his ex-wife whilst in the company of his new girlfriend whom he wanted to impress. The ex-wife said:

> I don't care what you do now. I don't care if you go and die somewhere. I've got my baby, and that's all I want. I don't want you. I don't want your family. I don't need you and I don't need your family either. Why don't you go and catch a disease and die of it?

This woman also had the pleasure of telling his new girlfriend that he would be hitting her soon too. These experiences are relatively rare compared with their opposite, where women live in fear of being found or continue to be harassed and assaulted and may even fear death.

While leaving may be difficult and take some years to achieve, in the end the decision can be easy. 'I just got up one morning and I thought, "Oh fuck this, I'm going." So I went around to my sister's and got in touch with Women's Aid.' Leaving can be hard, and can raise ambivalent emotions, 'The moment I sat in the [police] car I thought, "This is wrong." Because of him I have to leave my mum, my dad, my brothers and sisters.' Women's problems do not cease on the point of leaving as the continuing support of men by families, friends, acquaintances can be joined by that of agencies, particularly at the point of leaving. There can be a lack of awareness or minimizing of the importance in the lives of women and children of home-based violence amongst agency staff who share the same cultural values and ambivalence about men in families as women's families, friends and other acquaintances.[5]

Out-of-control men, however, can be feared. Media representation and public opinion lurch between the binary opposition of kind and caring son, husband, father and that of sex fiend, beast, violent hooligan or dangerous criminal (Hanmer and Saunders, 1993). Although women are in the greatest danger from men with whom they live, out-of-control men are portrayed and understood as 'other' or unlike those whom we know. To demand social responsibility for men in families is to reverse this understanding, but to do so will challenge the uniquely privileged position of men in families. Creating similar expectations for men and women in relation to appropriate behaviour in family life[6] inevitably involves a loss of social and personal privileges for men. This would be a major social transformation. We should not be surprised that after twenty-five years of women's campaigning and direct services to women this remains a demand yet to be achieved.

NOTES

1 Direct services to women began with the provision of refuges through Women's Aid groups in 1971. Refuges provide accommodation for women and their children who leave violent situations, and there are national associations in England, Northern Ireland, Scotland and Wales. Rape Crisis help lines and other services, and Incest Survivor groups are also provided by women for women.

2 Paula Wilcox (1996) *Social Support and Women Leaving Violent Relationship*, PhD thesis, University of Bradford, explores the informal support available to, and needed by, women who have been rehoused as a result of violence from the men with whom they previously lived.

3 This research, Violence and the Stress-Coping Process: Project 1, was funded through the Economic and Social Research Council's Initiative on the Management of Personal Welfare, 1991–93 (L206252003).

4 This analysis assumes women want to alter the relationship and believe they need the help of others to do so. One of the sixty women interviewed did not conform to this pattern. She believed others could not help her or him and that she had to do it herself. She did not intend to leave the relationship, but used the refuge from time to time for temporary relief as changes in his behaviour were too slow. Although the statutory authori-

ties were only just beginning to become aware of her, the conflict she experienced between her desire to continue the relationship and the possibility that her children might be taken from her drove her into the refuge on this particular occasion.

5 For example, in a comment on the Panorama interview by Princess Diana, the psychologist Oliver James said:

> What I find worrying is that, through her interview, Diana will have encouraged a lot of discontented women to blame a man or their relationship instead of seeing that they have problems. A lot of these women will make a tragic mistake, divorce and destroy their children's lives, as a result of what Diana has said. One would have liked her to have thought more widely and offered that insight to the nation.
>
> (Walk, 1995: 4)

6 For example, a woman who by leaving for a holiday before her ex-cohabitee appeared to look after the children took a chance that he could turn up as promised. She was jailed for a year when he did not. Judge Wickham said, 'What you did was a serious crime against your children, putting your personal pleasure before their welfare. You took a chance – good mothers don't take such chances.' Although seen as a good mother, this did not mitigate her offence. The judge took the view that, 'if you are not punished for leaving your children there will be widespread sense of outrage that justice has not been done and a real risk that someone else will take the law into his or her own hands'. There was, of course, no criticism of or charges against the ex-cohabitee and father (*The Independent* 15 November 1995: 5).

REFERENCES

Binney, Val, Harkell, Gina and Nixon, Judy (1981) *Leaving Violent Men*, London: National Women's Aid Foundation.

Borkowski, Margaret, Murch, Mervyn and Walker, Val (1983) *Marital Violence: The Community Response*, London: Tavistock.

Dobash, Rebecca Emerson and Dobash, Russell (1980) *Violence Against Wives: The Case Against the Patriarchy*, Shepton Mallet: Open Books.

Edwards, Susan (1989) *Policing 'Domestic' Violence: Women, the Law and the State*, London: Sage.

Hague, Gill and Malos, Ellen (1993) *Domestic Violence: Action for Change*, Cheltenham: New Clarion Press.

Hague, Gill, Malos, Ellen and Dear, Wendy (1995) *Against Domestic Violence: Inter-agency Initiatives*, Bristol School for Advanced Urban Studies, University of Bristol.

Hanmer, Jalna (1995) *Policy Development and Implementation Seminars: Patterns of Agency Contact with Women*, Research Paper No. 12, Research Unit on Violence, Abuse and Gender Relations, University of Bradford.

Hanmer, Jalna and Saunders, Sheila (1984) *Well-Founded Fear: A Community Study of Violence to Women*, London: Hutchinson.

—— (1993) *Women, Violence and Crime Prevention*, Aldershot: Avebury.

Harne, Lynne and Radford, Jill (1994) 'Reinstating patriarchy: the politics of the family and the new legislations', in Audrey Mullender and Rebecca Morley (eds) *Children Living with Domestic Violence*, London: Birch and Whiting.

Hearn, Jeff (1995) *Policy Development and Implementation Seminars: Patterns of Agency Contacts with Men Who Have Been Violent to Known Women*, Research Paper No. 13, Research Unit on Violence, Abuse and Gender Relations, University of Bradford.

Hester, Marianne and Radford, Lorraine (1996) 'Contractions and compromises: the impact of the Children's Act on women's and children's safety' in Marianne Hester, Liz Kelly and Jill Radford (eds) *Women Violence and Male Power*, Buckingham: Open University Press.

Independent, The (1995) 'Mother of three jailed in home-alone case', 15 November: 5.

Maynard, Mary (1985) 'The response of social workers to domestic violence' in Jan Pahl (ed.) *Private Violence and Public Policy: The Needs of Battered Women and the Response of the Public Services*, London: Routledge & Kegan Paul, pp. 125–41.

Mirlees-Black, C., Mayhew, P. and Percy, A. (1996) *The 1996 British Crime Survey England and Wales*, London: Home Office Statistical Bulletin.

Mooney, Jan (1993) *The Hidden Figure: Domestic Violence in North London*, London: Middlesex University (London, Islington Police and Crime Prevention Unit, 1994).

Parliamentary Select Committee on Violence in the Family (1975) vol I (together with the proceedings of the committee), vol II Evidence, vol III, Appendices, London: HMSO.

Walk, Penny (1995) 'Feminist guru who made up Diana's mind', The News Review, *The Sunday Times*, 31 December.

Wilcox, P. (1996) *Social Support and Women Leaving Violent Relationships*, Ph.D. thesis, University of Bradford.

Chapter 6

Men will be men
The ambiguity of men's support for men who have been violent to known women

Jeff Hearn

Support – that is, personal, emotional and social support – is often seen as a good thing. Social support can provide empathy, time, advice, resources, options and sometimes solutions to people's problems. There is now a very large literature that considers the various ways in which social support can assist people through life, and particularly through life crises, and help those people towards positive experiences and outcomes, or at least more positive ones than those who do not receive such support (see, for example, Cohen and Syme, 1985; Titterton, 1989, 1992). This is all very well, and at one level of analysis social support is to be recommended. After all, we become human through the social. And it is our social relationships and social relations, including those of social support, that form us. In this respect at least Marx was quite right. People, although he usually meant men, may create history, though not in conditions of their own choosing (Marx and Engels, 1970; Marx, 1977b). In this social context, the individual is not 'responsible for [social relations] whose creature he socially remains, however much he may subjectively raise himself above them' (Marx, 1977a: 21). People are the product of the historical ensemble of social relations rather than a particular or single determining relation (Marx, 1976; Marx and Engels, 1970; Sève, 1978). While Marx emphasized the negative and destructive aspects of social relations under capitalism, and especially the social relation and social experience of alienation, he could have also developed a materialist theory of social support. Indeed arguably, Marx's theory of class formation and progression of a class-in-itself to a class-for-itself lays the basis for such a theory. The theme of the collective benefits of class solidarity are vital in the development of workforce, trade-union and community organization, and class consciousness. Thus, while much of the work on social support has been developed within a relatively narrow social-psychological theoretical frame, there is nothing in itself that makes the notion of social support antithetic to more sociological, political or materialist analyses.

This chapter addresses the ambiguities and complexities of men's support for men who have been violent to known women. It draws on a research project on men who have been violent to known women,[1] and has been linked to, but is separate from, a research project on women who have experienced violence from known men, directed by Jalna Hanmer (1993, 1996). This chapter's focus on the evaluation of *men's* support for men is not to diminish the place of women in supporting, challenging and changing men; nor the relation between women and men who are involved in this process; nor, of course, the impact of men's violence on women (see Chapter 5, this volume).

As discussed elsewhere (see Williams *et al.*, forthcoming), a central feature of the programme was the development, evaluation and indeed critique of what Titterton (1989, 1992) called the 'new paradigm' of welfare. This paradigm emphasized variation, diversity and mediation in the delivery and receipt of welfare services. As such, it was developed in contrast to the so-called 'old paradigm', which focused on the commonalities between or collectivities of welfare recipients. In presenting this contrast, Titterton drew heavily on US social psychological literature on the mediating place of coping resources and social support in determining the welfare outcomes for individuals and groups. He thus presented a stress-coping–social-support model of life events and thus welfare.

In Titterton's (1989) review of the management of personal welfare, as seen through the lens of the 'new paradigm' and the stress-coping–social-support model, the only reference to the study of men's violence to known women was that by Mitchell and Hodson (1983). Its results broadly confirmed the positive benefits for the women of greater personal resources, active coping styles, social support from friends and family, and institutional responsiveness in coping with the violence. The project on women's experiences of violence from known men was a direct replication of the Mitchell and Hodson study. The project on men's experiences was a direct application of that study to men who had been violent to known women.

The application of the stress-coping–social-support model to men who have been violent to known women needs some explanation.

Indeed, I should say at the outset that as a researcher I had some doubts about its applicability to such men, and was extremely interested to find out if such a model worked empirically. This partly stemmed from the inadequacies of the *stress model of violence*, put forward, for example, by Peterson (1980), who argues: 'conjugal violence is a response to either private or structural stresses'. Among several problems with this approach is why it is men who perpetrate more violence to women rather than vice versa, when women as members of a subordinated group are likely to experience more private and structural stresses.[2] If the model is to be broadly useful it needs to be applicable to a wide range of situations. If the model is meant to apply only to those in a clear 'victim' position then this needs to be stated. Thus men who have been violent to known women present an interesting test for the model. They are clearly people with problems, yet they are not victims in the usual sense of that word. What they have done has caused problems for others (women, children, indeed some men); they also have problems of their own. Rather than dismissing the model out of hand, much of its application to men has involved discriminating between which elements are relevant and which are not. This has mainly entailed, first, placing the model in a much broader societal context, and second, refining the elements in relation to the particular character of the problem under discussion. In particular, men's support for men who have been violent to known women constitutes one form of resource for those men; like other resources, it is often profoundly ambiguous in its meanings and effects (Hearn, 1996d: 108).

A number of previous studies of men who have been violent to known women have emphasized the importance of men's support for one another in perpetuating this violence. These include a variety of studies by DeKeseredy (for example, 1990), which stress the way 'male peer support' reproduces men's violence: 'Peer support refers to the attachments to male peers and the resources that these men provide which encourage and legitimate woman abuse' (p. 130). DeKeseredy identifies these attachments and resources as social integration, informational support and esteem support. He also cites a number of studies that have found a strong relationship between the frequency of abusers' contacts with their friends and female victimization. Meanwhile, other studies have stressed the non-assertiveness of men who batter compared with men who are non-batterers (for example, Hotaling and Sugarman, 1986; Maiuro *et al.*, 1986), and indeed the relative depression of batterers (Maiuro *et al.*, 1988). This chapter considers the ambiguity of men's support for men, drawing primarily on the interviews with men.

QUESTIONNAIRE MEASURES

The basic testing of the model of stress-coping–social-support was conducted through questionnaire measures (as in Mitchell and Hodson, 1983). In addition, semi-structured interviews were conducted with the men giving their accounts of what they had done, why they had done it, and with what consequences. The questionnaire responses were analysed to evaluate the relevance of social support in affecting how men 'cope with' – or more accurately, reproduce or move away from – their own violence.

Social support was measured in five main ways:

(a) the empathic responses of his friends;
(b) the avoidance responses of his friends;
(c) the contact with family and friends accompanied by his partner;
(d) the contact with family and friends unaccompanied by his partner;
(e) the number of his supporters, with whom he could be when he wanted to relax or have fun.

There are three broad types of correlations (or lack of them) that may be observed. First, there is the question of the connection between the amount of violence and the presence or absence of social support. The results here may, if not fully contradict, then at least complicate the positive association of 'male peer support and woman abuse', summarized by DeKeseredy (1990). In general terms, greater violence reported by men, as measured both quantitatively and qualitatively, was moderately correlated with greater social isolation. The amount (quantity) and level (quality) of violence was negatively correlated (to a statistical significance of less than 0.05) with the number of people to whom the man could talk about how he was feeling or personal problems and the number of people with whom the man could be when he wanted to have fun or relax. There was also a similar degree of positive correlation between the level (quality) of violence and the presence of empathic responses of friends to discussing the man's violence. A slightly lower positive correlation was found between empathic responses of friends and the amount (quantity) of violence, though this was still significant (p < 0.05). This may suggest that for some men strong friendships involve empathic support for their violence.

While social isolation, from friends and family, may for some men tend not to inhibit their violence, it is the nature or quality of that 'support' that is crucial. Indeed, the level of violence correlated positively with *both* empathic (0.26) and avoidant (0.24) responses from men's friends to his violence. It is likely to be the nature of men's contact with his friends rather than the volume as such that is most significant. The importance of the *qualitative* nature of social support is reinforced by the finding that the actual amount of the man's contact with family and friends – both accompanied and unaccompanied by his partner – was not significant at all.

Second, there are connections between social support and the coping responses of the man concerned. A similar pattern was found here. No significant correlation was found between coping responses and the extent of contacts with family and friends, accompanied or unaccompanied. On the other hand, all forms of coping – active behavioural (dealing with problem by conscious action), active cognitive (actively redefining or rethinking the problem), and avoidant (escaping from dealing with problem, for example, through drink, smoking, food and so on) – correlated strongly with both empathic and avoidant responses of the man's friends, and with the number of the man's supporters. Thus again it is quality of social support networks not their quantitative size.

Third, social support may be linked to the adjustment or 'wellbeing' of the men. Generally very little correlation was found with measures of self-esteem, depression and sense of 'mastery'. However, the number of the man's supporters was significantly correlated with the man's 'wellbeing' – positively with self-esteem and 'mastery' and negatively with depression. So in terms of the man's own wellbeing number of friends may well be important; however, in terms of changing his behaviour towards or away from violence, the quality of those relationships may be far more important.

THE INTERVIEW ACCOUNTS

Social support can of course help men to change. It depends, however, on the nature of that support. If a man who has been violent to a known woman has a close social network, whether of a community, family or other type, that condones or encourages violence to women, then it is likely that that closeness is itself likely to assist him in maintaining that violence. On the other hand, if the man concerned has a close social network that opposes violence to women, then that closeness is likely to assist him in moving away from that violence.

While the questionnaire information gave only the most general indications of the relationships that existed around social support, qualitative data from the interviews provided a clearer picture of the form of men's support for men. I shall now summarize the main ways in which men spoke of their relation with other men in the open-ended, semi-structured interviews.[3] The following groups of relations with men are considered throughout this chapter:

- men family members
- men friends
- men in agencies
- men in men's programmes.

MEN FAMILY MEMBERS

In most cases men reported that men family members either do not know about the man's violence, or choose to ignore it, or to defend the man – socially, emotionally, even physically. It is rare for men of the man's *own* family of origin to take a lead in opposing the man's violence. However, men from the woman's family do sometimes take initiatives, but these themselves may often be rebutted by the man or his supporters.

A man who reported about thirty examples of his violence was able to say without any hint of contradiction: 'I think my father . . . I don't think he actually knew that I used to be violent to her. I actually think that he knew that we didn't get on at times.'

A more cautious decision appeared to have been taken by the family of a man who had been violent to women 'loads' of times: 'our family minds their own business. If he clouts his wife, he clouts his wife. If I clout mine, I clout mine.'

An apparently different response was described by another man:

Q.　Did any of your family or any of your friends know about the violence?

A. Two of my brothers knew. You know, they was blaming me
for it, but they know different now. They've read everything
what she's put down in statements and they know now that
99 per cent she started it.

The major attention from men family members came from those of
the woman's family of origin, usually fathers or brothers. A man
who was imprisoned for multiple assaults on the woman described
rather dolefully: 'They [her brothers] could come up at any time
because like I were having a lot of trouble with her brothers.
I never got on with her brothers and that. It were just any time.
Places where I went . . .'

This was understood as significant inconvenience to the conduct
of his relationship with the woman on his own terms. This man also
reported how the woman's father had attacked him with a hammer,
and that 'since that hammer attack I've been violent when I've had
drink or if someone's threatened me . . . like if people you know lift
their arms up right quick, I'm sort of nervous of them'. Violence
from a family member is connected with the man's violence to
the woman. In contrast, a man on probation who was conscious
of his problem of violence described how

Her father in particular tried to buy me off with a cheque book,
with money, to leave his daughter. She come from a nice respectable background, and it still worries me now. But I feel I've got it
[his violence] under wraps. I feel it's still under the surface there,
but obviously I'm going to still work on myself and get it sorted.

A much more aggressive response to a similar problem was from
this 50-year-old man who had a long history of assaults on women:

Why don't they [her family/parents] just keep out of it. My
mother never interferes with us, my sister doesn't, and whatever.
They never interfere. I resent that [their interfering] with [from]
her family, I told her that. If I get old fella [her father], and
I've asked him to get round table and we'll talk it out. I've
told him and told her, and I said, 'If I meet him, I'll push him
down to floor. . . .' Oh yes, I want to give him a good beating.
Oh yes, there'd be no mercy.

A number of other men reported clear violent or potentially violent conflict between men from her family and himself, together
with his supporters. For example:

she [his ex-wife] came back with her boyfriend in a van. I know he came to physically beat me senseless. . . . Luckily my brother was there. . . . Well, he came to the door and my brother wouldn't let him in, I mean he were going to flatten him, which he would have done.

Rarely, men family members do involve external agencies. One man referred to the intervention of the woman's father: 'He's caused a bit of aggro in the past, very much so. . . . He's had me locked up for violence . . . and I took it out on [was violent to] her.' This kind of intervention through agencies like the police by men in the family was unusual; more common was either direct intervention with the man himself or little or no action.

MEN FRIENDS

Men interviewed reported a somewhat similar pattern of responses from men friends to that described from men family members. However, with men friends' direct intervention against the man's violence was even more unusual. Men reported that their men friends either did not intervene at all or gave active support to the violence. (This refers to men friends encountered outside the context of men's programmes, who are discussed separately below.) For example, a man who reported his extensive violence in the context of a complex mixture of addiction, depression, insomnia and suicidal thoughts was asked: 'Obviously your family and your friends know about what happened [his violence]. How have they reacted over it?' He responded: 'Brilliant. Not one person has turned against me. Obviously in these cases some people turn right against you, call you all sorts. But not one person has turned against me. Everybody I know.'

Similarly, a man who had stabbed his wife reported:

they [his friends] said, 'You've done nothing wrong against us or our families, you're still the same person as you were before.' They said: 'What you've done, you've done something wrong, yes. And any man would have done something more or less similar, maybe not the same thing, or maybe not even anything related, but they would have fought for their children, sort of thing.' They said, 'And when children are involved in any sort of relationship or a man and a woman argument, it's a case of domestic and anything can happen.'

Some men did have a large circle of friends, but chose not to use their friends to talk about their or one another's violence. They might, for example, be friends and meet primarily for drinking or playing sport or watching sport. The agenda there was different; it was not generally something as intimate or disclosing or embarrassing or ambiguous as his violence to his wife. On the other hand, in some cases the existence of male friendship networks was continued through an agreement, whether explicit or implicit, not to 'interfere' with other men's private business.

As a man who had been imprisoned for various acts of violence to women, including indecent assault, explained:

> And like my mate were with me when all this [indecent assault] has gone off. He's even turned round to me and said, 'You've done nowt.'
> Q. Right. But he was there.
> A. Yes, he says he were there.
> Q. So was he a witness?
> A. Police wouldn't have him as a witness for me. They wouldn't have him as a witness.
> Q. If you had have called him as a witness, what would he have said in court?
> A. He'd have probably said what he said to me, that nowt happened.

Another man, with a very extensive history of violence to both women and men, gave a more detailed account of his relations with men friends:

> Q. How about your friends? Did they know about the violence?
> A. I think a few but – I've got different types of friends like, I've been in crime a few years now, I have friends that are criminals and I have friends that aren't criminals you see. So the friends that are criminals, they know exactly what I'm like, but there's people that I associate with when I go out to clubs and that, that don't know . . .
> Q. So the ones who know, how do they react?
> A. They just don't get involved. I've been in my [man] friend's house when he's been violent towards his girlfriend. I just do not get involved. If my friend got involved, I'd be violent with him. I actually chased somebody with a knife before –

Rob, this lad in our house before, when he actually tried to stop something.

Q. What happened then?

A. She was shouting about my colour in front of him and I actually just went to get her and he jumps in front of her and says 'Don't Bill, just leave it till later'. And I said, 'Are you going to get out my way Rob?' And he said, 'I'm not getting out of way' and I went and got a big carving knife to chase him out the way. But I didn't even hit her after that. I just chased him off. Didn't chase him out the house, just sort of out the bedroom. . . . Banished her to the bedroom.

Q. So it's almost like an unwritten rule that if you're around when one of your mates is being violent to his girlfriend, you keep quiet.

A. You don't get involved. I don't get involved, so I don't expect them to get involved with mine. That's how it is. But there's these people that will get involved. Like if people know that I've been bad to her as in striking her and things, I've also been good to her.

Not only do men friends not generally get involved with their or one another's violence, but if they do attempt to intervene that may itself be resisted, sometimes with the threat of further violence. An important part of such a structuring of men's friendships is the assumption by most men that 'friends' and 'mates' themselves refer to men not women.

Occasionally men report more ambiguous relations with men friends. In giving an account of his control of the woman, including her movements and social life, a man who also reported many physical assaults explained:

One guy [friend] said to me before 'You're just a cunt to her.' I was in a nightclub one day and she said something to me – I can't remember what it was – but I'd sent her out of the nightclub and sent her home and he'd said to me – 'I am a cunt to her'.

In a small number of interviews, there were accounts of positive encouragement rather than non-involvement. One man specifically reported the part played by another man, a friend of the woman, in his violence:

Colin [the man friend] were saying nothing. . . . He was just standing there encouraging me more than owt. I realize that now. He were there saying, like, 'Go on, go on', you know like encouraging me. And it excited me as he were encouraging me. He said, 'Go on, do it, do it, do her in', you know like that. Not sort of saying 'Kill her', not saying them words, but he was saying like you know 'Do it'. And that in a sense made me even go worser, because I was pulling the belt round her . . . doing her neck. She went like unconscious, well basically, and then I hit her and kind of just picked her up and just kind of threw her over the kind of little wall and I just went. And literally she were screaming hysterically and Colin went kind of white. And then I stood still for a while and then just shaking, and then realized that I'd probably just killed her. . . . She came round. You know like she were coughing, spluttering, she'd gone blue or something. . . . I can't remember totally offhand now, but it were like right to the very edge, but I stopped, summat stopped me. Thank God, it did, you know.

Somewhat similarly, some men have a positive expectation that their men friends will be violent. This may be taken for granted, and accordingly absence of violence is viewed with suspicion: 'But I mean I know men who couldn't be violent even when it's probably better for them and the woman. I think because they're not fully developed people. I'm a bit wary of men who are never violent.'

MEN IN AGENCIES

Men in agencies are often in an ambiguous relationship to men who have been violent to known women. Agencies are involved with men through both the provision of services – for example, counselling, medical, welfare services – and the exertion of control, primarily in the shape of the criminal justice system. Almost all of these agencies are controlled by men as managers and policy-makers (Hearn, 1994, 1995, 1996d), although in the medical and welfare sectors especially much of the work in contact, both professional and administrative, is performed by women. Even so, almost all of these agencies can be usefully understood as 'men's agencies'. Within such agencies, men staff, whether managerial, professional or administrative, are likely to maintain dominant forms of agency policy and practice, or work within the dominant interests and definitions of men, or both. If agency policy and practice is itself constructed within such dominant interests and definitions, then men in the agency are likely to be under double pressure to perpetuate those practices. Where agency policy and practice are in contradiction with men's dominant interests and definitions, men in the agency may be able to use either as a reference point for their actions, or may act in ambiguous or contradictory ways or differently at different times.

In general, men were most appreciative of the support that they received from individual men in agencies who operated relatively autonomously, with their interests in view and with the ability to offer what appeared to be individual services. In this sense, the major contrast was not so much between men in the criminal justice system and men in the welfare system, as between men in agencies who sought to control men often as part of a particular agency category (principally police officers but also prison staff and some social workers in relation to child protection) and men in agencies who sought to give more individualized service to men (principally probation officers, doctors, solicitors, counsellors).

Men's constructions of the supportiveness or otherwise of particular contacts with agencies were related to the interaction of men's own predisposition to continue or discontinue his violence and the nature of the agency contact itself, as seeking to challenge or (implicitly or explicitly) maintain his violence. Men generally constructed contacts with agencies and contacts with men in those agencies as either helpful, neutral ('a waste of time'), or difficult. For most men, contacts with men in agencies were helpful and supportive and they provided some service without challenging his violence too directly. This could include medication for, say, depression or assistance with not getting charged. Interestingly, solicitors were rated on the questionnaire returns as slightly more helpful to the men than counsellors.

Doctors and solicitors were particularly valued by men in terms of their ability and willingness to give individualized treatment or assistance, or what is defined by men as such. Contacts with doctors/GPs and with solicitors, in relation to violence, were reported by 29 and 37 men respectively. GPs tended to focus their attention to addiction, depression, counselling, occasionally self-harm and child abuse, and sometimes referral on to more specialist psychiatric or psychological services. Typical examples were the following that focused on treatment for depression and drugs respectively.

Just recently I've got a doctor because I've never really bothered with doctors, and I've told him about me not getting
work and how depressed I've been getting about the violence,
so he put me on tranquillisers, you know to calm me down,
you know, slow me down. Actually I've got them in a box
and I keep them at home, and if I feel that I'm going to start
going, they're always there. I know that sounds crazy but it's
like putting a wall there to stop me from going any further.
So I'm taking note that way.

Q. And how do you feel about that response from your doctor?
A. Oh, I feel good about it. Like he's prepared to do that, yes.
He's concerned, I feel that he is concerned about me, even
though I hardly know him, and I've only just got to know
him sort of thing.
Q. Was your doctor aware of that violence?
A. Well he knew I got violent when I were off them [drugs].
Q. So have you talked to him about that?
A. Yes, I told him.
Q. And how do you feel about how he responded?
A. Well like all doctors they're all right with you.

Another man described events following his arrest for indecent
assault:

Q. And how did you feel about the solicitor?
A. The solicitors were good. What hurt me more than anything
was you know, when I was locked up, a doctor comes, you
know when you've been charged with indecent assault and
that, and does all tests and that. You know, I didn't like that
at all. . . . But I had to agree to it, because I'd nowt to hide
you see. I agreed to it straightaway. But my solicitor were brilliant. I've still got the same one.

In a more routine case of assault, the charge for which was in due
course dropped, the man expressed his appreciation as follows:

my solicitor, he said, you should have got in touch with me
sooner. You should have told me sooner what had happened
and what was happening. You know just come down and see
me whenever. . . . I've known him since I were a kid so I can
relate to him, you know, talk to him straightaway. So he knew
straight off like. He just said I should have come sooner, or I

should have waited to give a statement till he come to police station.

For most of the men, the test of a good solicitor in their view is whether he (or she) can get the charges dropped or can assist the obtaining of an acquittal or a lesser charge or sentence. 'He, well he's a good lawyer is mine. He handled it very well, but as I say, the police backed it up [continued with the charge], and they did me in a sense. She dropped the charges, but the police weren't going to drop the charges.'

However, the positiveness of such support as perceived by the men needs to be viewed with great caution. Follow-up interviews and other contacts with doctors and solicitors themselves revealed a more complex picture. Solicitors generally saw these cases of domestic violence as relatively unimportant parts of their work, and relatively routine tasks to be dealt with and dispensed with. Doctors and GPs rarely intervened directly against men's violence: they generally defined the prime problem in terms other than the violence to known women (Hearn, 1995). Indeed, there were a number of examples where the man considered that discussion of his violence had been part of the consultation but it had not been known of or noted by the doctor. In the space of the few minutes of a typical consultation there is room for considerable misunderstanding between patient and doctor over the significance or even the presence of violence as a problem. It is perhaps partly for this reason that men can often see doctors as valuable support even though, and perhaps because, they may do little, if anything, to confront the violence directly.

Men's perceptions of probation and probation officers were much more variable and were reported in diverse ways. In some cases the man was extremely grateful for the support of the officer – support that did not necessarily mean working directly on his violence. 'He's a great fella, I think a lot about him. That's what our lass says to me, she says, "You're not on probation, you'd think you were the way you what is it . . . the way you keep ringing Mr Tapper up."'

On the other hand, some men saw the attentions of individual probation officers as intrusive and potentially controlling.

I don't really like probation officers to tell you the truth because they delve into your lives. They dig in and stuff like that. They just pry. For example, my probation officer he said to me, he said, 'When you get out [of prison], if you want to go and get anything back off of Trudy', he says, 'I'd advise you not to go to her house, but to come to me and I shall liaise with whoever is her probation officer'. . . . Why shouldn't I just go round to her door?. . . . But they're telling me that I can't. I've got to go through it this way.

However, in general men's accounts of their contacts with such individual workers (doctors, solicitors, probation officers), with whom a more continuous relationship could be developed, contrasted greatly with those of men's contacts with police, with whom meetings were much more intermittent and lacking in continuity. Several men reported having a series of contacts with the police over their violence to women, that had not led to arrest, charging or cautioning, at least not to their knowledge. These sometimes, but far from always, referred to violence before 1988 when the policy of West Yorkshire Police towards domestic violence changed to one of prosecution along the same lines as violence elsewhere. Other men referred to the police as behaving reasonably, dealing with the arrest in a routine and non-vindictive way ('They just took me in'), only getting involved if the woman was willing to maintain her statement ('We're not getting involved unless we know that you're going to carry it through'), or even condoning the violence ('I would've done the same myself'). All of these responses from the police were seen as helpful and supportive by the men.

However, the more usual view from the men was to see the police as a hostile and indeed dangerous force that was not helpful and supportive to the men. There were several reports of police being liable to do violence or actually doing violence to the man. This was particularly so for men who spoke of their regular and intense assaults on women. In some cases, the initial violence from the man to the woman was swiftly transformed to violence between the man and the police.

After a series of major attacks on both men and a woman, a man reported:

Gone in my garden, got my dog out of't pen and gone back up to this [his girlfriend's] house. And all the police have been there and they've said like I set a pit bull on them. So they've done the usual thing, they've set about me, they've brayed me with truncheon things they've had.

Another man who, unusually, had been imprisoned for his violence to women gave a similar account:

A. They'd give me what I'd been giving them and then they'd throw me out.

Q. What, beat you up?

A. Yes . . . I still feel bitter against them [the police], because of the way they treated me and that. They deformed me for life.

Q. How do you mean they deformed you for life?

A. Broke my fingers, broke my nose, and I've lost use of my finger because of them. And when I complained, they just covered it up.

Q. Covered up?

A. It's been covered up somewhere along line. When my solicitor, once I got sentenced, he didn't want to know.

Some men expressed their antagonism to the police in terms of clear anger and resentment.

A. I felt that it was a bit over the top, because she got a crack, and she grabbed hold of little David. Kid was involved funnily enough, not the kid getting hurt, but he was in the middle of it. That's how it all came out. I felt the police went over the top, blew it out of proportion. It was all blown completely out of proportion because of what Esther said. I was a man of six foot odd, weighed 200 and odd pound, so she kind of blew it like I was some sort of bloody monster. I was a big fella or whatever. And I totally broke down in police station. I made a voluntary statement straightaway. I shouldn't have done but I did, and they let me out, you know, basically there were nowt more further said.

Q. How do you feel then about the police, about what they did?

A. I felt unjust, I felt angry. Angry, not in that kind of anger, mad anger. I felt that they just blew it out of proportion. I felt disgusted with it. I thought, 'They're going overboard here a bit.' You know, grievous bodily harm, where it was just like a crack you know. But I butted her to keep her away. She had a knife to me by the way. She was prepared to show violence towards me, which shocked me really, because usually it could have gone on worse than that. It could have gone out of control but it didn't. Maybe because she put up obstacles in front of me to threaten me so it kind of stopped me dead in my tracks. She tried to have a knife to my chest or my neck. So it were like self-defence I felt. And the police over-dramatized it. Over-blowed it by saying grievous bodily harm.

Another man argued his anger at the police for being arrested and charged was counterproductive.

A. Why should I get locked up? Man and wife. I don't go round, what is it, I don't go round slavering [silavaing] round at their wives. They want to just keep out of it when I get, what is it, in one of those moods. It's no good controlling me because, why lock me up, and let me out? They know it's still there. It's no good them locking me up. They're defeating themselves because I'm locked up and I'm getting worse. When I get out. They've locked me up to cool me down. They haven't cooled me down at all.

Q. So you're saying it gets you even more angry?

A. Course it does. Oh, it doesn't half. Of course it does. They're taking my freedom away, to them. But don't forget while they're taking it away they're supposed to see that I'm going to calm down. I'm not. I'm scheming it up in my mind to get it more and more, you know what I mean.

Q. You take that out on your wife when you get out then?

A. Well, most of it will maybe come out on her. But mostly I'll just turn to the drink and just get stupidity with it. I turn to drink before I turn to her.

The key issues as perceived by most men were how to avoid arrest, charging and prosecution, and how to avoid physical violence from the police. Most men thus see the police as extremely unsupportive to them; this is all the more so because many men do not distinguish between charging and prosecution, and assume that the police rather than the Crown Prosecution Service are totally responsible for the decision to prosecute. Men's anger to the police can often incorporate more general resentment to the prosecution, the Courts, magistrates and judges and the criminal justice system more generally. Such perceptions may obscure the way in which the operation of the police and the criminal justice system reproduce the dominant construction of men. In that sense police antagonism to men who have been violent to known women may actually assist in making men more dangerous to women. This paradox is, of course, most clearly illustrated in the treatment of some men in prison.

> I'd like her [his probation officer] to try and help me more to get parole so I can get out of here. So I can try and help myself and get myself sorted, instead of leaving me in prison, where I see violence going on every day. It's been no help to me. They sent me to a dispersal unit where I've seen people getting scalded in water, and getting brayed with bed legs, and I've just had no effect from it after so long. It just felt as if it were a natural thing. And I had to get away from that. I mean, I don't know what it's supposed to do, prison, for people who have been in trouble with violence. There's more violence goes off in prison than there is anywhere else. It's doing nowt for us is it? Not doing nowt at all.

Thus antagonistic non-support can contribute to support for men and men's violence both structurally and individually.

Finally, in this section, it is important to acknowledge the attempts of some men to seek assistance for their violence whilst in prison. As one man imprisoned for his violence to women bemoaned:

A. I think there should be more help for us!
Q. What sort of help would you look for? I mean what would you say it should be?
A. Well no one's given advice or anything on it. I mean there should be more advice given to you when you come into prison, so there should be more help when you're out in the community.
Q. What sort of people have you asked for help?
A. I've asked probation for help. I asked the judge the day he sentenced me for help instead of sending me to prison. I've asked the prison in general for help.
Q. And what sort of help do you think it is that you ought to be offered?
A. Counselling. Summat to find out why my behaviour is like it is.

He continued:

> They [Probation Officers in prison] haven't got a lot of time for us to be quite honest. They see too many people, and they just don't seem to have the time for you. I've asked for help and been refused it. I'm just powerless, there's nowt else I can do

to get help. I'd like to know why I, what is it, why I behave like this.

He concluded that he needed to attend a men's programme after serving his sentence.

Another man who had served imprisonment for his violence reflected on his experiences on moving away from violence.

What started frightening me about it [his violence], and I talked to people about it, a lot cleverer people than myself. And they advised me to seek help because it were concerning me. And when I went to the last prison sentence I did, I went to —— Prison, where I learnt a great deal about it. I did start doing group therapy and I was a pretty good success at it. I didn't want to leave in the end, because I felt it were doing good for inmates. I'm talking about murderers, IRA, mixing with all the worse ones you could possibly meet. And in a daft way, I could understand where they were coming from. Because I'd lived that kind of life, but as for violence, I don't really rightly know even now what triggers me off. I'm calming it a lot better. I don't blow up. I can put it in the dustbin where it belongs, and I think that's because I've met somebody important who you've just seen today [a woman partner]. Who's just come into my life and like my life is just starting to fall into place and I feel, deep down in my heart, I've got some good qualities. Though I still feel guilt and I feel ashamed of what I did. And I've kept to that promise that I'd never hurt anybody. And thank God I haven't.

He also reported 'going to this programme for your anger' in prison, and planned to go to a men's programme on release.

MEN IN MEN'S PROGRAMMES

Men's accounts of the involvement or lack of involvement of other men as friends or agency staff stand in clear contrast to those that refer to other men met in men's programmes devised to work against violence. In examining the latter accounts it is often difficult to disentangle men's relations with other men in the programme, and their experience of the programme more generally, including their evaluations of the usefulness or otherwise of the programme, and their assessment of the programme leaders. In all, nineteen of

the sixty men interviewed were referred from the men's programmes. An additional man referred from another agency had
had some previous contact with one of the programmes. Three programmes co-operated in this research in the referral of men. Of
these, two were the source of seventeen of the nineteen men.
These both used a cognitive-behavioural model of intervention, as
summarized in the programme booklet, *Be safe!* (Waring and
Wilson, 1990). In one programme, the model was not specifically
feminist or pro-feminist (see Waring and Wilson, 1992); in the
other a more feminist-influenced approach was in use. The third
programme used an adaptation of the Duluth Power and Control
model (Pence and Paymar, 1990). Interestingly, women were
involved as leaders in all three programmes, in collaboration with
men in two cases. The key feature of such men's programmes is
that, unlike all the other agencies with which men have contact,
they have as their central task the countering of men's violence to
known women (Hearn, 1995, 1996d).

Some men had had a long history of contact with other agencies
and interventions before going to the men's programmes. Sometimes these previous contacts were dismissed as unhelpful: 'before
I went to [men's programme], I went to psychiatrists, psycho-
therapists, psychoanalysts, the doctor, Relate, Marriage Guidance
Council, they've all been totally useless.'

Virtually all the men had some positive remarks to make about
the programme; only one dismissed the experience as a 'complete
waste of time'. This positiveness cannot of course be taken as
evidence of success in stopping violence.[4]

Several men spoke about their initial joining of the programme
and their reaction to the men there.

Q.   How do you feel about the initial response of the group?
A.   Pleased in the sense that I felt I could get somewhere but I was
     scared shitless the first time. Very daunting. I mean I've got
     over that part of it now but . . . the hard part is sitting down
     in front of god knows how many people you don't know and
     trying to tell them what a naughty boy you've been. . . .
     Very daunting at first. [Clear emotion in voice]
Q.   How about when you first made contact though?
A.   The group itself, I found it a bit daunting to come along the
     first time. I must admit that I was having second thoughts
     on the actual day – it was a Thursday – and I was having

second thoughts about . . . not about having to go through the process, admitting what you've done to somebody and trying to do something about it, 'cos ultimately I wanted to stop doing what I was doing. I was just a bit afraid of going the first time, I suppose. It must be like the first day at school, I suppose, I wasn't too sure about what it would involve. But once I came along and . . . actually coming and admitting to people what you've done was like taking a weight off me altogether. And once I'd actually done that and to sit with other guys and realize that they re not two-headed monsters, they're just normal-looking people from all walks of life, from, like, schoolteachers to civil servants, to policemen. You realize that it's not just a problem that's confined to any particular class or racial or any other class system. It cuts right across the whole society. And after that I used to really enjoy coming to the group. I always felt . . . just before coming, I was always a little bit iffy, you know, but then once I'd been, it was great.

A key theme for many men's appreciation of the programme was the opportunity to talk. Sometimes this was expressed by the man simply in terms of allowing him to talk more about his violence, almost regardless of listening, interaction or response from other men. One particular man paralleled his account of talking in the group with that of expressing emotion – as a means of stopping his violence:

I keep on coming here . . . instead of bottling things up, to talk out, to talk about things. . . . It's teached me talk about things instead of bottling it up. I'm finding now that I can talk about my problem where I couldn't before. And I also feel I'm making better steps overcoming, controlling what the cause has been with me [considered by him to be his upbringing].

More usually, men referred to talking as a more reciprocal process through which they realize their similarity with other men:

getting my gripes off my chest and then somebody else giving me say advice or listening to somebody else giving you an idea of how to deal with a situation . . .

like swapping your ideas. The idea that you're sort of in a group and they re giving ideas to you, and you might sit and think yes, well, that's a good idea, I might try that next time.

Well, there's others [other men] very similar you know. Who's been through, some still split up from their wives or girlfriends. . . . And it's people who's in the same boat who can understand it, you know. I can relate to them you know. Sort of I don't feel ashamed to come straight because they've done the same sort of thing. How to avoid doing it in the future. Putting this programme into practice.

For some men, this initial feeling of similarity with other men was contrasted with a subsequent realization of their difference from other men. For example, a man who reported fairly persistent violence on 'loads' of occasions described the process as follows:

I recognized, well I had it confirmed I wasn't alone. I wasn't the only one walking the streets, you know being violent towards a woman. In fact I was staggered at the figures that they showed us, just how common it is, if you believe the figures, and obviously it's in my interest to believe them. I mean I was just staggered. So that was comforting. . . . It was also helpful in as much as I would hear someone in a very similar situation give a totally different viewpoint to it, and I could say I agree, I disagree.

Another man who admitted 'loads' of violence described a rather comparable progression in his relations with other men:

A.   It's almost like a safety net if you like.
Q.   Did you find it difficult at first to talk things out [in the group]?
A.   Not particularly, no. A lot better than I expected. I expected to hear things from people who were in the same boat, but the first week you were given some background information outside the group. . . . It's a lot easier [to speak] than you expect. . . . Some of it's putting what was in my head on paper, and some of it's actually giving you the practical things to structure your self-control. There's some useful practical skills come out of it, and I guess it's the actual people coming together. It wasn't something that ever bothered me in terms of I felt like a freak or something, but there's something about knowing that it's a problem across a broad section of people. There is a group side of things that is quite valuable. I think the most important thing is the structure of the programme for me although I feel quite a lot of it doesn't relate directly [to him].

Another man elaborated on this theme of difference from other men in a more direct way:

> Looking back, even now after the first three weeks of going I think I'd learnt as much as I ever was going to do. Most if it were circumstantial [superficial?] to that. It were the same thing, week in, week out. I realized that at a very early stage. You know, I benefited greatly from it for the first three weeks as much as going for the rest of the year but I never got a chance to put it into practice [the woman had left him]. Not with her anyway. . . . I thought that the fact of me going there would make her realize that I were doing something positive. And bring her back. But I was only using it as an excuse at the time, I must admit. I was only going there to sort of impress, I think, that I was doing something. I were only going there as a guise I think. . . . I got some benefit out of it . . . I got a lot of benefit out of it. But going there and comparing myself with some of the others, I'd say I'd lost a lot more [the woman] but I wouldn't say I were as motivated as a lot of them that were there. You know, they sort of do worse things. I think I probably weren't as bad as them. . . . I realized that I wasn't quite as bad as I thought I were, because I'd say we'd had about six fights in fifteen years.

Thus an interesting, and in some ways, paradoxical relation is often constructed between men's similarity with one another and men's sense of difference from other men. Many men appear to be comforted by their similarity with other men, especially in the initial stages of the programme. This can be used by the man either to move away from violence or to continue his violence. Subsequent feelings of difference from other men can also be a means of deciding to stop violence (because other men are not doing that) or to carry on with it (because of denial that he is like other men). These feelings of similarity and difference themselves feed into more general ways of being men – of maintaining bonding with other men, and of asserting independent autonomy from other men, respectively.

A few men spoke extremely positively about the whole experience of their men's programme. One man with a history of fifteen years of violence, who attended a programme for 18 months, concluded as follows:

I finally got to the point where I am today, where there is no violence whatsoever. There is a certain amount of unwanted verbal abuse, but that is entirely down to me. It is entirely through a slovenly attitude, letting myself slip into irrational thinking rather than thinking well it's your own insecurity. . . .

I recognize that the violence was all about power, about wanting, I had to have my way, and by any means I would get my way. And usually the quickest means was violence. At the same time I always used to think that I never got my own [way] but in effect I did. I always got my own way. . . .

I realize now that in the past 18 months my life has done a complete turn-around. I no longer, well I say no longer, I want to have power, there are times when I allow myself to regress when I shouldn't do. But I'm not willing now to let things ride as I did before. . . .

And I'm generally taking life less seriously than ever I have done before because the attitude I have now is that life is to be enjoyed, and as long as you don't hurt anybody else, which is ironic in what behaviour I've displayed in the past fifteen years, it doesn't matter what you do. I'm actually now getting to a stage where I'm not in overt but in covert ways, trying to philosophize with the people I work with, and trying to guide people through things I've learnt through the group [men's programme]. . . . Taking responsibility for my own actions rather than laying the blame with anybody else.

Another man who said he had been violent about fifty times described the programme in the following terms: 'I'm now living back with my wife. . . . So now I'm quite happy at the moment. The only reason I think is because she's noticed a great change in me since I've been coming to the group [men's programme] and, well, I mean I'm as happy as a pig in it.'

He had recently graduated to become a co-facilitator for some group sessions: 'I couldn't praise the group enough, I really couldn't.'

The question of social support is especially important in formulating practical responses and opposition to men's violence to known women – for example, the organization of men's programmes and other focused interventions against men's violence. In such interventions there is typically a tension between support of men, both between men and from the facilitators to the men, and confrontation of men, from both the facilitators and one another (Lees and Lloyd, 1994: 38–9). Within this tension, there are certainly ways in which peer support between men can be positive in turning men away from violence.

In trying to change men through the development of men's programmes and similar interventions, one element of the process of change is that of social support between the men in the group. However, different models of intervention put a different emphasis on the significance of this support, and its place in both the intervention and the group process more generally. In more cognitively based interventions, the establishment of a supportive group process is often seen as necessary to begin the intervention.

Saunders, in his review of cognitive and behavioural approaches, summarizes this element as follows:

> In a group setting, the men can be taught to praise one another by making specific reinforcing comments both for reports of progress during the week and for acquiring skills during the session. This peer support appears to be one of the strongest forms of reinforcement the men can receive, and they report that it is a very useful part of the group experience (Gondolf, 1984). The support is one of the ways the men decrease the strong dependence for praise and acceptance they often have on their partner. The men's overdependence on others can be lowered even more if they learn to praise themselves, a skill explained by some cognitive therapists.
>
> (Saunders, 1989: 82)

On the other hand, Gondolf (1989: xi) suggests that: 'We may need a variety of ways to interrupt men's violence and bring safety to women. . . . Those batterers in deep denial and resistance may be more likely to respond to the didactic confrontation of the feminist approach.'

CONCLUSIONS

Men's support for men is one of the prime ways in which men are produced and reproduced as men. It is a routine way of men affirming to each other that men are men and men will be men. Understanding the nature of men's social support for men who have been violent is both a theoretical and a practical question. Theoretically, it raises the complicated issue of how we conceptualize social support, especially for the (relatively) powerful. Practically, it raises the equally complicated question of how support to such men *should* be given by men. To give support to men who have been violent without condoning or colluding with that violence is difficult. It is an especially difficult issue for men giving support to men. Behaving appropriately with men who have been violent to women remains a problem in many situations: in the community, in families, in professional interventions and the development of policy, and indeed in doing research.

How are men to support men to stop being violent without supporting their violence?

These questions, both theoretical and practical, problematize the extent which social support can necessarily be considered a 'good thing', as is generally assumed in much of the US social psychological literature on the subject. The concept of social support needs to be re-evaluated critically. It is not a unified concept. This is partly a matter of the differential experience of women and men in relation to the problem of men's violence to known women. For example, *a lack of intervention* by friends, family or agencies is likely to be non-supportive for women but is likely to be supportive, or at least experienced as supportive, for men. The notion of 'family support' is unclear when considered in relation to violence and abuse, as the family is the site of both the source of the problem and any would-be 'support'. Much of this critique resolves around the ungendered usages of the concept of social support in many previous studies (Hanmer and Hearn, forthcoming), and the need for a gendered analysis of social support, particularly in relation to men's violence and abuse.

So, let us try to conceptualize the relationship of men's support for men and the reproduction or countering of violence. First, it is necessary to understand men as members of a powerful social group or category. The literature on social support generally fails to deal satisfactorily with power relations and particularly what might be meant by social support for the *relatively* powerful. The simple answer to this is to see men's social support as just that – our giving support to the powerful. Thus men's social support is comparable to the *support* that the members of other powerful groups might have and receive for one another. This is well documented in the literature on elites, power networks, coalitions, cabals, state formation and many other concepts that are the stuff of what is usually called political science. However, such studies do not generally consider individual men as husbands and fathers, themselves generally relatively individualized in their own homes, as part of political science. While the powerful provide support for one another in numerous formal and informal ways, for men who have been violent to known women the support is generally by informal modes. On the other hand, more formal relations between individual men and men in agencies can also be understood as means of social support between those who are relatively powerful. These relations may inhibit change, facilitate change, or even reproduce violence through the operations of state agencies.

Second, men's particular social relations are simultaneously a means of increasing men's power, and reducing and limiting that power. Men who are involved in social networks are on the one hand able to exercise influence through those networks and towards the members of the networks, and on the other are controlled by the social relations and social relationships of those networks. Conversely, men who are socially isolated do not have networks over which they exert influence but they are also not constrained by those networks. Men without friends, as claimed by a considerable number of the men interviewed, are both socially less powerful and socially more powerful. They are more powerful in several senses. First, they do not pre-emptively have to modify their behaviour to ameliorate others. Second, whatever they do does not meet with responses and reactions from others. A third possible implication is that this may also indirectly affect the isolation of women, and their ability to gain support. For all these reasons, isolated men may be able to be violent to women with few consequences.

Third, many men's relationships with one another are characterized by contradictions of both support from and competition with one another. Patriarchal and fratriarchal relations between men can be characterized by two contradictory features: collectivism and peer social support (fratriarchal); and hierarchical individualism and competition (patriarchal). Men routinely support one another, prefer men's opinions to women's, and favour courses of action that favour men, whilst at the same time expecting, even demanding, that men stand up for themselves and engage in 'give and take' (Hearn, 1985; Collinson, 1992). While the fratriarchal element makes for a basic quantity and level of social support between men, the patriarchal element makes the quality of that support suspect, even shallow or threatening. Patriarchal and fratriarchal structures are both inhabited by men and account for the particular form that men take. These structures are themselves systems of dominance and in that sense they produce and account for men's violence to women, children and men. To put this slightly differently, men's violence does not just occur within patriarchal and fratriarchal contexts, it is itself part of those contexts (Hearn, 1996b). Men's support for men is one of the ways men's violence is produced and reproduced, and in turn how patriarchy (DeKeseredy, 1990) and fratriarchy are produced and reproduced (also see May and Strikwerda, 1994).

Fourth, there is the specific character of the support or network (or networks) of support within which men live. These might be characterized as more or less intense and cohesive, and as more or less supportive of men's violence. Thus one might envisage, for example, an intense, cohesive network that is strongly supportive of men's violence or its opposite, a more diffuse, less cohesive network that is opposed to men's violence. Other networks may be ambiguous or contradictory in their relation to support for or opposition to men's violence. This gives six broad types of specific network of social support.

Fifth, particular men are more or less integrated into or isolated from these particular networks of support. For example, an individual man might recognize that he lives in a cohesive network but feel strongly isolated from it. In such a situation the man may continue his violence fatalistically as if he has no real willpower of his own. This contrasts with a situation where there is a cohesive network that is supportive of violence (as noted above) and into which the individual feels strongly integrated. In that scenario the man may continue with his violence as he feels he has the 'moral duty' to do so. He may even feel he is being violent for altruistic reasons, to control others so that they behave as they should do and as recognized by the community. A third alternative is for men to do violence when they are strongly integrated into a less cohesive social situation. Here violence may be done and justified for particularistic and narrowly egoistic reasons rather than on grounds that stem from a wider moral community. His violence is seen as an individual choice arising from individual circumstances with an individual woman. It may even be seen as part of an individual journey through life, a necessary evil. Some men may find themselves in a less cohesive social network and they themselves may be weakly integrated into it. This is the social situation of anomie. It is assumed by the man that his violence 'just happens';

it is not particularly sought by him. He is unsure, unclear about why he is being violent. His violence is anomie. It confuses him. It may be associated with drink, drugs and severe personal difficulties in other areas of life.[5]

Sixth, there is the exact nature of different forms of supportive or non-supportive interaction that men may experience from others, in this context particularly other men. This may be the diffuse support of ordinary life or it may be specifically directed towards his violence. It may be the kind of support that avoids the subject of violence and colludes with the reproduction of violence. Or it may be empathetic with the man's situation; this could in some situations be a means to changing the situation, but perhaps more likely such empathy might be taken by the man to mean consent to his violence. Alternatively, interaction and intervention can be clearly initiated on the basis of opposition to violence. Men's violence can be challenged and changed by men. The support that is at issue here is that which may support the man in his attempts to change his behaviour away from violence.

It is clear from this research that what might be meant by men's social support (and indeed lack of support) of men who have been violent to known women is various. Such 'support' by friends, family or agencies might include:

1 passive non-intervention *against* a man who wishes to continue his violence (for example, ignoring of the problem by the family);
2 active intervention *in favour of* a man who wishes to continue his violence (for example, encouragement from friends);
3 active intervention *with* a man who wishes to discontinue his violence (for example, men's programmes).

In contrast, 'lack of support' by friends, family or agencies might include:

1 passive non-intervention *with* a man who wishes to continue his violence (for example, 'sending to Coventry');
2 active intervention *against* a man who wishes to continue his violence (for example, police arrest);
3 passive non-intervention *against* a man who wishes to discontinue his violence (for example, undermining of men's motivation to change).

There is clearly a lot of room for interpretation and misinterpretation of the interactions between men. For example, almost any sign of friendly concern that is not overtly condemnatory or confronting can be interpreted by some men as giving support to him or even condoning his violence. The agreement from friends and family to talk about the problem can easily be interpreted by the man or by others as supportive of the man. Men's discussions with family or friends may avoid the topic, may empathize with the man, or may confront the man, or of course involve some combination of responses. A problem is that it is not always clear what empathy might mean when giving social support to the peer who is responsible for their own problem – in this case, men who have been violent to known women. Most importantly, there is the question of what non-avoidant, non-empathic responses of friends to men might look like.

Alternatively, withdrawal of concern or interaction may be taken by the man that the other man is not interested in him or his violence. This may be temporarily disconcerting or even hurtful but again it can be re-interpreted as disinterested or condoning of his violent behaviour. Theoretically, withdrawal of social interaction can of course be a punishment leading to behaviour change; but in practice, this would usually have to be conducted on a relatively wide scale by a variety of friends and acquaintances for there to be a clear effect. More likely, severe 'sendings to Coventry' might cause a man to think about moving house or locality.

Men's discussions with friends and family have to be considered critically in terms of the literature on social support. When someone is in a position of disadvantage – as, for example, a woman who has received violence from a man – discussions with family and friends may avoid the topic or may focus on the topic in an empathetic way. Just talking about the problem might be equally empathetic in some cases. With men such discussions may be more ambiguous. The agreement of friends and family to talk can easily be interpreted by the man or by others as supportive of the man.

In evaluating men's support for men is that men's personal relationships with one another it is necessary to be clear that those relations can take widely differing forms – from remote and sexist male bonding against women to intimate and transforming. Many men, specifically many heterosexual men, may maintain supportive social contacts with other men but these are often not intimate friendships (see Miller, 1983; Strikwerda and May, 1992; Nardi, 1992). The men interviewed defined themselves as heterosexual in a taken-for-granted way (Hearn, 1996a). For many heterosexual men, intimacy between men friends may be constrained and circumscribed by homophobia. Significant, but limited, friendships between men may mean that male heterosexuality is characteristically homosocial, and even homosexual (Irigaray, 1985).

Finally, it is very important not to treat this question of social support or networks of support in too deterministic a way. Individual men may stand out against a pro-violent support network or may indeed continue with violence despite networks that oppose violence.

ACKNOWLEDGEMENTS

I am grateful to Roger Barford, John Davis, Philip Raws and David Riley for conducting interviews; Linda Arbuckle for administering the Project; and Jalna Hanmer for collaboration on Project 1. I would also like to thank Lynne Gerrard for typing the script, and Lisa Price and Paula Wilcox for bibliographic information.

NOTES

1 ESRC Project L206 25 2003. The project on men involved interviewing sixty men who had been violent to known women. Questionnaires were completed and accounts were obtained. Men were interviewed from a number of sources, principally men who had been arrested by the police, men who were in contact with a probation officer, men who were in prison, and men who were in men's programmes. A number of men were also recruited from other welfare agencies and from the community who were not currently in contact with agencies. Because of the methods of the access that were used, most of the men (fifty-seven) were white, and as such this chapter is mainly about white men (including English, Irish, Jewish and Scottish men). One hundred and thirty follow-up interviews and other research contacts were also carried out with agency staff who had dealt with the individual men and where the men's permission was granted. For summaries of the whole project, see Hearn 1993, 1995, 1996c, 1996d, 1998.

2 The exact relationship of the 'stress–coping–social-support' models, as proposed by Mitchell and Hodson (1983) and Titterton (1989, 1992) amongst others, and 'stress as cause of violence' models (Gelles, 1972; Straus et al., 1980) is complex and far from clear. However, in simple terms in the first case, violence is conceptualized as a stress that may or may not be coped with; in the second, other stresses are assumed to lead to the violence. The inadequacies of the second model, particularly in terms of its treatment of gender, do not necessarily invalidate the first but do certainly cast doubt on its general applicability.

3 The analysis of transcripts was conducted by extracting those parts in which men gave accounts of their relations with and support from other men. The main features were then summarized and illustrated by relevant quotes and other information.

4 An evaluation of the effectiveness of men's programmes has recently been completed by Dobash *et al.* (1996).

5 This formulation draws on Durkheim's (1952) classic study of suicide.

REFERENCES

Cohen, S. and Syme, S.L. (eds) (1985) *Social Support and Health*, Orlando, FL: Academic.

Collinson, D.L. (1992) *Managing the Shopfloor*, Berlin: de Gruyter.

DeKeseredy, W.S. (1990) 'Male peer support and woman abuse: the current state of knowledge', *Sociological Focus*, 23(2) (May): 129–39.

Dobash, R.P., Dobash, R.E., Cavanagh, K. and Lewis, R. (1996) *Research Evaluation of Programmes for Violent Men*, Edinburgh: Scottish Office.

Durkheim, E. (1952) *Suicide: A Study in Sociology*, London: Routledge & Kegan Paul, first published in French, 1897.

Gelles, R.J. (1972) *The Violent Home*, New York: Sage.

Gondolf, E.W. (1984) *Batterers Anonymous: Self-help Counselling for Men who Batter Women*, San Bernardino, CA: B.A. Press.

—— (1989) Foreword, in P.L. Caesar and L.K. Hamberger (eds) *Treating Men who Batter: Theory, Practice and Programs*, New York: Springer, pp. ix–xiii.

Hanmer, J. (1993) *Violence, Abuse and the Stress-Coping Process, Project 1. End of Award Report to the ESRC*, Bradford: Violence, Abuse and Gender Relations Research Unit, University of Bradford.

—— (1996) 'Women and violence: commonalities and diversities', in B. Fawcett, B. Featherstone, J. Hearn and C. Toft (eds) *Violence and Gender Relations: Theories and Interventions*, London: Sage, pp. 7–21.

Hanmer, J. and Hearn, J. (forthcoming) 'Gender and welfare research', in F. Williams, J. Popay and A. Oakley (eds) *Welfare Research: A Critique of Theory and Method*, London: UCL Press.

Hearn, J. (1985) 'Men's sexuality at work', in A. Metcalf and M. Humphries (eds) *The Sexuality of Men*, London: Pluto, pp. 110–28.

—— (1993) *Violence, Abuse and the Stress-Coping Process Project 2. End of Award Report to the ESRC*, Bradford: Violence, Abuse and Gender Relations Research Unit, University of Bradford.

—— (1994) 'The organization(s) of violence: men, gender relations, organizations and violences', *Human Relations*, 47(6) (June): 707–30.

—— (1995) *It Just Happened: A Research and Policy Report on Men's Violence to Known Women*, Bradford: Violence, Abuse and Gender Relations Research Unit, University of Bradford, Research Paper No 6.

—— (1996a) 'Heteroseksuaalinen Väkivalta Lähipiirin Naisia Kohtaan Sukupnolistunnt Väkivalta Miesten Kertomuksissa', *Janus* (Finland), 4(1): 39–55.

—— (1996b) 'Men and men's violence to known women: the lure and lack of cultural studies approaches', Paper at Crossroads in Cultural Studies Conference, University of Tampere (July). Mimeo, University of Manchester.

—— (1996c) 'Men's violence to known women: historical, everyday and theoretical constructions', in B. Fawcett, B. Featherstone, J. Hearn and C. Toft (eds) *Violence and Gender Relations. Theories and Interventions*, London: Sage, pp. 22–37.

—— (1996d) 'Men's violence to known women: men's accounts and men's policy developments', in B. Fawcett, B. Featherstone, J. Hearn and C. Toft (eds) *Violence and Gender Relations: Theories and Interventions*, London: Sage, pp. 99–114.

—— (1998) *The Violences of Men: How Men Talk About and How Agencies Respond to Men's Violences to Known Women*, London: Sage.

Hotaling, G.T. and Sugarman, D.B. (1986) 'An analysis of risk markers in husband to wife violence: the current state of knowledge', *Violence and Victims*, 1: 101–24.

Irigaray, L. (1985) *This Sex which Is Not One*, New York: Cornell University Press, first published in French, 1977.

Lees, J. and Lloyd, T. (1994) *Working with Men who Batter their Partners*, London: WWM/The B Team.

Maiuro, R.D., Cahn, T.S. and Vitaliano, P.P. (1986) 'Assertiveness deficits and hostility in domestically violent men', *Violence and Victims*, 1: 279–90.

Maiuro, R.D., Cahn, T.S., Vitaliano, P.P., Wagner, B.C. and egree, J.B. (1988) 'Anger, hostility and depression in domestically violent versus generally assaultive men and nonviolent control subjects', *Journal of Consulting and Clinical Psychology*, 56: 17–23.

Marx, K. (1976) *Preface and Introduction to a Contribution to the Critique of Political Economy*, Peking: Foreign Languages Press.

—— (1977a) *Capital*, Vol. 1, London: Lawrence & Wishart.

—— (1977b) 'The Eighteenth Brumaire of Louis Bonaparte', in D. McLellan (ed.) *Karl Marx: Selected Writings*, Oxford: Oxford University Press, pp. 300–25.

Marx, K. and Engels, F. (1970) *The German Ideology*, London: Lawrence & Wishart.

May, L. and Strikwerda, R. (1994) 'Men in groups: collective responsibility for rape', *Hypatia*, 9(2) (Spring): 134–51.

Miller, S. (1983) *Men and Friendship*, Bristol: Gateway.

Mitchell, R.E. and Hodson, C.A. (1983) 'Coping with domestic violence: social support and psychological health among battered women', *American Journal of Community Psychology*, 11(6): 629–54.

Nardi, P. (ed.) (1992) *Men's Friendships*, Newbury Park, CA: Sage.

Pence, E. and Paymar, M. (1990) *Power and Control Tactics of Men who Batter*, Duluth: Minnesota Program Development, first published 1986.

Peterson, R. (1980) 'Social class, social learning and wife abuse', *Social Services Review*, 54(3): 390–406.

Saunders, D.G. (1989) 'Cognitive and behavioral interventions with men who batter: application and outcome', in P.L. Caesar and L.K. Hamberger (eds) *Treating Men who Batter: Theory, Practice and Programs*, New York: Springer, pp. 77–100.

Sève, L. (1978) *Man in Marxist Theory and the Psychology of Personality*, Hassocks, Sussex: Harvester, first published in French, 1974.

Straus, Murray A., Gelles, Richard J. and Steinmetz, Suzanne K. (1980) *Behind Closed Doors: Violence in the American Family*, New York: Anchor/Doubleday.

Strikwerda, R.A. and May, L. (1992) 'Male friendship and intimacy', *Hypatia* 7(3), (Summer): 100–25.

Titterton, M. (1989) 'The management of personal welfare', Glasgow: Department of Social Administration and Social Work, University of Glasgow.

—— (1992) 'Managing threats to welfare: the search for a new paradigm of welfare', *Journal of Social Policy*, 21(1): 1–23.

Waring, T. and Wilson, J. (1990) *Be safe! A Self-help Manual for Domestic Violence*, Bolton: MOVE.

Waring, T. and Wilson, J. (1992) 'The management of denial in a group programme for domestic violence', *Counselling*, 3(1) (February): 37–9.

Williams, F., Popay, J. and Oakley, A. (eds) (forthcoming) *Welfare Research. A Critique of Theory and Method*, London: UCL Press.

Chapter 7

Male carers in marriage
Re-examining feminist analysis of informal care

Gillian Parker and Julie Seymour

In 1983, an article in *Community Care* stated that 'for a husband to care for his wife in her early incapacity in old age is exceptional, both in the necessity for the wife to receive care, and in his readiness to undertake it' (Froggatt, 1983: 21). In the subsequent decade, analysis of national surveys has shown that male carers, rather than being exceptional, make up a significant proportion of those providing informal care for family members (Arber and Gilbert, 1989; Parker and Lawton, 1991). While early feminist critiques of informal care have focused on the impact of community care policies on women (Dalley, 1983; Finch, 1984), such figures suggest that men must now be included in such research and analysis (Parker, 1993).

The bulk of research on caring has tended to focus on the relationships between children and parents (Lewis and Meredith, 1988; Beresford, 1994). As the following section will show, much male caring takes place within the context of a marital relationship, and as a result has been excluded from scrutiny. Two recent qualitative studies which rectify this balance have examined the position of spouse-carers (Parker, 1993; Seymour, 1995)[1] and will be reported in this chapter. The first study involved long-term carers, where one spouse had been caring for the other for at least four, and in some cases, up to twenty, years. The second, concentrated on couples in relatively new caring situations – that is, within the first 18 months of the onset of physical impairment or chronic illness of one spouse. There is also an increasing literature on the situation of male carers in same-sex relationships, largely focusing on issues arising from HIV and AIDS (Shelby, 1992; Small, 1993). However, within this chapter, we will be concentrating on male carers in heterosexual relationships. The main issues addressed

Male carers in marriage
Re-examining feminist analysis of informal care

Gillian Parker and Julie Seymour

In 1983, an article in *Community Care* stated that 'for a husband to care for his wife in her early incapacity in old age is exceptional, both in the necessity for the wife to receive care, and in his readiness to undertake it' (Froggatt, 1983: 21). In the subsequent decade, analysis of national surveys has shown that male carers, rather than being exceptional, make up a significant proportion of those providing informal care for family members (Arber and Gilbert, 1989; Parker and Lawton, 1991). While early feminist critiques of informal care have focused on the impact of community care policies on women (Dalley, 1983; Finch, 1984), such figures suggest that men must now be included in such research and analysis (Parker, 1993).

The bulk of research on caring has tended to focus on the relationships between children and parents (Lewis and Meredith, 1988; Beresford, 1994). As the following section will show, much male caring takes place within the context of a marital relationship, and as a result has been excluded from scrutiny. Two recent qualitative studies which rectify this balance have examined the position of spouse-carers (Parker, 1993; Seymour, 1995)[1] and will be reported in this chapter. The first study involved long-term carers, where one spouse had been caring for the other for at least four, and in some cases, up to twenty, years. The second, concentrated on couples in relatively new caring situations – that is, within the first 18 months of the onset of physical impairment or chronic illness of one spouse. There is also an increasing literature on the situation of male carers in same-sex relationships, largely focusing on issues arising from HIV and AIDS (Shelby, 1992; Small, 1993). However, within this chapter, we will be concentrating on male carers in heterosexual relationships. The main issues addressed that more than 90 per cent of elderly married people who needed help with domestic or personal care received this from their spouses. Further, among 'severely disabled' elderly people living with just their spouse almost a half were women being looked after by their husbands. Similarly, recent analysis of 1985 GHS data suggests that as many as 12 per cent of all men – that is, some 2.5 million individuals – are involved in some caring activities (Parker and Lawton, 1991).

When such general figures are examined more closely, a clearer picture emerges of the particular ways in which men are involved in informal care. Key issues here are co-residence and the type of relationship between the carer and cared-for person. Men are more likely than women to be caring for someone in the same household. Male carers are also significantly more likely than are female carers to be caring for spouses and parents-in-law rather than friends and neighbours. Finally, except when caring for a spouse, men are less likely than are women to provide personal care, such as help with bathing, dressing or toileting (Parker and Lawton, 1991). Hence, the kind of informal care carried out by men as a group is different, both in its content and in relation to those who receive it, from that provided by women. Nevertheless, male informal carers must be acknowledged and recognized by researchers and welfare practitioners.

In order to clarify understanding about male carers in relation to female we need to be able to answer three different sorts of questions: about the *prevalence* of caring responsibilities among men; about the *nature* of caring activities carried out by men; and about the *impact* of caring on men.

PREVALENCE OF CARING

Re-analysis of the 1985 GHS has shown that although similar proportions of men and women in the population at large identify themselves as carers, their 'risk' of becoming carers is lower. Thus, for example, the likelihood (odds) of being a carer if one is a married man is 0.15 compared to that of 0.22 for a married woman. Similarly, the odds for all never-married men is 0.08 compared with 0.11 for never-married women, while the figures for ever-married (divorced, separated or widowed) men and women are 0.12 and 0.18 respectively (Parker and Lawton, 1991). However, the 'risk' of being a carer varies by age and marital status. Ever-married men aged 30 to 44 and never-married men aged 45 to 64 are particularly unlikely to be carers compared to women. By contrast, single men aged 30 to 44, and married or ever-married men aged 65 or over, are almost as likely to be carers as women in the same sub-group. Ever-married men aged 16 to 29 (admittedly a rather small group) are actually *more* likely to be carers than women in the same circumstances.

THE NATURE OF CARING

As already outlined above, men are less likely than women to be main carers, more likely to be caring for a spouse or parent-in-law, more likely to be looking after someone in their own household, and less likely (except when caring for a wife) to be providing personal care. Although the *average* number of hours of care they provide is lower than for women, the proportion caring for long hours (30 or more per week) is the same as for women (14 per cent). However, many of these factors interact: for example, all main carers care for longer hours; certain types of caring relationships more commonly take place in the same household; and so on. By controlling for the nature of the relationship between people and for the level of responsibility they have – that is, by comparing like with like – many of the differences between male and female carers disappear. The main difference that does remain – except in relation to those caring for spouses – is that women are still more likely than men to be providing personal care. However, although being a male carer reduces the likelihood of being involved in personal care, multi-variate analysis shows that the nature of the carer's relationship to the person being helped has more influence on the type of care provided than does sex of the carer (Parker and Lawton, 1991). Hence, as Rose and Bruce (1995) state of their study of elderly spouse-carers, 'where the material circumstances make it both possible and necessary, and partners share an ideology of love and duty, then gendered constructions of caring must give way to the pragmatics of coping'.

THE IMPACT OF CARING

Studies of parents caring for disabled children and of offspring caring for elderly parents have consistently demonstrated that women suffer greater effects, particularly economic ones, than men as a result of caring (Baldwin, 1985; Nissel and Bonnerjea, 1982). However, these studies were comparing men and women *within the same caring situation* and where one person (the woman) was almost always more heavily involved than the other. In the majority of such cases, it could be argued that the relative responsibilities of men and women merely replicated those that already existed, and for the same reasons. Women take the bulk of 'hands-on' responsibility, partly because that is what women 'normally' do, growing out of their responsibility for childcare, but also because they would be unable to equal the earnings power of their male partners if *they* stayed at home to care.

Simply making a comparison of labour-market activity between all male carers and all female carers tells us little about any differential impact of caring. Male and female carers as groups are different in age and marital status, in the relationship to the person they are helping, in their caring histories and so on. Any straight comparison between them thus confounds the possible impact of caring with a number of other factors which may or may not have anything to do with being a carer. At its most obvious, for example, comparing the employment patterns of male and female carers of working age would show that men were more likely to be in paid work than women; but how do we judge the extent to which responsibility for this difference can be laid at the door of caring rather than at the door of all the other factors that make men's and women's work patterns different? Again, re-analysis of GHS data allows us to throw some light on this. The 1985 survey results suggest that once the effects of marital status and having a dependent child are controlled for, women who are also carers are only slightly less likely than their peers to be in paid work. By contrast, men's labour-market participation is significantly affected by caring responsibilities, even when marital status and dependent children are taken into account (Parker and Lawton, 1991). When female carers are in paid work, whether or not they are working part- or full-time, is, again, more influenced by their marital status and having dependent children than by their caring activity. For men, it is caring that increases their chances of being in part-time work rather than their marital or family status. In other words, women's labour-market activity is suppressed by a relatively small amount by caring, because it has already been suppressed substantially by marriage or, more substantially, by the presence of dependent children. Men do not experience this more general depressive effect but do seem to experience a substantial impact as a result of caring.

Much of this difference may be accounted for by the importance of spouse-caring among men, and particularly among those providing intensive types of care. To understand this we have to look at the alternative options that members of a family or household have when one of their number needs assistance with everyday activities.[2]

In heterosexual, two-parent households with a disabled child, decisions about who should care for that child are taken within a normative framework that, by and large, deems childcare women's work. However, as we have already argued above, it also takes place within a structural framework which, for the majority, makes it impossible for women to command a similar level of financial resources within the labour market. In the absence of any moves towards redressing these balances, it makes at least financial sense for women to be carers when other forms of support are inadequate. Similarly, when couples take on the care of elderly, frail parents or parents-in-law, the sacrifice of the woman's job is likely to have less financial impact than would that of a man. By contrast, when a spouse is disabled, few choices are available. Younger disabled people, in particular, are poorly supported by services which would enable them to meet their daily living needs without their partners becoming involved. As a result, non-disabled partners can find their labour-market activity severely affected. In-depth research suggests that in such circumstances, *male* partners have more difficulty adapting their paid work to caring responsibilities because of the relative lack of flexible and/or part-time jobs for them (Parker, 1993). As a result, when their partners need a substantial amount of support, they seem more likely to suffer once and for all effects on their paid work. Alternatives to the non-disabled partner becoming involved in providing support are limited, unless either partner earns sufficient to buy in other forms of support. Given that disabled people are widely discriminated against in the labour market, and that there is a strong relationship between low income and disability, this is not an option for many.

Having explored the extent to which men do provide informal care and having shown that it is concentrated within marriage, we will now consider whether men and women differ in their experiences of caring.

MALE SPOUSES' EXPERIENCE OF CARING

Personal Care

Many writers have assumed, either directly or by default, that the intimate nature of marriage would make the giving and receiving of personal care between spouses unproblematic. For example, Borsay (1990: 114) has suggested that 'the management of disability in marriage is smoothed by ageing and the suspension of conventions pertaining to bodily care'. Similarly, Ungerson's writing suggests that personal care between people of the opposite sex is problematic only when it involves blood relationships (Ungerson, 1983). This leads her to argue that women looking after male relatives *other than their husbands* 'may find themselves in exceptionally trying circumstances' (1983: 75). She makes no mention of men providing personal care to women and whether or not this could be expected to be more or less 'trying' if provided to a wife.

In fact, the situation in relation to giving personal care within marriage is complicated. First, as outlined earlier, men caring for disabled or frail elderly wives *do* provide personal care. The 1985 UK GHS data on informal care show that male carers as a whole are less likely than women to be providing personal care; 16 per cent of male carers report this type of care-giving compared to 25 per cent of female carers (Parker and Lawton, 1991). Among the main carers of spouses, however, there are no differences between the proportions of men and women providing personal care. Second, qualitative research has challenged the idea that providing personal care in marriage is unproblematic. Among long-term spouse-carers, for example, the performance of personal care tasks can create problems in the sexual relationship of the couple. However, the main problems are created not so much for the carers, who tend to get used to providing personal care after a time, but rather for the person receiving this type of assistance. In relatively new caring situations, Seymour (1995) found that husbands were less likely to be involved in personal care than were wives. Her small-scale study found that three of the seven male carers interviewed had refused to carry out such tasks or had arranged for another, female, informal carer to perform them for payment. There were no similar findings among the female spouse-carers. Again, however, these arrangements seemed to have their origin as much in the sensitivities (actual or assumed) of the women who required assistance as in any reluctance in their partners to carry out the tasks, as the following response illustrates:

INTERVIEWER   Do you have to help her at all with these sorts of things [personal care]?

MALE   No, she likely wouldn't want me helping her, it's a bit like that I think. . . There are *certain barriers*, whether you like it or not.

(Our italics)

As suggested, some short-term male carers felt unable to provide cross-sex personal care for their wives and considered same-sex carers, who may have been merely acquaintances, more suited to the task. Hence one man's neighbour visited his wife to:

MALE   Give her a good strip wash, which is something better than I can. . . . . She was a nurse and she gives her a better do than me, more private.

Such comments would appear to echo Ungerson's (1983) discussion of personal care as subject to pollution taboos and hence more likely to be performed by women. Yet some male carers in both the long-term and newer caring relationships carried out, and had done for some time, significant personal tending tasks. The spouse most heavily involved in personal care among the long-term spouse carers was a man: he inserted his wife's catheter, changed her urine bag, carried out manual evacuation of her bowels, and helped during menstruation. In the absence of adequate supportive services he and his wife had no alternative; she hated being helped by him in this way while he had, to a degree, resigned himself to it. Among the more recent carers, too, personal care-giving to wives 'stood out' as something unusual initially, but for some, at least, had become part of the routine by the time of interview:

MALE   I automatically do it and you get to live with things.

This carer and his wife both explained the ease with which he undertook personal care as arising from their former habits of not locking the bathroom door and having conversations with each other while one partner bathed. This suggests that individual marital patterns of privacy may intersect the more general sexual stereotyping of tasks resulting in the performance of personal tending by some male carers. On the one hand, 'being married does not magically dispose of the embarrassment we are brought up to feel about our bodies and nudity, or the psychological difficulties that come when we feel that we are challenging "normal" boundaries' (Parker, 1993: 16). On the other hand, 'giving and receiving personal assistance can be an expression of love' when carried out by choice and aided by suitable resources (Morris, 1993: 10).

If we move from a concentration on personal care to a wider consideration of the role of carer, we can again examine whether the experiences of male carers differ from those of their female counterparts.

Overall experience of being a carer

Parker (1993) has suggested that the differences between male and female spouse carers have their basis in social structures predicated on gender. Structural inequalities and gender roles lead to varying material and practical conditions for male and female carers. Financially, the lack of flexibility in the male labour market, as mentioned above, provides little part-time work for male carers, while indirect discrimination in the benefit system results in lower benefits for disabled women. As a result, male spouse-carers may be materially worse off than are female carers in a similar position. However, the gendered dynamics of power in marriage and the ability of men to assert their needs may put them in a more powerful position than their female counterparts.

At the level of feelings, however, there may be more similarity between male and female carers than has been previously suggested might be the case. In the study of long-term spouse-carers, around a half of those who were supporting a disabled partner spoke of a duty or responsibility to care and men were just as likely as women to explain their continued help and support of their partners in this way. Similarly, Rose and Bruce (1995) noted of the elderly spouse-carers they interviewed that, 'like women, men expressed feelings of sadness and resignation, frustration and anger'.

Which men become carers?

Earlier we looked at selected characteristics of men – their age and marital status – that might increase their 'risk' of becoming carers. Beyond these, however, there are also issues about personality or emotional predisposition that might influence some men to take up or continue relationships that include caring responsibility. Perhaps some men *develop* a more caring side in response to experience. For example, does the fact that most male carers are spouse-carers indicate that involvement in an intimate adult relationship allows men to develop this aspect of their abilities? Applegate and Kaye (1994: 165) suggest that the experience of caring by male elder carers can 'potentiate nurturant capacities' that men are usually socialized to suppress. That is, being a carer allows men to develop a 'caring' nature. Certainly, some of the male long-term carers indicated a development of this sort, as this quotation suggests:

> It helps you kind of perhaps understand each other a little better and it makes you realize. . . .
>
> It's made me think when she's been ill, you know, more about *her* which is what you should do anyway, really, well or ill, but we don't. . . .

Alternatively (or perhaps as well), it may be that marital status, the combination of co-residence and an intimate relationship, prevents men from 'opting out' of caring responsibilities. In other caring relationships, men seem able to negotiate their non-involvement, especially if a female candidate is also available (Finch, 1989; Finch and Mason, 1993). For example, some fathers absent themselves from caring for their disabled children by having extremely long working days (Baldwin, 1985). Marriage may be the context where, for men, emotional concerns and normative behaviour ('In sickness and in health') exert their strongest influence.

A third possibility, which may increase as second and third marital relationships become more prevalent, is that the requirement or desire to care is a contributory factor in the formation of some new partnerships. Seymour found that, in two cases, the fact that the male partner was 'that sort of person' – that is 'caring' – had been significantly instrumental in the initiation of the relationships. This was stated explicitly by one woman, whose onset of chronic illness coincided with the formation of her new relationship, and was confirmed later by her partner, who said:

MALE   I like looking after her, I enjoy looking after her. . . . I can't think of anything I could advise anybody else on, apart from just be caring, be gentle and just be patient, you know.

These examples would suggest that, for some men, having a 'caring' nature makes them more likely to become a carer. Notably, both cases were co-habitations rather than marriages, and all partners had been previously divorced, perhaps indicating a non-traditional view of married life.

To conclude this section, it would appear that while the material and practical aspects of caring are mediated by gendered employment structures and concepts of appropriate task performance, at the level of feelings and emotions, however, there are fewer differences between male and female spouse-carers.

Welfare services' involvement with male carers

This section will focus particularly on the 'visibility' of male carers to welfare practitioners. This includes whether they are perceived as available to provide care, and if so, the extent to which service provision is influenced by the gender of the recipient. Men, as carers, seem paradoxically to be both invisible and 'ultra-visible' to welfare practitioners. They may be invisible when gendered assumptions by welfare workers exclude them as potential sources of informal care. Twigg and Atkin (1994: 136) cite the tradition in the home-help service of 'domestic help to elderly people being withheld where there was a female relative in the locality but not where there was a male'. In contrast, those men who *are* identified as carers may be 'ultra-visible' due to the gendered nature of most caring tasks. This could result in the provision of services for male carers which were not available to female carers, either to allow men to continue in the labour market (Atkin, 1992) or to substitute for their wives' domestic labour. Both Parker (1993) and Seymour (1995) found that the lack of substitute male labour (gardening, decorating, maintenance) offered by welfare services often meant that female carers were overwhelmed by the sheer volume of tasks they were now required to perform. In the long-term carers study it seemed that it was easier for husbands to accept welfare services which substituted for their wives' domestic labour, while female carers often considered the provision of such domestic labour as inappropriate. Indeed, some women found it insulting to be offered such assistance. However, it was also the case that men were more likely to articulate a perceived *right* to services (even if they or their wives were not currently receiving any). By contrast, women used notions of 'deservingness' in relation to services, and this usually meant that 'someone else' was more deserving than they were, echoing Gilligan's (1982) moral reasoning.

The issue of gender and service provision is further complicated by the relationship and location in which most male caring takes place. Arber and Gilbert (1989) stressed that for elderly people, the co-residence of carer and cared-for person, and the age structure of the household were more important factors influencing the amount of welfare support received than was the gender of the carer. Co-resident carers were least likely to receive welfare services and this was particularly so where the household contained younger people. Similarly, secondary analysis of the 1985 GHS shows that most of the variation in service receipt between carers is explained by the age of the person being helped, whether or not they are a relative of the carer and living in the same household, and the type of care being provided. Male carers are slightly more likely than females to be receiving a service of any sort, but service provision to people being cared for by a relative in the same household is at such a low level that this small difference is of minimal importance (Parker and Lawton, 1994).

This suggests that, in the very situations where men are most likely to become carers (residing with their spouse), they are, regardless of their sex, least likely to receive welfare support (Anderson, 1992; Parker and Lawton, 1994). This is exacerbated in the case of young spouse-carers (Parker, 1993; Seymour, 1995).

CONCLUSION

This chapter has shown that, while gender is a key factor in shaping the experiences of male carers, it is mediated by other aspects of their situation. Crucially, the fact that the site of most male caring is the marital relationship makes their emotional experiences very like those of female spouse-carers. It also means that complex dynamics affect the provision and receipt of welfare services to male spouse-carers which to some extent offset their previously supposed gendered advantages.

Do these findings result in a need to reconceptualize earlier feminist analyses of community care? How can we incorporate this recognition of both the numbers of and the lack of welfare support for male carers in discussions of informal care? Clearly, it has started with an acknowledgement of their significant presence. The caveat should always be made however, that, as a group, they are less involved than women in the 'labour' of caring, particularly the provision of personal care. Parker's research, however, suggests that for male spouse-carers the 'love' of caring is also a key dimension.

The earlier separation of these two aspects of caring (caring 'for' and caring 'about' – see Graham 1983) and the exploration of the former aspect, usefully served to highlight the sheer volume of work involved. While not losing sight of this emphasis, it would now seem appropriate to refocus on the second aspect of caring, the emotional dimension of caring 'about', to develop work on male carers further. This would expand on the Scandinavian literature of the 1980s which was concerned with the relational aspects of caring (Waerness, 1984) and which, in Britain, has already been further developed by Rose and Bruce (1995). For, as Twigg and Atkin (1994) remind us, caring takes place within a relationship and it is becoming increasingly inappropriate to consider the carer in isolation from the cared-for person. This return to the 'duality' (Twigg, 1994) of the caring situation may prove a particularly fruitful development in the study of male carers.

NOTES

1 This research was supported by a grant from the Economic and Social Research Council.
2 This examination of options has to take place within a context where alternative sources of support for older and disabled adults which would enable them not to have to rely on family members for support are not widely available.

REFERENCES

Anderson, R. (1992) *The Aftermath of Stroke: The Experience of Patients and their Families*, Cambridge: Cambridge University Press.

Applegate, J. and Kaye, L. (1994) 'Male elder caregivers', in C. Williams (ed.) *Doing Women's Work: Men and Non-traditional Occupations,* London: Sage.

Arber, S. and Gilbert, N. (1989) 'Men: the forgotten carers', *Sociology*, 23(1): 111–18.

Atkin, K. (1992) 'Similarities and differences between carers', in J. Twigg (ed.) *Carers: Research and Practice*, London: HMSO.

Baldwin, S.M. (1985) *The Costs of Caring*, London: Routledge & Kegan Paul.

Beresford, B. (1994) *Positively Parents: Caring for a Severely Disabled Child*, London: HMSO.

Borsay, A. (1990) 'Disability and attitudes to family care in Britain: towards a sociological perspective', *Disability, Handicap and Society*, 5(2): 107–22.

Briggs, A. (1983) *Who Cares?* Chatham, Kent: Association of Carers.

Dalley, G. (1983) 'Ideologies of care: a feminist contribution to the debate', *Critical Social Policy* 8 (Autumn): 72–81.

—— (1988) *Ideologies of Caring*, Basingstoke: Macmillan.

EOC (1980) *The Experience of Caring for Elderly and Handicapped Dependents*, Manchester: Equal Opportunities Commission.

Finch, J. (1984) 'Community care: developing non-sexist alternatives', *Critical Social Policy*, 9 (Spring): 6–18.

—— (1989) *Family Obligations and Social Change*, Oxford: Polity Press.

Finch, J. and Mason, J. (1993) *Negotiating Family Responsibilities*, London: Routledge.

Froggatt, A. (1983) 'In sickness and in health: husbands as carers', *Community Care* (20 October).

Gilligan, C. (1982) *In a Different Voice: Psychological Theory and Women's Development*, Cambridge, MA: Harvard University Press.

Graham, H. (1983) 'Caring: a labour of love', in J. Finch and D. Groves (eds) *A Labour of Love: Women, Work and Caring*, London: Routledge & Kegan Paul.

Lewis, J. and Meredith, B. (1988) *Daughters who Care: Daughters Caring for Mothers at Home*, London: Routledge.

Morris, J. (1993) *Community Care or Independent Living?* York: Joseph Rowntree Foundation.

Nissel, M. and Bonnerjea, L. (1982) *Family Care of the Handicapped Elderly: Who Pays?* London: Policy Studies Institute.

Parker, G. (1993) *With this Body: Caring and Disability in Marriage*, Buckingham: Open University Press.

Parker, G. and Lawton, D. (1991) 'Further analysis of the 1985 General Household Survey Data on informal care', Report 4: 'Male carers', Working Paper DHSS 849, York: Social Policy Research Unit, University of York.

—— (1994) *Different Types of Care, Different Types of Carer*, London: HMSO.

Rose, H. and Bruce, E. (1995) 'Mutual care but differential esteem: caring between older couples', in S. Arber and J. Ginn (eds) *Connecting Gender and Ageing: A Sociological Approach*, Milton Keynes: Open University Press.

Seymour, J. (1995) *The Negotiation of Coping: Disablement, Caring and Marriage*, York: Social Policy Research Unit, University of York.

Shelby, R. D. (1992) *If a Partner has Aids: Guide to Clinical Intervention for Relationships in Crisis*, New York: Harrington Park Press.

Small, N. (1993) *AIDS: The Challenge – Understanding Education and Care*, Aldershot: Avebury.

Twigg, J. (1994) 'Carers, Services and Professionals', Paper given to Caring for Carers: Implications of Recent Research SSI Regional Dissemination Event, York (9 December).

Twigg, J. and Atkin, K. (1994) *Carers Perceived: Policy and Practice in Informal Care*, Buckingham: Open University Press.

Ungerson, C. (1983) 'Women and caring: skills, tasks and taboos', in E. Garmarnikow, D. Morgan, J. Purvis and D. Taylor (eds) *The Public and the Private*, London: Heinemann.

—— (1987) *Policy is Personal: Sex, Gender and Informal Care*, London: Tavistock.

Waerness, K. (1984) 'Caring as women's work in the Welfare State', in H. Holter (ed.) *Patriarchy in a Welfare Society*, Oslo: Universitetsforlaget.

Chapter 8

'I'm just a bloke who's had kids'
Men and women on parenthood

Sue Clarke and Jennie Popay

This chapter focuses on men's and women's accounts of parenthood. It begins with a review of the existing literature on fatherhood, looking particularly at three key themes: cultural images; the practice of fathering; and the social meanings attached to fatherhood and parenthood. The chapter then presents data from a small-scale study of men's and women's perceptions of the experience of parenting and considers the implications for future research. The word 'parenting' is used alongside 'mothering' and 'fathering' despite a recognition that it is problematic. It can, of course, be used to render invisible the gendered nature of childcare in the domestic sphere. However, 'fathering' and 'mothering' are also problematic in the context of this chapter in that they both denote the gender of the parent and carry assumptions about the nature of labour, responsibilities and meanings associated with being a mother or father. Given that this chapter is explicitly about gender division in parenting, we hope to transcend the limits language can impose.

IMAGES OF FATHERHOOD IN A HISTORICAL CONTEXT

There is a widespread view that in the last two decades there has been an increasing interest in fatherhood, and a significant transformation in the ideology of fathering towards a more caring, nurturant model. However, although, as Lewis and O'Brien (1987a: 4) have noted, '[i]n each generation some authors feel that men are breaking new ground', historical research does not support the notion of linear change. For example, on the basis of an analysis of popular magazine articles from 1900 to 1989, Atkinson and

Blackwelder (1993) argue that fathers have been presented as both instrumental and expressive actors for at least a century (see also LaRossa and Reitzes, 1995). In his survey of US historical research, Marsiglio (1995a) reaches the same conclusion, and suggests that social constructionist perspectives have shown how the specific types of fatherhood images to which people are exposed in their lives vary according to socio-historical context, culture, social/ ethnic/class background and religious affiliation. Similarly, Stearns (1991: 49), examining fatherhood in West European and American society since 1600, argues that this has been marked by 'diversity and tension'.

This said, as Williams notes in Chapter 3, the current emphasis on fatherhood within popular culture and social, political and policy discourse can be argued to be new. Fatherhood, she suggests, is in part a lens through which men's other identities – particularly as workers and husbands/partners – are signified. Whilst this has opened up discursive space to include the private domestic world of men, she argues that the space has been captured by representations of both 'good' and 'bad' fathers which are underpinned by a traditional (albeit reconstituted) heterosexual gender order rather than representations which allow for plurality in identities and roles.

CULTURAL IMAGES OF FATHERHOOD

Marsiglio (1995a), reviewing largely North American literature, summarizes the ways numerous researchers have explored the meaning and changing nature of what he terms the symbolic representations, ideologies and the cultural/sub-cultural images of fatherhood. Particular attention has been paid in the literature to a set of 'conflicting cultural standards' identified by Furstenberg (1988, 1995) – what he calls the 'good dads/bad dads complex'. These polarized images, he argues, represent the involved and nurturing father versus the uninvolved, 'deadbeat' father retreating from his paternal obligations. Other authors have suggested that the 'good dad' in contemporary culture also retains the notion of the 'good provider' (Silverstein, 1996). These opposing images are reinforced in the social and political arenas by, for example, fathers' rights' groups and mothers' groups involved in divorce and custody struggles. Similarly, in the political sphere (Moss, 1995a: xvi), government rhetoric surrounding the establishment and activities of the Child Support Agency reinforces the image of the 'good provider' and the dichotomy between this image and that of the absent, 'deadbeat' father.

Marsiglio (1995a, 1995b) speculates that media coverage of social problems said to be associated with high divorce rates and out-of-wedlock childbearing and greater public awareness of sexual abuse of children has led to the increased prominence of negative stereotypical images of fathers. In contrast, it is argued that images of nurturant, caring fathers have been increasingly portrayed in films, magazine articles and advertising. Segal (1990), for example, suggests that by the 1980s Hollywood, in films such as *Kramer vs Kramer* and *Ordinary People*, was creating fathers who were '*more* sensitive, and *more* nurturing, than their self-centred, ambitious wives'; and that subsequent films such as *Three Men and a Baby* showed 'the new interest in fathering and fatherhood' (1990: 29). However, other authors have pointed to the ambiguous – or even disparaging – nature of many of these apparently positive images. Burgess and Ruxton (1996: 5), for instance, note, in connection with the UK media, that 'when men are portrayed with babies, they are normally ridiculed . . . or their involvement with the child is seen as developing from an abnormal situation . . . and almost never are father and child seen gazing at each other, face-to-face'. Similarly, Burman (1994: 100) argues that while late 1980s childcare magazines started to include articles on or about fathers, this was often done in ways which 'confirmed men's peripheral role',[1] re-affirming male reluctance and emphasizing traditional roles.

Whatever the nature of visual images of fathers in popular culture, the media debate about contemporary fatherhood remains limited. On the basis of his analysis of coverage of fathers and fatherhood in UK daily and Sunday papers over one month in June 1994, Lloyd concludes that '[t]here was very little comment about what fathers are supposed to be, no guidance about how to be a father in the 1990s, with any pointers faltering after breadwinner and the general call on men to "take more responsibility"' (1995: 50). He argues from this that sharing of family responsibilities between men and women, reconciliation of employment and family life for men and women and the role of men and fathers as carers 'have failed to establish themselves on the public agenda in Britain in the 1990s' (1995: 51).

Ethnicity and class are also important in the construction of fatherhood images and ideology. By focusing on cultures other than the dominant white culture of the United States/United Kingdom some studies set out to demonstrate the Anglocentric bias of traditional social science literature. Mirandé (1991), for example, demonstrates the enormous diversity of ethnic minority families in the United States. He argues that, while programmes such as the *Cosby* show ostensibly depict 'black families', the dominant model of the family employed is still the Anglo-American ideal. Silverstein (1996) similarly argues that gender and ethnicity should not be assumed to be homogeneous variables, but rather understood to act both independently and interactively depending on context. McAdoo (1988) also argues that ethnicity and class have been wrongly conflated in the construction by whites of stereotypical images of the 'irresponsible' black father.

On a similar note, Marsiglio (1995a) suggests that the relationship between class and fatherhood is unclear in the literature. However, he cites Griswold (1993) as observing that social class has continued to play a major role in shaping fatherhood imagery. In particular, Griswold suggests that the 'new fatherhood' image is middle class:

> part of a middle-class strategy of survival in which men accommodate to the realities of their wives' careers and the decline of their breadwinning capabilities . . . pushing a pram . . . becomes . . . a public symbol of their commitment to a more refined, progressive set of values than those held by working-class men still imprisoned by outdated ideas of masculinity.
>
> (Griswold, 1993: 254; cited in Marsiglio, 1995a: 5)

Commenting on current research on cultural images of fatherhood, Lewis (1995: 65) argues that 'we need to know more about why fathers are depicted in particular ways rather than just the descriptions of a small selection of texts'. He goes on to suggest (p. 63) that we are 'in a period of reassessment. Fatherhood seems to be under the public gaze and we do not fully approve of what we see'.

FATHERING PRACTICE AND CHILD DEVELOPMENT

Another prominent theme in the literature on fatherhood is the nature and extent of men's involvement in childcare and domestic labour. Much of this research highlights the importance of macro socio-economic and technological changes in shaping fathering practice – including, for example, changes in work and family patterns and changes in family size and structure (Lewis and O'Brien, 1987a; Moss, 1995a). The argument that this has resulted in profound changes in men's involvement in parenting is, however, problematic. Additionally, whilst roughly 10,000 articles had been published by 1994 on how fathers influence child development (Lamb, 1994), there is little consensus regarding these effects.

There appears to be a general consensus that women spend more time on, and take more responsibility for, childcare than men, regardless of employment status (see Lamb, 1986; Brannen and Moss, 1987; Horna and Lupri, 1987; Kimmel, 1987a; Barnett and Baruch, 1988; Parke, 1988; Segal, 1990; Hall, 1994; Ishii-Kuntz, 1994; White, 1994; Brayfield, 1995; O'Brien and Jones, 1995). This is broadly supported by empirical research on the division of domestic labour and household work, though the detailed picture remains somewhat confused. Overall research suggests that, depending on household type, women's employment status and age of children, men's contribution to parenting labour alternates between a quarter and a third (Jump and Haas, 1987; Bronstein, 1988; Warde and Hetherington, 1993; Hall, 1994; Ishii-Kuntz, 1994; Silverstein, 1996). Their contribution to overall responsibility has been reported to be negligible (Lamb, 1986).

There is also consensus in the literature that men are potentially just as competent as women in parenting, and as capable of being nurturant. Silverstein (1996), reviewing the literature, states that research findings have not documented gender differences in competent parenting. She cites Lamb's (1987) review of research on parental caretaking in Western cultures as demonstrating that neither fathers nor mothers are 'natural' caretakers – that both parents learn 'on the job' (see also Hanson, 1986; Lamb, 1986; Marsiglio, 1995a; Burgess and Ruxton, 1996).

As already noted, the literature on fathers' influence on child development is now considerable and the impact of divorce and remarriage is a prominent theme. However, as Marsiglio (1995a) argues, research findings in this field are mixed. There is support for the idea that it is the *quality* of the child's environment that is of most importance (see, for example, reviews in Lamb, 1986; Lamb *et al.*, 1987). Similarly, Samuels (1995) argues that there are no inevitable negative psychological consequences of lone parenthood or parenting carried out by two or more persons of the same sex. Although Burgess and Ruxton (1996: 2) state that the absence of fathers is 'a source of stress' within families, they are careful to argue that, in terms of the effect on children's well-being, it is difficult to isolate different influences on negative outcomes, such as poverty, racism and maternal failure (1996: 2 and 69). They cite a meta-analysis of ninety-two American and British studies which suggests that parental conflict is one of the strongest influences on negative outcomes. Phillips (1995) also argues in her discussion of boys that the worst father is not one who is missing, but one who 'teaches him to be bad'; that losing, for example, a violent or abusive father would not be a great loss to a child. These findings contrast with the arguments of those authors who seek to link the absence of fathers with criminal and anti-social behaviour in young males (Dennis and Erdos, 1992).

Researchers have considered factors that might constrain or facilitate paternal involvement such as social class, ethnicity, cultural differences, family characteristics and structure (including age and gender of children), timing of fatherhood, personal life histories, personal motivation, beliefs, values, macro-structural changes (such as employment patterns), organizational culture and social policy. Sandqvist (1987:157), for example, has argued that the low take-up of parental leave and benefits in Sweden may be due to a number of factors, including negative reactions at work; 'inertia of tradition and habit' for both men and women; and a multitude of reasons for the fathers from 'reluctance to give up privileges to deep-seated problems of identity and personality' (see also Carlsen, 1995; Haas and Hwang, 1995). Similarly, Bowen and Orthner (1991), in a review of research, find workplace organizations to be ambivalent towards parenthood in an attempt to foster practices promoting organizational performance and success; and that organizational cultures reinforce traditional fatherhood roles.

In the context of an overall picture of relatively low participation for fathers in general, the literature suggests that paternal arrangements are so diverse that, as Bradley (1985: 151) argues, 'commonalities' of fathering behaviour are difficult to find. O'Brien and Jones (1995: 27) similarly note the 'confusing and complex' picture of fatherhood at a private, relational level:

[i]n any one day one may hear about, see or personally experience diverse forms of fathering – from men in the local park
carrying their babies in slings discussing feeding and sleeping
practices, to men who find it difficult to fit in any time with
their children and have little knowledge of their children's interests never mind food preferences. It appears that different models
of fatherhood and fathering are being negotiated in the home, in
the work-place and more widely across generations.

(See also Parke, 1988; Segal, 1990; Bozett and Hanson, 1991a: 265;
Burman, 1994.)

THE 'MEANING' OF FATHERHOOD

A third major theme within the literature on fatherhood is the
meanings men and women attach to fatherhood and parenthood.
There have been a number of noteworthy studies which have
explored men's and other family members' perceptions of fatherhood: O'Brien and Jones (1995), for example, describe a 1990s
UK project, 'Inter-generational Perceptions of Fatherhood', which
is aiming overall to look at the meaning of fatherhood for contemporary children and their parents. Other UK studies have focused
on 'dual-earner' households (Brannen and Moss, 1987) and samples
of middle-class couples (see, for example, Backett, 1987). North
American research has been more extensive and has focused on a
wide range of social groups including African-American fathers
and feminist couples (see, for example, Connor, 1986; Daniels and
Weingarten, 1988; Daly, 1993; Hall, 1994; Blaisure and Allen,
1995; Furstenberg, 1995; and Allen and Doherty, 1996). There has
also been some research in Australia (see, for example, White, 1994).

One theme that emerges consistently in these studies is the disparity between stated beliefs and actual behaviour: Brannen and
Moss (1987), for example, found that while lip-service was paid
to an egalitarian ideology, women in 'dual-earner' households
were still doing the bulk of the work and bearing most responsibility; Backett (1987: 87) argues from her data that 'respondents perceived frequent contradictions between beliefs in . . . fair and
mutual parental involvement, and what actually happened'; and
O'Brien and Jones (1995), in their report on the first phase of the
'Inter-generational Perceptions of Fatherhood' project focusing
on the attitudes of young people (average age 14.9) to fatherhood,

found a 'degree of mismatch' between the young people's attitudes and values, and reported behaviour concerning the responsibilities of fatherhood (see also Warde and Hetherington, 1993; White, 1994; Blaisure and Allen, 1995). Interestingly, a qualitative study by Bertoia and Drakich (1993) of members of Canadian fathers' rights groups also found a contradiction between the movement's public rhetoric and the fathers' subjective, individualized accounts. They conclude that the fathers' rights activists have co-opted the language but not the spirit of equality; that their rhetoric of equality conceals their wish not for an equal sharing of childcare and responsibility after divorce, but for equal access to their children, information and decision-making.

The actual meanings and definitions attached by men to fatherhood, and their personal experiences of fathering, are themselves unclear from the literature. Methodological difficulties in conducting and interpreting research, and the limitations of current research paradigms, are important here (McKee, 1982; Lamb, 1986: 7–9; Backett, 1987; Marsiglio, 1995a: 13–14; Burman, 1994). Additionally, however, as Lewis (1986: 15–17) comments, although meanings attached to being fathers and husbands are changing, few researchers have turned their attention to the question of what it means to be a father and a husband. Although there has been a ground-swell of research and empirical studies, we still have little knowledge of how most men perceive fatherhood. More recently, White (1994) has similarly noted that little attention has been paid to how fathers interpret and define what being a father means to them. In the next section we seek to make a modest empirical contribution to this field.

A SMALL-SCALE, QUALITATIVE STUDY OF MEN'S AND WOMEN'S ACCOUNTS OF PARENTING

During 1987, as part of an ESRC[2] study of patterns of health and illness in households with dependent children, separate, in-depth, semi-structured interviews were conducted with mothers and fathers in fourteen two-parent households in the Greater London area (other households in the sample involved either one parent raising children alone or one of the two parents was not available for interview). During the interviews, respondents were encouraged to talk about their experience of parenthood and their views about the domestic division of labour within the household. Using this dataset, the subjective perceptions of men and women about parenthood and gender divisions can therefore be explored and compared between women and men within the same household.

Clearly, there have been important social changes since these interviews were conducted. In order to add a more recent dimension to the picture they provide, similar interviews were conducted with women and men in two further two-parent households in the North West of England during 1996 – making a total of sixteen households. Households were selected through two different approaches. The majority were drawn from a larger sample used during a survey of household living standards undertaken in 1985, whilst a few were obtained through a snowballing technique.

These sixteen households reflect a number of cross-cutting dimensions of diversity. The age of children, for example, ranged from new babies to adult children (though all had children living in the household), whilst household size varied from five resident children to one. Household income ranged from in excess of £500,000 per annum (excluding income from investments) to households living on means-tested social security benefit. Employment patterns and domestic divisions of labour were similarly diverse, including men involved full-time in childcare, mothers employed for a wide range of hours (including households where both parents were in full-time career posts, referred to as 'dual-career'), households with neither parent in paid employment and full-time housewives/mothers where the father was employed full-time. Though the majority of the women and men interviewed were white, the sample does include a Gujurati couple and a black British couple. A number of the people involved had remarried. Finally, the social class background of the sample was also diverse, including children of hereditary lords and schoolteachers, as well as people who had experienced considerable material disadvantage during their childhood.

The households can be classified into three broad groups in terms of their material circumstances: high income (over £60k), middle income (£15–59k) and low income (<£15k). The middle-income group clearly covers a wide range of income levels. To a considerable degree, although not entirely, these income groups also reflect the social class backgrounds of the women and men involved. The sample includes two low-income households (one with both parents unemployed, one with the man in full-time work and the woman working part-time); seven middle-income households (including one in which the man was the main carer but had a part-time job, one dual-career, two in which the woman worked part-time and the man full-time and three with single male earners); and seven high-income households (six with a single male earner and one 'role reversal').

Men's and women's accounts

In some senses material circumstances had a powerful influence on the experience of parenthood. In the high- and upper-middle-income households, for example, people had access to a wide range of 'labour-saving' devices and in many instances were able, when they so wished, to buy in additional help with childcare and domestic labour. Importantly, however, not all of these households had help with childcare (though most had part-time cleaners). In the main, these parents did not worry about providing physically for their children. In the low-income households, however, domestic work was more labour-intensive. For example, parents had to walk or use public transport for shopping and they made more shopping trips for essential items because there was no freezer (though this does not mean that overall these women and men spent more time doing domestic work and childcare). Concerns about absolute shortages of money were prominent in the interviews with men and women in these households – though, as discussed elsewhere (Popay, 1991), in all of the households, regardless of income level, money was not generally considered to be important to one's ability to be a 'good parent'.

Broadly speaking the analysis revealed three patterns of accounts among these households, although within these groups there was also considerable diversity both between women and men and among each gender group. These three groups can be characterized along two dimensions. First, and perhaps predictably, they differ in terms of the nature and degree of men's involvement in childcare, ranging from a 'traditional' division of childcare and domestic labour in one group to a more egalitarian division at the other extreme. More interestingly, however, and linked to the gender division of labour, they differ in the ways in which the discourse around new fatherhood is invoked. One group of men and women, as we shall show, invoke the rhetoric of 'new fathers' with enthusiasm, but the extent to which and ways in which this is driven through into fathering practice is less obvious. For this reason we refer to

these as the 'nouveau traditionalists'. The second group make no
rhetorical allusions to the 'new fathers' discourse, nor are they
explicitly pursuing greater equality in the domestic division of
labour. Rather, these women and men are 'pragmatists' – shifting
the gender division of labour in the context of household employment patterns which severely constrain both partners' time. The
third group are more explicitly egalitarian at both a rhetorical
and practical level.

The nouveau traditionalists

The accounts of men and women in nine of these households contained many elements of the stereotypical images of breadwinner
father and full-time nurturant mother (these included five of the
seven high-income households, three of the middle-income households and one low-income household). The men in these households
identified a 'provider role' as a key aspect of fatherhood. This
included, in particular, the provision of financial resources and
'the best education possible'. In some accounts the interwoven
nature of these themes was apparent. As one senior executive noted:

> I think you have to be prepared to put the monetary resources
> into the children . . . if you look at the money side of it . . . it
> would be easy for us to say 'Don't spend any money on educat-
> ing the children we will go on holiday'.
>
> (H/H4)

The responsibility of fatherhood could be forcefully expressed. One
father in a high-income household, for example, talked of the 'awe-
some responsibility of providing education and protecting them in
the future' (H/H3).

These men had little experience of routine childcare and domestic
labour – leaving that domain almost entirely to their partners.
However, alongside 'traditional' elements, their account of fatherhood also contained a different, and for them complementary,
dimension, invoking, at a rhetorical level, the 'new man/father' discourse. Good parenthood was frequently described, for example, as
an ability to put the children first before one's own needs – also a
prominent theme in women's accounts. For these men, fathers
were felt to have a vital role in loving and nurturing their
children – providing an upbringing which would guide them and

help them to develop to their full. As one director of a small company described it:

> I mean I've just been terribly involved with them. I mean I'm you know, very very interested in them. I mean I'm interested in what they do, anything they do really. . . . I mean one tries to encourage them to develop really.
>
> (H/H17)

Fatherhood was also described as a source of pleasure and fulfilment. And, although they have been presented here in a somewhat fragmented way, inevitably these different elements of fatherhood were normally bound together:

> Well, I think it is about providing for them, getting involved with everything they do, showing them things when I am doing things, . . . I don't know, basically enjoying them I suppose. Babies are a bit boring but I have got used to them. . . . I have got more time for Jean now – she makes me laugh.
>
> (H/H13)

These men therefore articulated a clear role for themselves as fathers in the nurturing of their children, in the context of their primary responsibility for earning income which frequently involved long hours away from the home and little involvement in the direct labour of parenting on a day-to-day basis. In this context, though some noted that they would like more time with the children, they felt overall that they were fulfilling their responsibilities at least adequately and often very well. They frequently provided a robust defence of their position in relation to day-to-day contact and involvement with parenting. Asked about whether he spent enough time with his teenage children, for instance, a senior manager commented thus:

> Well, during the week I'm just not around . . . but I don't feel that I've neglected them . . . it's meant that I've taken a different attitude to what I do at the weekends. I mean, for example, . . . I've stopped playing golf because I didn't have enough time to do that. I had no time to do the garden, participate in their recreation activities at the weekend and have recreation activities myself. If I were playing golf all day Saturday and Sunday then I guess I would be saying I'm neglecting my input to them but over their schooling career I've always been around

you know at some stage during the week, if they've had home-
work problems or school problems . . . and, of course, I am
chair of the school governors.

(H/H4)

Another senior executive, who spent substantial periods away from
home, argued similarly that although he would like to spend more
time with his family, if he was criticized he would 'fight my corner
like an alleycat because I feel I do all I can as a father, as a husband
and as a man' (H/H3).

Similarly, a father in a low-income household commented that
his wife complained that he didn't do enough around the house,
and argued that: 'I think she is being unreasonable when she says
it. She says she works 24 hours a day but the kids are in bed so
she hasn't got them for the rest of the evening so she's in the
same boat as me then' (H/H13).

A number of these fathers felt that, in general, men needed to
learn to show their emotions more easily to their children and
others. As one man expressed it: 'Men are the loneliest people in
the world.' However, although their accounts of fatherhood
picked up on key themes in the contemporary debate about the
'new father', only one of these men explicitly linked his perspectives
on, and experience of, fatherhood to this debate. Commenting on
the pressures he felt men as fathers experienced in society, he said:

men have every right to complain about women seeing them as
success symbols. I feel I'm that in the family. On the one hand
they may well say . . . 'Why are you involved in your work so
much?' but in the next breath you know, it's the school fees,
and I say, 'Well, going to private school certainly wasn't my
idea', and now they've got friends that go skiing and . . . it esca-
lates the level that this success machine has just got to keep
going. Any complaints they might have about me being preoccupied with work these days get short shift.

(H/H18)

As already noted, a number of these men were in their second
marriages and they spontaneously contrasted their greater involvement with fathering now and their belief in the importance of a
nurturing role for fathers, with their behaviour as fathers in their
previous relationships. A key influence was allocated to their present partners in shaping their new, more involved fathering prac-

tice. One man, for example, who talked of his young 'love children' in contrast to his children from his first marriage, tied this closely to his second wife's attitude towards parenthood, noting: 'I've had to learn a lot from her . . . how to be with children' (H/H3). Similarly, a second man spoke of the birth of his children to his first wife compared to those with his second:

> I just didn't understand what was going on, I was neither that close to the mother nor aware of myself, so that when Jane had John it was completely totally different . . . because Jane was a completely competent person compared to my first wife. Then to have her educate me . . . about birth, about feelings about children, about plans for children, about ambitions for children, every aspect of that I think she led me.
>
> (H/H18)

For some of these men their accounts suggest that the private world of fatherhood provided a contrast with, and/or refuge or distraction from, the stresses and strains of the public world of paid employment and other formal activities (such as membership of professional associations). But in an important sense it would appear that for these men it is the public world of paid employment which provides their major reference point in life. As one man vividly described it:

> Interestingly I believe being a parent enables one to leave the office behind one. You can leave the office with a series of problems going round in your mind, you walk in the front door here and you're confronted with a totally different set of problems, you know, can't do the homework, teachers being unreasonable, ill, or whatever it may be, or you know, row between mother and children . . . and that I find gets me out of the work. I think if I hadn't got that I might well sit here still worrying about the problem I took away with me from the office. And that means that when I go back in the office the next day, I think I'm fresher. The more responsibility I've taken with the company, the more it has meant that I have had less time with the family . . . but I don't think that's been an adverse effect.
>
> (H/H4)

Other men suggested that it was the responsibilities of fatherhood that drew them more firmly into the world of paid employment.

One man, for example, talked of his greatest fears as being his: 'capacity to deliver, like insurance policies, education plans . . . how do I provide for them and still not bust my gut and end up killing myself' (H/H3).

All but one of the women in these households were involved fulltime in childcare and domestic labour (though two of the women in the middle-income households did work around six hours a week). These women all emphasized the importance of a mother's care of children, particularly in the early years, and the status and value of motherhood, and most (though not all) were strongly resistant to women combining paid work with motherhood – even on a parttime basis. Not surprisingly, most of these women were very resistant to the use of nannies, despite in most instances having household incomes which were more than adequate to support full-time help with childcare – seeing them as disruptive of the essential mother–child relationship. In some instances these attitudes were linked back to the women's own experience of being cared for by a nanny in their childhood:

> One thing I feel terribly strongly about is . . . I don't like people with careers and families. I know they say, 'Oh, I'll go round the bend and I've got nanny.' No, I would be terribly sad if either of our daughters did that because I think it's a responsible decision that you take and you must give yourself to your children . . . a mother, yes a mother more than a father. I just don't feel it is natural having somebody else doing your job . . . my mother had nannies for us . . . she was always giving them the sack because she was a super mother and she couldn't stand it, they'd be doing things she didn't like.
>
> (H/H4)

Where nannies were employed, the women stressed the importance of their controlling the detailed planning of, and their constant presence in, their children's lives. As one woman commented:

> I couldn't get a job where I hardly see them . . . my nanny doesn't have sole charge. I like to know what is going on at different times even if I don't want to take them to every party and every swimming lesson.
>
> (H/H5)

Similarly, another woman noted that:

As a journalist I saw this whole market being created of two career households and the children being put in crèches or left with childminders, au pairs, anything to get the children off one's hands. I was very shocked by this. I was not having a baby to be looked after by somebody else.

(H/H17)

Like their male partners, alongside the 'traditional' perspectives on motherhood evident in these women's accounts – albeit that in the high- and middle-income households some aspects of maternal labour were done by paid cleaners and nannies – some of these women also echoed aspects of the contemporary discourse around fatherhood, motherhood and parenting. There was, for example, some suggestion that women felt a need to justify full-time involvement in motherhood in the context of contemporary feminist debates about women's rights to be more than mothers. They did this through a dual call to the natural nature of maternity – as vital to healthy child development and a central part of being a woman – and by drawing on metaphors of paid labour. In some instances the language of the labour force was used directly. A mother of two teenage children in a high-income household, for example, explained how she had negotiated an allowance for herself from her husband:

I've always found it difficult to, I was financially independent before, to rely on a husband and he's always said, 'No, you're doing a good job of work, that's why I'm here to pay you to do this.' And I've accepted it and then I think, I feel useless, I didn't have any money of my own. So I went to him and said, 'Look, I can't go out to work. . . . I think I'm worth at least £50 a week. . . . I will take a slight cut in my housekeeping (which he had just put up) and I'll have two accounts and one you will pay like my wages. I think I'm worth that.'

(H/H4)

Others did not draw directly on imagery from the world of paid employment but stressed how much work they did. Asked if they had paid work, for example, these two women in higher-income households answered:

No, not paid work, it does not mean I am idle though. I am fortunate in being a supported parent and I think that is actually a good thing to be and I feel no guilt or anything about it. I also get involved in things that are like an extension of being a parent, chair of the play group and a school governor. I haven't gone to sleep.

(H/H17)

No, the children have always been my main job. I've never liked to farm them out. We've been lucky financially, so that's enabled me to do it the way I want to. I haven't had to work, but I've done a lot of other things, like setting up committees.

(H/H18)

As many of the quotes above highlight, most of these women also stressed the strength of their partner's commitment to parenthood, frequently noting what 'good fathers' their partners were and how they would do more if they could. In the context of her husband's long absences from the home, for example, one woman commented that:

John is away a lot so I take the responsibility. . . . I mean a lot of the time I am a single mother really. . . he would like to be more important and when he comes home he will jump back into his father's role.

(H/H3)

The wish to present partners in a good light was not, however, evident in all the households in this group. In the lower-income households, for example, women were more likely to feel that their partners could do more than they did. Asked whether she thought the work of looking after the children and home was fairly shared, for example, one mother who worked part-time, said:

He don't do any housework, he does help with the washing up sometimes and he does a little bit of cooking . . . it does get me down sometimes because he don't, I mean I do all the decorating and I have to do the garden when I get time to do it, he doesn't do anything like that at all. But he will do the shopping. I usually do the main shopping on Friday but he usually gets a few bits for me. I don't think I could cope with a full-time job and everything else at the moment. He would have to help a lot more. I would like to have the money a full-time job brings but I do like to have a few hours at home as well. It's things like cleaning windows as well, which he doesn't do. He's amazing really (*Laughs*).

(H/H10)

And another commented:

The housework, well I do that. I mean I'm here. But I would like sometime for him to take them away for the day. He does take them out sometimes on a Saturday afternoon to his mum's for about 2 or 3 hours, but then he's going to his mum's, you know, he's going to somewhere where there's somebody who can help. But I just wish sometimes, you know . . .

(H/H13)

Despite the obvious enthusiasm for full-time motherhood amongst most of the women in this group there was also ambivalence about aspects of the experience. As the above quotation illustrates, a number of these women reflected, for example, on the lack of time they had for themselves. This was particularly evident in the accounts of women in lower-income households, albeit not confined to these. The mother of two young children in a lower-middle-income household commented, for example: 'Well, by 6 o'clock I am glad when Pete comes home because at the time you are a mother you are never by yourself' (H/H14).

Some appeared to be defensive about not having paid work and uncertain of the worth of what they did. A woman in a high income family, for instance, voiced her guilt at being paid to stay at home with children and, when prompted as to why she felt guilty, replied that:

It's not using intellect at all. Somebody stupid could do this job. No, on second thoughts, the emotional side, the dealing with the children, what I'm saying is it takes a little bit of brain power, but not a lot.

(H/H17)

The pragmatists

Two of the middle-income households (one at the higher and one at the lower end of the range) differed from those described above in that the women and men involved were both in paid employment (the men full-time and the women part-time) and, in the context of these employment patterns, they were attempting to reform the 'traditional' practice of fathering and mothering. However, this was not presented as a conscious attempt to pursue greater equality between the partners (as it was in the third group of households described below) but rather as a pragmatic response to their situation. As one of the fathers put it:

> Children should wherever possible be brought up with a full-time parent and in this case it was Lucy . . . it crossed my mind to work part-time but that never really became a serious possibility, probably because I didn't want to I suppose, I don't know.
>
> (H/H25)

As in other households, these men spoke of the importance of the 'provider role' in fathering in terms of financial security, of the need to nurture and love children, and of the pleasure and satisfaction of watching children grow up. In contrast to men in the 'nouveau traditional' households, they also spoke of their direct involvement in childcare and domestic labour on a day-to-day basis: both partners were working and so both had to contribute to looking after the children and running the household. As one of these two fathers commented:

> I often think that our life is so busy, so full of stuff to do that neither of us particularly want to do, that the person best able to do it is the one best equipped to do it . . . these are not things, responsibilities that have been allotted or discussed and given to each partner, they have arisen from the circumstances, the fact that Lucy works two days a week means that she is able to take the children to school and gets more involved with that side of things.
>
> (H/H25)

In the context of what were perceived to be severe time constraints, this man felt that he should perhaps do more childcare than he was doing at the moment:

> I feel that I should be getting involved with the children. I do a bit of that in passing anyway. I often think I could be a better father. . . . I think I should get more involved . . . but Lucy seems to be doing such a good job.
>
> (H/H25)

However, the other father, who worked from home, had a different perspective:

our arrangements are entirely fair, Sara does more than me but then I would rather employ more people to do the work. She won't do that. I would like to have a live-in nanny, but she doesn't. I respect that, it's her home, but she has to accept the consequences.

(H/H8)

This comment points to an important contradiction in men's accounts, which was apparent across many of the households in this study: whilst on the one hand men may speak of the need for them to be actively involved in parenting this was frequently tempered by a form of resistance. For example, in one of these two households, the father who worked from home felt that men should be more directly involved in childcare and described how he did this on a daily basis. But, as he went on to say:

I give the children breakfast. I give Tom breakfast every morning and sometimes Dick. I don't mind the children thumping around me and making a nuisance of themselves although I resist being asked things like 'Can you be in tomorrow morning to look after Dick?', because I don't know what important things might come up, but I do actually do it.

(H/H8)

Similarly, the father in the second household described how he resisted his wife's attempts to involve him in discussions about childcare issues:

We sort of discuss things. . . . Lucy tries to discuss things but I would rather think about other things. . . . When she tries to discuss these things with me . . . many things influence how I react but I do think 'You know all about that kind of stuff and for you to brief me on what is going on, train me for that week perhaps, is pointless because I could be doing something else. . . . You know what you are doing, I have complete faith in you, so you don't need to discuss it with me'.

(H/H25)

As another extract from the same interview indicates, these men were not unaware of the contradictions inherent in their position:

I can't get my head around childcare arrangements . . . a steel shutter comes down in my head. . . . I can deal with computers and . . . I guess I just don't want to know I suppose . . . I just trust her which isn't exactly fair I suppose.

(H/H25)

Perhaps because they were more involved on a day-to-day basis, these two fathers also appeared more circumspect than fathers in the 'nouveau traditional' households about the pleasures of parenthood. As one father noted:

I find spending time with the children less exciting than perhaps I should. . . . I get bored. When they were younger I read to them regularly but almost as soon as I started reading I started to yawn. . . . I don't know what it is really . . . I don't think I particularly enjoy playing with them.

(H/H25)

In this context it is interesting to note that both of these men suggested that whilst they spent social time with the children, these activities tended to be the things they liked doing.

A final prominent theme in the accounts provided by these men was that parenthood was different for women than for men. Highlighting the sense of responsibility he felt was associated with parenthood, the father who worked from home went on to argue that his wife took the responsibility more seriously than he did, perhaps because she was younger than him or because he was brought up to be 'very laid back about life in general'. The other father noted that:

what I actually believe is that despite how liberated in general men seem to become, it is still the woman who goes towards looking after the children. Whether that is biological or what it is . . . no matter how much men become involved in becoming a parent they have to go a heck of a long way to become as totally emotionally. . . as much involved with the children as the mother does.

(H/H25)

Both of the women in these households were employed part-time. However, their experience of employment appeared somewhat different. The mother in the lower-middle-income household, for example, noted that she was working for financial reasons and would ideally prefer not to be employed. However, she was not so much expressing a wish to be a full-time mother as to have more free time for herself:

> I wouldn't be in work at all if I had a chance. I enjoy my work and it keeps me in adult company but in the week I'm happy with my own company. I like being my own boss, it is not to do with me wanting to be with children but not wanting some-body controlling my time.
>
> (H/H25)

In contrast, the woman in the second, upper-middle-income household commented that:

> I love to work, but I don't like to work. . . . I like to be with the children, but I have my own interests so, and I enjoy what I do, so I don't really do it for the money. I do it because without it I'd go crazy. But I know I run my life round them and I do very little that I want to do and I work which is selfish, I suppose, in one way, but they are my first priority, and I wouldn't go out, for instance.
>
> (H/H8)

Both of these women did the bulk of the childcare in the household but both also felt that their husbands did their share. One noted, 'we share everything really', whilst the other commented that she thought she had 'an incredible partner'. Despite this they did recog-nize shortcomings in their partners in particular, and fathers in general. These themes were in fact apparent in women's accounts in many of the households in this sample, not just these two. There were a number of different facets to these comments. It was suggested, for example, that men did not do the technical aspects of childcare as well as they might. For example, there were minor concerns that fathers did not bother to find matching clothes, or to cook proper meals. More significantly, there was some concern that men neglected the social relationship aspects of child-rearing:

> if Pete were bringing them up alone they would never have any-body home for tea. It would never occur to him to socialize the children, they would never go to swimming lessons or things like that. Socializing the children is fairly boring . . . and he wants his life to be uncomplicated. If circumstances changed he would take things on, . . . he wouldn't grumble, but as it is he can currently

afford to take one step back . . . he would do it if it happened but he wouldn't organize it.

(H/H25)

Egalitarians

The men and women in the final five households differed from the two described above in that they reported that they were explicitly pursuing equality between themselves in the way they practised parenting. The employment patterns and income levels in these households were diverse. In one household both parents had full-time professional careers (upper-middle-income); in two the fathers were providing the greater part of the childcare and domestic labour (although one of these men had a part-time evening job in a club), whilst the mothers had full-time employment (one high-income, the other upper-middle-income); in another both parents were unemployed; and in the fifth the father worked full-time and the mother was undertaking a further education course (high-income).

The men in these households all articulated a clear commitment to equality between themselves and their partners in parenting. As a working-class father with a full-time employed professional partner put it:

> at the end of the day most people still think it's a woman's job to bring up the kids and a father stays in the background, maybe for discipline or the odd night of babysitting . . . that's the general view that I get from the lads . . . my own view is it should be 50/50. I think the father should be there to give support all the time . . . generally give kids what they need. I don't think it should be one person's responsibility for everything . . . it puts too much pressure on the other person. At the end of the day you're going to fall out. If you've had the child you should share the responsibility of bringing them up together.

(H/H26)

Although the nature of their involvement varied, men in these households were more involved in all aspects of parenting than those in other households in the sample. In three cases the men were taking much the greater share of childcare and domestic labour at the time of the interviews. Although these arrangements also appear to have arisen for pragmatic reasons, rather than on ideological grounds, without these situations arising, it was reported, parenting would have been shared.

In one household, for example, both the man and woman worked full-time with professional careers. They had a full-time live-out nanny and initially the mother had been the one to get home for the nanny to leave at the end of the day. More recently, however, she had got a new job some distance from home and he hadn't yet found a new post. The mother was therefore staying away some evenings or working long days and he was doing much more of the childcare and domestic labour.

> We had always assumed that Tricia would work and indeed that I would . . . but I think that since she has been in Cookson the division of work is probably fairer . . . we look at our diaries each week and work out who's coming home early. I mean most of the work is in the evening and then at the weekend we work out what's to be done and then decide whether we are going to do it or not.
>
> (H/H1)

Despite their commitment to equality and greater involvement in parenting, and like the men in the pragmatic households, all but one of these men were less than enthusiastic about the routine labour involved in parenting. In one high-income household, for example, the father had lost his job when the second child was born. They had had mixed experiences of nannies with the first child (not his) and the woman's business was beginning to do very well. They therefore decided that he should stay at home to look after the children. At the time of the interview he had been doing this for five years and reported that: 'I am grateful to have had that time, it's certainly been extremely different for me and a nice experience to have lived through, a tough one but nice' (H/H2). Despite this positive comment, however, in many ways this man's account of his experience of being a full-time mother/ housewife was far from positive, strongly echoing women's experience reported in other research. When asked in what sense the experience had been tough, for instance, he replied:

> mental stress, physical stress, complete change of routine, especially for a man. Talking to other men basically it's not a situation that they would, nobody envies, I mean none of my male colleagues envy what I do . . . from having a completely

structured day in an office . . . and dealing with sane logical adults, suddenly having an 18-month-old baby requiring all that attention . . . I found the whole thing very stressful. I just found that everything had suffered, my appearance and how I felt about myself.

(H/H2)

At the time of the interview both children had gone to school full-time and he was considering looking for a part-time job. However, again reflecting the experience of many women, he expressed a lack of confidence in his ability to do this. Commenting that he felt 'somewhat redundant' now, he went on to note that he was 'in many ways, mentally sterile . . . just the boredom, the constant boredom and tedium of doing the same jobs over and over again . . . which nobody appreciated'.

Another man, in an upper-middle-income household, staying at home to care for his 9-year-old son whilst his partner worked full-time, also commented on the difficulties he had experienced when his child was young:

I like to do more things with him now than I did before. Before he went to school full time he was at home more and it got to be a bit of an effort sometimes to keep him occupied. Sometimes all you wanted to do was sit down and relax, rejuvenate, but you had to be all the time with him and you used to think it was never going to end . . . but now it's more enjoyment than hassle.

(H/H26)

In the other high-income household, the father had accepted responsibility for providing and organizing 50 per cent of the childcare, although the woman did not have paid employment. They also attempted to share other aspects of domestic labour more or less equally. In practice, however, the father bought in childcare on a regular basis so that he could fit his parenting responsibilities in with his employment. As he commented:

whether I spend an equal amount of time . . . the answer to that is 'no I don't', although I should do. And the agreement we have between us is that I should. Although we do divide the week up into periods when she is off and so if I can't do it, I get somebody else to look after them, pick them up from school, look after them till, er, six in the evening, that sort of time period.

(H/H11)

In this household they had clearly agreed that they should be equally involved in all aspects of parenting, though both also noted that in the early years, linked to breastfeeding, it is likely that the mother will have a closer relationship with children than the father and both acknowledged that they still hadn't achieved equality.

In the four egalitarian households described so far the women were the most circumspect about motherhood of all of the women in this sample. This is not to say that they did not value motherhood or report considerable pleasure and satisfaction from their children. They did. However, their accounts also testify to the guilt women could feel over their decision to combine motherhood and paid employment and over the loss they could feel regarding time for themselves:

> for me being a mother is about never being able to finish a conversation, having to sit on the edge of the bath whilst he has a poo to discuss the meaning of life and what happens when people die. A total change in my lifestyle. Thirty-eight years without anybody depending on me to be there . . . and now a total change in time, space, freedom. . . . I now have little time for me, my friends.
>
> (H/H26)

In some respects these women presented themselves as different from other women. One mother, for example, noted that she was

> not a natural mother. I can't give myself totally to the kids. They get as much time at the weekend as other children do during the week and we hardly ever go out. There is the stereotype of people who put children first in front of everything else but I'm not like that. . . . I get irritated if I try to do that.
>
> (H/H1)

Another woman described her decision to work full-time as the 'natural' thing to do, but went on to note that she was:

> in a position to do what I want . . . it's not the same for other people. . . . I have been very lucky in being financially secure, mobile, articulate, middle class, know what I am entitled to.
>
> (H/H26)

Only in one of these five households was parenting presented as a completely unproblematic experience for the man (and indeed for the woman). Both parents were previously in unskilled employment but had been unemployed for a long period, although they earned a little extra money from a cleaning job that they did together. Their accounts of how they organized the domestic labour, including childcare, were more or less identical and idealistic. They reported doing most work together, having generally good relationships with their two teenage children who, in the main, did things they were asked to do (though there did appear to be some tensions around cooking, cleaning and tidying up). They organized regular family conferences during which major decisions about household expenditure were taken on a democratic basis. Parenthood for this couple was a source of considerable pleasure and pride in a world which was denying them material comfort and in which other ways of obtaining satisfaction were severely restricted. If they were concerned or ambivalent about aspects of their experience of parenting, they clearly did not wish to share these with the researcher.

The ultimate responsibility

Although the women in the 'egalitarian' households recognized that their partners were more involved than most men, like some other women in this study, they were also guarded in their praise of the men in their lives and/or of men in general. Across the sample, there were men and women who spoke of important ways in which men's involvement in parenting – even when at home all day caring for children – was more circumscribed than that of women. In one of the 'role reversal' households, for instance, the woman did all the cooking when she got home, and in all sixteen households, regardless of the division of day-to-day childcare, the women had ultimate responsibility for long-term planning, for organizing their children's social time, and if they were in employment they 'made up' for lack of time spent with children during the week at the weekend. This compensation strategy was not so apparent in the households where men worked full-time and women cared full-time for children.

In some senses, even when men had the major caring responsibilities these were described rather like a job specification – involving specified times for work to start and end and clearly defined tasks to be performed. Women's sense of responsibility, in contrast, transcended the physical time they spent with children. One woman pointed, for example, to her partner's more relaxed attitude towards discipline and behavioural problems, commenting that this sometimes made her feel that she shouldered more responsibility for 'getting this right'. Another felt that, whilst her life had changed completely since the birth of her son, that of her partner, who was at home full-time caring for him, probably hadn't changed as much. Commenting in general on the notion of 'new fathers', she added:

> I think what new fathers do is choose the nicer elements to get involved with and it's still women who have responsibility. . . . They may share care but women still do the worrying, planning, anxiety about whether what they are doing is right, is the child going to turn out right, what's going to happen in 6 months' time. . . . Jack is very supportive but he doesn't do the worrying. I don't think he does the worrying . . . that to me would be the new man . . . they have so much further to go.
>
> (H/H26)

CONCLUSIONS

Despite some caveats – for example, the small size of the sample involved and the relative lack of cultural diversity amongst the respondents' 'voices' – this research does highlight a number of important issues around the meanings fatherhood and motherhood have for men and women in contemporary Britain.

In the context of the earlier literature review, the diversity in the accounts of the experience of fathering, mothering and parenting and in the patterns of childcare and domestic labour described in these sixteen households is important. The relationship between income group and occupational social group within these households has not been explicitly explored in the analysis. Predictably, the achieved social class and social class of origin of these men and women provided a complicated picture. However, in general, there was a close relationship between the achieved social class of the men and women involved and the income of the household, with one or two notable exceptions. For example, in one of the upper-middle-income households in which the mother was employed full-time and the father was doing day-to-day childcare, the mother was a professional and the father was unskilled working-class. The study findings suggest that working-class men are not necessarily 'imprisoned' by outdated ideas of masculinity, but neither are all middle-class men seeking new experiences in the realm of fatherhood. Additionally, there is an indication from these data that men do feel that they are under pressure to be more involved in family life than they were in earlier marriages and/or than their fathers were, as Lewis and O'Brien (1987a) have argued. However, whilst a concept of more involved and nurturing fatherhood is apparent in the subjective accounts of some men, the extent to which this is working through into individual practice remains to be explored more closely.

Women's ambivalence about the experience of mothering is also important. Such ambivalence appears to be equally evident in the accounts of women who, at the same time, espouse a strong moral and personal commitment to full-time motherhood as it is among women who have chosen to combine motherhood with paid employment. The need to draw on metaphors from the world of paid work to justify full-time involvement in motherhood points up this ambivalence.

One of the most consistent findings from existing research is that whatever the employment status of parents, women retain ultimate responsibility for childcare and for emotional labour (Russell and Radin, 1983; Lamb, 1986; Backett, 1987; Barnett and Baruch, 1988; Delphy and Leonard, 1992; Duncombe and Marsden, 1993; Warde and Hetherington, 1993; O'Brien and Jones, 1995; Holland et al., 1996). The study reported on here supports this finding. Even where the men in the study households were shouldering a considerable proportion of the physical labour of parenting and housework, the women still felt themselves to have full-time responsibility for children's welfare in a way not evident in the men's accounts. And the men in general concurred with these views. The complex ways in which this division of responsibility is 'negotiated' between women and men and the factors that shape these negotiations is arguably one of the most important questions remaining to be addressed by research in the field of parenting.

Men's accounts of parental 'responsibility' appear to be more 'bounded' than women's accounts, particularly in relation to the moral, social and emotional responsibilities involved. Women carry the 'worry' and 'manage' the enterprise of parenting, albeit, as Delphy and Leonard (1992) argue, from a position of oppression. But the nature of this oppression may differ in important ways. It is unlikely, for example, that it will be the same across social groups. Many of the women in the higher-income households in this study had unearned income of their own, at times very substantial. The key role of ideology in binding these women into motherhood would therefore appear to be critical. For other women, where financial independence is contingent upon paid employment, or where money is in desperately short supply, the situation is perhaps more complex. Cultural diversity can also be expected.

For many women, however, there was a sense in which they did not 'trust' their partners to do a good enough job of parenting – and their partners often agreed with this assessment, noting that the women were justified in these concerns. Women's expressed attitudes in this regard have been argued to be a device to ensure that they retained power over the domestic realm (Backett, 1987; Russell, 1987; Burman, 1994; Lewis, 1995). However, it might also be conceptualized as a strategy adopted to 'protect' the well-being of their children in the context of men's relative and perhaps learned incompetence.

As noted at the beginning of this chapter, much has been written about the changing nature of men's involvement in the domestic world. Segal (1990) has commented on the dangers of reasserting the importance of fatherhood in the context of male dominance. At the same time, however, she argues for the importance of men's involvement in childcare and nurturing 'as a crucial factor . . . in the forging of "masculinity" into something less coercive and oppressive to women' (1990: 57). (See also the discussion in Silverstein, 1996.) In this context, Burman (1994: 97–8) suggests there is a need for new theoretical and methodological paradigms to theorize the growing visibility of men as fathers. To date in fatherhood research theorizing about the interrelationship between the 'private' world of the family and the 'public' world outside has been limited. Women's ambivalence concerning the active participation of fathers in childcare and their own involvement in mothering reminds us that these worlds cannot be separated. Neither has there been any consistent attempt to theorize adequately the difficult relationship between agency and structure – the ways in which mothers and fathers negotiate and shape their experience of parenting within wider structures of power and control in society. However, a number of studies have attempted to locate their analyses in wider theoretical perspectives (Backett, 1987; Delphy and Leonard, 1992; White, 1994).

The study described here supports the notion that motherhood is mandated and fatherhood discretionary (Lutwin and Siperstein, 1985; Parke, 1988: x; Daly, 1993): that men 'opt in' and women have to 'opt out' of childcare. As Daniels and Weingarten (1988) argue, for many men fatherhood provides moments of pleasure bracketing tedious work days. Men are basically enabled by their hierarchical position in the family and in the outside world to make choices concerning their involvement which influence the lives of the rest of their families, thereby by and large maintaining 'their privileged positions' (Delphy and Leonard, 1992: 190–2; see also Backett, 1987; Holland *et al.*, 1996.) As one of the respondents succinctly puts it, he is 'just a bloke that's had kids' who can, to a large extent, control his experience of fatherhood. For the women involved in this study, the transition to motherhood was a more profound and transformative experience for which the social 'script' was more tightly written, leaving little room for interpretation.

NOTES

1 Role theory, and the concept of the 'sex role', is extensively applied in the fatherhood literature. The term 'role' has been reproduced in this chapter as appropriate. Role theory and terminology is, however, now the subject of some debate, with critiques developed by, for example, Connell (1995).
2 This research was conducted by Jennie Popay whilst at the Thomas Coram Research Centre at the Institute of London as part of an ESRC funded Centre programme.

REFERENCES

Allen, W.D. and Doherty, W.J. (1996) 'The responsibilities of fatherhood as perceived by African-American teenage fathers', *Families in Society: The Journal of Contemporary Human Services*, 77(3): 142–55.
Atkinson, M.P. and Blackwelder, S.P. (1993) 'Fathering in the 20th century', *Journal of Marriage and the Family*, 55(4): 975–86.
Backett, K. (1987) 'The negotiation of fatherhood', in C. Lewis and M. O'Brien (eds) *Reassessing Fatherhood*, London: Sage, pp. 74–90.
Barnett, R.C. and Baruch, G.K. (1988) 'Correlates of fathers' participation in family work', in P. Bronstein and C.P. Cowan (eds) *Fatherhood Today*, New York: Wiley, pp. 66–78.
Bertoia, C. and Drakich, J. (1993) 'The fathers rights movement – contradictions in rhetoric and practice', *Journal of Family Issues*, 14(4): 592–615; rptd in W. Marsiglio (ed.) (1995) *Fatherhood*, Thousand Oaks, CA: Sage, pp. 230–54.

Blaisure, K.R. and Allen, K.R. (1995) 'Feminists and the ideology and practice of marital equality', *Journal of Marriage and the Family*, 57(Feb.): 5–19.

Bowen, G.L. and Orthner, D.K. (1991) 'Effects of organizational culture on fatherhood', in F.W. Bozett and S.M.H. Hanson (eds) *Fatherhood and Families in Cultural Context*, New York: Springer, pp. 187–217.

Bozett, F.W. and Hanson, S.M.H. (1991a) 'Cultural change and the future of fatherhood and families', in F.W. Bozett and S.M.H. Hanson (eds) *Fatherhood and Families in Cultural Context*, New York: Springer, pp. 263–74.

—— (eds) (1991b) *Fatherhood and Families in Cultural Context*, New York: Springer.

Bradley, R.H. (1985) 'Fathers and the school-age child', in S.M.H. Hanson and F.W. Bozett (eds) *Dimensions of Fatherhood*, Beverly Hills, CA: Sage, pp. 141–69.

Brannen, J. and Moss, P. (1987) 'Fathers in dual-earner households – through mothers' eyes', in C. Lewis and M. O'Brien (eds) *Reassessing Fatherhood*, London: Sage, pp. 126–43.

Brayfield, A. (1995) 'Juggling jobs and kids: the impact of employment schedules on fathers' caring for children', *Journal of Marriage and the Family*, 57(May): 321–32.

Bronstein, P. (1988) 'Marital and parenting roles in transition: an overview', in P. Bronstein and C.P. Cowan (eds) *Fatherhood Today*, New York: Wiley, pp. 3–10.

Bronstein, P. and Cowan, C.P. (eds) (1988) *Fatherhood Today: Men's Changing Role in the Family*, New York: Wiley.

Burgess, A. and Ruxton, S. (1996) *Men and their Children: Proposals for Public Policy*, London: Institute for Public Policy Research.

Burman, E. (1994) *Deconstructing Developmental Psychology*, London: Routledge.

Carlsen, S. (1995) 'When working men become fathers', in P. Moss (ed.) *Father Figures*, Edinburgh: HMSO, pp. 53–61.

Connell, R.W. (1995) *Masculinities*, Cambridge: Polity Press.

Connor, M.E. (1986) 'Some parenting attitudes of young black fathers', in R.A. Lewis and R.E. Salt (eds) *Men in Families*, Beverly Hills, CA: Sage, pp. 159–68.

Daly, K.J. (1993) 'Reshaping fatherhood: finding the models', *Journal of Family Issues*, 14(4): 510–30; rptd in W. Marsiglio (ed.) (1995) *Fatherhood*, Thousand Oaks, CA: Sage, pp. 21–40.

Daniels, P. and Weingarten, K. (1988) 'The fatherhood click: the timing of parenthood in men's lives', in P. Bronstein and C.P. Cowan (eds) *Fatherhood Today*, New York: Wiley, pp. 36–52.

Delphy, C. and Leonard, D. (1992) *Familiar Exploitation: A New Analysis of Marriage in Contemporary Western Societies*, Cambridge: Polity Press.

Dennis, N. and Erdos, G. (1992) *Families without Fatherhood*, London: Institute of Economic Affairs, Health & Welfare Unit.

Duncombe, J. and Marsden, D. (1993) 'Love and intimacy – the gender division of emotion and emotion work', *Sociology: The Journal of the British Sociological Association*, 27(2): 221–41.

Furstenberg, F.F. (1988) 'Good dads – bad dads: two faces of fatherhood', in A.J. Cherlin (ed.) *The Changing American Family and Public Policy*, Washington DC: Urban Institute Press, pp. 193–218.

—— (1995) 'Fathering in the inner city: paternal participation and public policy', in W. Marsiglio (ed.) *Fatherhood*, Thousand Oaks, CA: Sage, pp. 119–47.

Griswold, R.L. (1993) *Fatherhood in America: A History*, New York: Basic Books.

Haas, L. and Hwang, P. (1995) 'Company culture and men's usage of family leave benefits in Sweden', *Family Relations*, 44(1): 28–36.

Hall, W.A. (1994) 'New fatherhood: myths and realities', *Public Health Nursing*, 11(4): 219–28.

Hanson, S.M.H. (1986) 'Parent–child relationships in single-father families', in R.A. Lewis and R.E. Salt (eds) *Men in Families*, Beverly Hills, CA: Sage, pp. 181–95.

Hanson, S.M.H. and Bozett, F.W. (eds) (1985) *Dimensions of Fatherhood*, Beverly Hills, CA: Sage.

Holland, J., Mauthner, M. and Sharpe, S. (1996) *Family Matters: Communicating Health Messages in the Family*, London: Health Education Authority (Family Health Research Reports).

Horna, J. and Lupri, E. (1987) 'Fathers' participation in work, family life and leisure: a Canadian experience', in C. Lewis and M. O'Brien (eds) *Reassessing Fatherhood*, London: Sage, pp. 54–73.

Ishii-Kuntz, M. (1994) 'Paternal involvement and perception toward fathers' roles: a comparison between Japan and the United States', *Journal of Family Issues*, 15(1): 30–48; rptd in W. Marsiglio (ed.) (1995) *Fatherhood*, Thousand Oaks, CA: Sage, pp. 102–18.

Jump, T.L. and Haas, L. (1987) 'Fathers in transition: dual-career fathers participating in child care', in M.S. Kimmel (ed.) *Changing Men*, Newbury Park, CA: Sage, pp. 98–114.

Kimmel, M.S. (1987a) 'Rethinking "masculinity": new directions in research', in M.S. Kimmel (ed.) *Changing Men*, Newbury Park, CA: Sage, pp. 9–24.

—— (ed.) (1987b) *Changing Men: New Directions in Research on Men and Masculinity*, Newbury Park, CA: Sage.

Lamb, M.E. (1986) 'The changing roles of fathers', in M.E. Lamb (ed.) *The Father's Role: Applied Perspectives*, New York: Wiley, pp. 3–27.

—— (1987) 'The emergent American father', in M.E. Lamb (ed.) *The Father's Role: Cross-Cultural Perspectives*, Hillsdale, NJ: Lawrence Erlbaum, pp. 3–25.

—— (1994) 'Paternal influences on child development', Paper presented at the Conference on Changing Fatherhood, University of Tilburg, Netherlands (May); cited in W. Marsiglio (ed.) (1995) *Fatherhood*, Thousand Oaks, CA: Sage.

Lamb, M.E., Pleck, J.H. and Levine, J.A. (1987) 'Effects of increased paternal involvement on fathers and mothers', in C. Lewis and M. O'Brien (eds) *Reassessing Fatherhood*, London: Sage, pp. 109–25.

LaRossa, R. and Reitzes, D.C. (1995) 'Gendered perceptions of father involvement in early 20th century America', *Journal of Marriage and the Family*, 57(1): 223–9.

Lewis, C. (1995) 'In conclusion: what opportunities are open to fathers?' in P. Moss (ed.) *Father Figures*, Edinburgh: HMSO, pp. 63–9.

Lewis, C. and O'Brien, M. (1987a) 'Constraints on fathers: research, theory and clinical practice', in C. Lewis and M. O'Brien (eds) *Reassessing Fatherhood*, London: Sage, pp. 1–19.

—— (eds) (1987b) *Reassessing Fatherhood: New Observations on Fathers and the Modern Family*, London: Sage.

Lewis, R.A. (1986) 'Introduction: what men get out of marriage and parenthood', in R.A. Lewis and R.E. Salt (eds) *Men in Families*, Beverly Hills, CA: Sage, pp. 11–25.

Lewis, R.A. and Salt, R.E. (eds) (1986) *Men in Families*, Beverly Hills, CA: Sage.

Lloyd, T. (1995) 'Fathers in the media: an analysis of newspaper coverage of fathers', in P. Moss (ed.) *Father Figures*, Edinburgh: HMSO, pp. 41–51.

Lutwin, D.R. and Siperstein, G.N. (1985) 'Househusband fathers', in S.M.H. Hanson and F.W. Bozett (eds) *Dimensions of Fatherhood*, Beverly Hills, CA: Sage, pp. 269–87.

McAdoo, J.L. (1988) 'Changing perspectives on the role of the black father', in P. Bronstein and C.P. Cowan (eds) *Fatherhood Today*, New York: Wiley, pp. 79–92.

McKee, L. (1982) 'Fathers' participation in infant care: a critique', in L. McKee and M. O'Brien (eds) *The Father Figure*, London: Tavistock, pp. 120–38.

Marsiglio, W. (1995a) 'Fatherhood scholarship: an overview and agenda for the future', in W. Marsiglio (ed.) *Fatherhood*, Thousand Oaks, CA: Sage, pp. 1–20; revised version of 'Contemporary scholarship on fatherhood: culture, identity, and conduct', *Journal of Family Issues* (1993) 14(4): 484–509.

—— (1995b) 'Fathers' diverse life course patterns and roles: theory and social interventions', in W. Marsiglio (ed.) *Fatherhood*, Thousand Oaks, CA: Sage, pp. 78–101.

—— (ed.) (1995c) *Fatherhood: Contemporary Theory, Research, and Social Policy*, Thousand Oaks, CA: Sage.

Mirandé, A. (1991) 'Ethnicity and fatherhood', in F.W. Bozett and S.M.H. Hanson (eds) *Fatherhood and Families in Cultural Context*, New York: Springer, pp. 53–82.

Moss, P. (1995a) Introduction to P. Moss (ed.) *Father Figures*, Edinburgh: HMSO, pp. xi–xxiv.

—— (ed.) (1995b) *Father Figures: Fathers in the Families of the 1990s*, Edinburgh: HMSO.

O'Brien, M. and Jones, D. (1995) 'Young people's attitudes to fatherhood', in P. Moss (ed.) *Father Figures*, Edinburgh: HMSO, pp. 27–39.

Parke, R.D. (1988) Foreword to P. Bronstein and C.P. Cowan (eds) *Fatherhood Today*, New York: Wiley, pp. ix–xii.

Phillips, A. (1995) 'The trouble with boys', in P. Moss (ed.) *Father Figures*, Edinburgh: HMSO, pp. 9–15.

Popay, J. (1991) 'My health is alright, I'm just tired all the time: women's experience of ill health', in H. Roberts (ed.) *Women's Health Matters*, London: Routledge, pp. 99–120.

Russell, G. (1987) 'Problems in role-reversed families', in C. Lewis and M. O'Brien (eds) *Reassessing Fatherhood*, London: Sage, pp. 161–79.

Russell, G. and Radin, N. (1983) 'Increased paternal participation: the fathers' perspective', in M.E. Lamb and A. Sagi (eds) *Fatherhood and Family Policy*, Hillsdale, NJ: Lawrence Erlbaum, pp. 139–65.

Samuels, A. (1995) 'The good-enough father of whatever sex', *Feminism & Psychology*, 5(4): 511–30.

Sandqvist, K. (1987) 'Swedish family policy and the attempt to change paternal roles', in C. Lewis and M. O'Brien (eds) *Reassessing Fatherhood*, London: Sage, pp. 144–60.

Segal, L. (1990) *Slow Motion: Changing Masculinities, Changing Men*, London: Virago.

Silverstein, L.B. (1996) 'Fathering is a feminist issue', *Psychology of Women Quarterly*, 20(1): 3–37.

Stearns, P.N. (1991) 'Fatherhood in historical perspective: the role of social change', in F.W. Bozett and S.M.H. Hanson (eds) *Fatherhood and Families in Cultural Context*, New York: Springer, pp. 28–52.

Warde, A. and Hetherington, K. (1993) 'A changing domestic division of labour? Issues of measurement and interpretation', *Work, Employment & Society*, 7(1): 23–45.

White, N.R. (1994) 'About fathers: masculinity and the social construction of fatherhood', *Australian and New Zealand Journal of Sociology*, 30(2): 119–31.

Chapter 9

'All jumbled up'
Employed women with unemployed husbands

*David Waddington, Chas Critcher and
Bella Dicks*

The troubled relationship between men and welfare examined in
this chapter is that stemming from male unemployment, on which
there is now a substantial body of literature. Using mainly quantitative studies, this research originally concentrated on measuring
men's experience of stress, classifying their coping strategies and
identifying sources of social support. However, there has been a
slow realization that male unemployment neither exists, nor can
be understood, as simply a problem for the man.

> Much of the psychological research on dislocated workers treats
> unemployment as a stressful event in the life of an individual. It
> is clear from the research we have conducted that unemployment
> affects not only individuals who lose their jobs but their spouses
> and families as well.
>
> (Liem and Liem, 1990: 200)

Despite this exhortation, it has remained true that little systematic
research has been done to assess the ways in which families are
affected by the unemployment of one of their members (Jackson
and Walsh, 1987: 194).

Redressing this imbalance has required more qualitative emphasis on how those affected interpret and describe their experiences.
Our approach is thus similar in its brief to a study of unemployed
men and their families in Kidderminster in the early 1980s:

> What then are the implications for families when the men's
> attachment to the labour market is broken? Does the loss of
> the economic provider role result in changes to the domestic
> division of labour? Are men freed to become more participative
> fathers and more active homemakers? How are the lives of

women and children affected by male unemployment? What is
the relationship between economic provision and power and
authority within the households? Does increased unemployment
herald a breakdown in patriarchal structures and enhance wives
spheres of authority?

(McKee and Bell, 1985: 388)

In keeping with other contributions to this volume, we are interested in how male troubles come to define the nature of the relationships between men and women. Our work on mining communities
(Waddington, Wykes and Critcher, 1991) has always insisted that
women's perspectives are as important and valid as men's. In this
chapter, we want to develop this concern by looking at interviews
with three couples where male unemployment had four quite
specific features. First, the man's unemployment had come about
as part of British Coal's extensive voluntary redundancy programme in the late 1980s. Second, these men had volunteered for
redundancy because they had serious health problems. Third,
these men were all at a particular stage in the life cycle: in their
mid to late forties with both dependent and independent children.
Fourth, and crucial for our interest in gender issues, in each case
the wife had a job, so that potentially they had taken over as the
principal wage earner.

Our interest is in exploring how these men and their wives, individually and together, work through the consequences of their
situation, especially the challenge posed to conventional gender
roles and identities. We will do this by looking in detail at the
accounts of three couples following the man's voluntary redundancy from the coal industry. In the next section, however, we
first place these case studies in the context of the wider literature.

NINE THESES ABOUT COPING WITH UNEMPLOYMENT

The literature on the factors shaping the social and psychological
impact of male unemployment is vast. We do not propose to summarize it here. Instead we have extracted from it nine theses which
can inform the analysis of our three case studies.

*1 Unemployment causes severe psychological harm to men, especially
in the long term.*

Warr (1985) has identified such harm in terms of reductions in: income; activity outside the home; goal-related activities in relation to others; scope for decision-making; the use and development of skills; the quality of social interaction; and prestige and social acceptability. There are increases in psychologically threatening activities, insecurity and uncertainty about the future. Warr suggests that severe symptoms of psychological ill health are observable in between 20 and 30 per cent of long-term unemployed men.

2 *There are identifiable variations in strategies for coping with unemployment.*

Considering why individuals vary in their capacity to cope with unemployment, Warr and Jackson (1987) distinguish between two basic kinds of adaptation. Resigned adaptation, they suggest, involves a process of psychological adjustment, where expectations of life are reduced to a level compatible with the status of unemployment. Constructive adaptation, in contrast, is argued to involve active attempts by the individual to cope with or offset the effects of unemployment, including the development of structured, purposive or meaningful activities, such as developing a political or leisure interest which acts as a substitute for paid labour.

Such findings appear to apply to unemployment in mining communities. Wass (1989, 1991) studied miners made redundant from Markham colliery in South Wales in 1985. She contrasted those who viewed redundancy as a form of early retirement, accepting closure as inevitable, using redundancy money to pay off mortgages and trying to remain active, with those suffering from ill health, unable or unwilling to find a substitute for work and depressed by continual rejection by employers.

3 *In occupational communities, unemployment poses a threat to the social identity of the male.*

Research suggests that in some sectors unemployment is not just the loss of paid work; it is a loss of the occupational status which underpins the local community. Joelson and Wahlquist's study of former Swedish shipyard workers emphasized how losing an occupational role in such a context can also mean the destruction of social identity. The unemployed found it difficult to meet their old friends, because one of the main things they had in common was lost (1987: 181). Similar conclusions have been reached in a series of studies of bankrupt farmers in America's Midwest (Farmer, 1986; Van Hooke, 1990; Wright and Rosenblatt, 1987).

4 Men's involvement in domestic labour following unemployment increases only marginally.

The immediate impact of male unemployment on a wife is that her husband is permanently around the house and not apparently contributing much. Evidence suggests that, following unemployment, male participation in domestic chores increases only marginally across a narrow range of possible activities (Binns and Mars, 1984; Laite and Halfpenny, 1987; McKee and Bell, 1985, 1986; Morris, 1988, 1992). The general tendency seems to be that unemployment fails to disturb established beliefs about which spouse should assume the responsibility for performing bread-winning, household maintenance or childcare activities (Liem and Liem, 1988: 99).

5 Unemployed men are hostile to their wives working if it means they are no longer the main source of income.

In a study of long-term unemployment on a Glasgow housing estate, Binns and Mars (1984) discovered that attempts by women to find paid employment outside the home were resisted by husbands, because they saw the woman adopting the role of principal income earner as a threat to their male identity.

6 Women's psychological reaction to their husband's loss of job is conditioned by his psychological reaction.

Quantitative studies have demonstrated that the level of male stress as a result of unemployment is the best predictor of the level of stress experienced by the wife. A study of the mental health of wives of redundant steel workers in Pennsylvania concluded that:

> Perhaps our most intriguing finding is that the effects of unemployment appear to be primarily indirect, or mediated by the distress of the person actually experiencing job loss; the husband's level of psychological stress better predicted his wife's symptoms than did his employment status *per se*.
>
> (Dew *et al.*, 1987: 181)

7 Having a job is generally likely to increase women's capacity to cope with an unemployed husband.

This proposition is derived from the literature on the effect of paid employment on women's well-being rather than from specific literature on unemployment. The general consensus (Nathanson, 1975; Brown and Harris, 1978) that paid employment improves women's psychological health has recently been qualified by identification of the conditions on which this depends, such as adequate childcare (Ross and Mirowsky, 1988) or the absence of other stressful life events (Parry, 1986). Focusing specifically on the role of paid work, Lennon and Rosenfeld support the argument that positive conditions in one sphere of life may compensate for negative conditions in another (1992: 324). In a review of findings about women, paid work and stress, Baruch et al. (1987) stressed the importance of the quality of the job and the practical support of husbands with housework. They concluded that having some degree of autonomy and control in both paid work and domestic labour was the most important factor in consolidating the beneficial effects of a job on women's mental health.

8 *Women's capacity to cope is enhanced by support from close relatives.*

The Pennsylvania study stressed support from close relatives as much more salient than that from friends or even spouses. Women most often cited mothers, fathers, sisters, sisters-in-law as relatives with whom they had most contact and to whom they felt closest (Penkower et al., 1988: 98).

9 *Families tend to maintain their existing division of labour and organization rather than undergo radical change.*

In considering family adaptations to unemployment, Jackson and Walsh (1987) demonstrate that accommodation responses, which involve substantial changes in the way the family is organized, are much less common than assimilation responses, which do not.

THE CASE STUDIES

The case studies to be presented here were collected during a research project on the social psychological impact of the contraction of the British deep-coal mining industry (Critcher et al., 1992; Dicks et al., 1993; Waddington et al., 1994). It was part of the Management of Personal Welfare Research Programme jointly funded by the ESRC and the Rowntree Foundation. During

1992, we used a combination of structured questionnaire survey and in-depth semi-structured interviews to study the impact of mining contraction on four South Yorkshire communities. We asked questions about their working, social and family lives and used objective and subjective measures of their psychological well-being. From the 400-strong survey sample we selected thirty ex-miners and thirty wives of ex-miners for follow-up interviews. These were mainly unrelated, but we chose to interview six married couples, in three of which the husband had taken voluntary redundancy. We focus on these three couples here. The husband was interviewed by a male researcher (David Waddington) and the wife by a female researcher (Bella Dicks). The interviews were conducted simultaneously in different rooms of the couple's house.

In the accounts which follow, we have organized excerpts and commentaries from the interview transcripts around four clusters: the husband's attitude towards redundancy and subsequent unemployment, including his state of health; attitudes towards the wife's job and the necessary adjustments, especially around domestic labour; the effects on their relationship, in the contexts of the wider family and sources of support; and finally the extent to which each of the partners perceived themselves as stressed and their strategies for coping. Our particular focus remains that of the women's experience, though, as we shall see, this was heavily structured by circumstances beyond their control.

Case study 1: Mr and Mrs Dear

Mr and Mrs Dear were in their late forties with two grown-up daughters, one married and one living at home, and a teenage son, also living at home.

Redundancy, health and unemployment

Both Mr and Mrs Dear regarded the pit closure programme as unavoidable, even desirable. As Mr Dear put it:

> It's just something that was going to come anyway. It's something that's happening all over the world. . . . I think the men used their head. I think they gave a fair amount of redundancy. Even the union men that were against it, most of them took it.

A number of worsening medical complaints (including back and elbow injuries and hypertension) had encouraged Mr Dear to take redundancy.

> The management I'd known till then had practically gone so, if I'd have got to the stage where I'd wanted a light job, I don't know if they'd have given me one, so I thought it best to finish. With the running about they're having to do now, I don't think I could have carried on.

Clearly in no desperate hurry to find a new job, Mr Dear occupied most of his time developing the building and concreting skills which had once been just a hobby. He was on the verge of starting his own business making coping stones. 'I've been buying a few moulds, just gradually building up different things and now I've got enough to have a little go. . . . Sometimes I don't have enough hours in the day for what I'd like to do.' Mrs Dear was pleased with her husband's venture.

> When he first finished – the first year – he seemed as if he didn't know what to do with himself but now he's much better. I hope the business takes off because it's something he likes to do and that would bring money in.

Women's employment and domestic labour

For Mrs Dear, going out to work as an assistant cook in a school canteen was a source of immense satisfaction:

> I enjoy the work. I especially like the cooking part. You get a lot of satisfaction when things come out well, especially if they look nice. At the moment I've been moving round and doing cook-in-charge jobs at different schools and meeting the girls there. I was a bit apprehensive at first and I couldn't sleep for the thought of going but after the first day it was all right and I've enjoyed it since.

Mr Dear recognized the value of his wife's work, both to herself and the wider family. It clearly mattered to him, however, that her wage had not yet become the family's primary source of income:

> She works damned hard from going out to coming home. She's the type who's always on the go. It's very important to her, she

really enjoys her work. I don't think she'd like to pack it in.
Moneywise helps a lot. You're not on top of each other all the
time and I think we need to be apart for so much of the day.
What she pays out now and what she used to do before I finished
work has never changed. She keeps her money; I pay exactly the
same as I used to before I finished.

At Mrs Dear's insistence, Mr Dear was virtually exempt from
housework:

He only doesn't do it because I get bored very easily when I get
home. And if I sit about, I tend to put a lot of weight on as well
and that doesn't help me. He used to clean up every day for me
and then I said to him, 'That's it: when I get home from work, I
want to start doing my own work', and that's how it got. If I'm
not in the house, I'm in the garden and if I'm not here, I'm over
at my daughter's doing something for her: either the windows or
a bit of ironing. If I ever had to sit still, it would come rather
hard. . . . Sometimes I get a bit tired but not really often. I've
always done it and that's the way I choose to look at it.

Marital and family relationships

Mr and Mrs Dear enjoyed a marriage in which they had come to a
mutual understanding about their relationship, so that open conflict
was unusual. Generally, they supported and were supported by
their immediate family. They always had some concern over their
older married daughter, who had suffered from birth from elephan-
tiasis, but they were consoled by the fact that she lived nearby, had
given birth to healthy children and had a caring and supportive husband. The only other source of recent stress had occurred two years
previously. Their younger daughter developed bulimia whilst at
university, after the two parents, Mr Dear especially, had openly
disapproved of her much older boyfriend. A year of tension
appeared to have been resolved by psychiatric counselling for the
daughter and a more tolerant attitude by the parents.

Stress and coping

Mr Dear recognized that he was healthier than when he had been at
the pit:

I think I've got less stress now than when I was working because you used to get tired at the pit. I've adapted to the pit top life now and I think I'm a lot better than I was. I worry about my daughter because she's disabled and you wonder what will happen to her when she gets older because she's only young now and she's already had a lot of bad times.

Mrs Dear associated occasional stress with changes at work; otherwise, there was the odd conflict over children:

Sometimes, when I move schools, then I get a bit worked up. If everybody's not getting on together and there's an atmosphere, that doesn't help. It's very rare Ken and me row and if we do it's usually over the kids.

Summary

Mr Dear had eagerly accepted the offer of redundancy, seeing it as an opportunity to escape an industry where his health made it increasingly difficult to survive. His medical conditions enabled him to rationalize his lack of employment. He had adapted by developing a consuming interest with the potential to earn money. He did not resent his wife working, though emphasized his continuing contribution to household finances. Mrs Dear enjoyed the advantage of a job which provided a lot of intrinsic satisfaction. An active woman, liable to become overweight, she refused to let her husband engage in housework. She welcomed the opportunity to help her disabled daughter with domestic chores. Mrs Dear was not unaffected by stress but she worried about her daughters or her work rather than her husband's unemployment. Had her husband's attitude to his unemployment or hers to her job been negative, their conjunction with family crises might have induced more stress than had actually been the case.

Case study 2: Mr and Mrs Kevans

Mr and Mrs Kevans were in their late forties with three grown-up, married daughters and a primary school age son.

Redundancy, health and unemployment

Mr Kevans had left the mining industry because he was 'sick and tired of management's attitude'. Though the decision to leave was technically his, he felt that, like many others, he was being deliberately pressured into leaving:

> Before the strike there were more happy lads down there; but after the strike you weren't doing your own job; you were getting mucked about all over the pit, doing every job but your own. The money was down, you couldn't earn any bonus and they said they wanted to get that heading going to get new faces to get the pit viable – and yet we were never working on it. It's all political: they just don't want our coal; they don't want our pits. They were just pushing us out anyway – with their attitude. They forced the men out, I don't care what anybody says.

Despite his resentment at what had happened in the industry, he was not unhappy to leave because he had been having health problems, as his wife explained. 'He was having trouble working in the end anyway because he'd got this injured neck. Knowing that he wasn't too good through the accident when it was time to finish made me feel better about the situation.' Though he would have preferred to have a job, his poor health restricted his prospects.

Women's employment and domestic labour

Like Mrs Dear, Mrs Kevans was employed part-time as a cook, working literally across the road in a social services day-care centre for the mentally impaired. She appreciated the responsibility of performing a socially useful role.

> The kitchen is the heart of the building. It's hard work, it's like an eight-hour job in four, so you haven't got a lot of time, but I enjoy my job and I've nobody telling me what to do. Here, you're the boss on the kitchen and it's up to you what people get. It's my domain, sort of thing. For most of the people there, that is their only meal of the day, so it's the satisfaction that they've had a good meal once they're there. You get some and you've never seen people eat like it! You do get attached to some of them.

Mrs Kevans was slightly discomfited by the fact that she worked while her husband could not:

> I like my job, so even if he was working I would still be working but I don't like the idea sometimes of me working and him not. It's a reversed role to what you're brought up to do. I think at first it was too much of a reversed role because I was used to coming home from work at two o'clock and cleaning up and doing what other jobs I had to do and now he's already done them. I know it sounds ungrateful but it just knocked me out of my routine altogether.

Mr Kevans made himself useful by looking after his infant granddaughter while his daughter worked part-time, and his own son after school. He saw none of this as any kind of challenge to his masculinity:

> It fits in nice with both of us, there are no disadvantages. There's the advantage of her bringing in a bit more money. We share the house together – well, I do what I can. I do the washing for her, I do the ironing, the sink's always clean. I can't do much heavy work in the garden but I'll cut the grass and that. I don't see why she should do it, when we're man and wife. You're a team and that's that. I've no qualms about doing women's work, none at all.

For her part, Mrs Kevans was another averse to being inactive. 'I just think I'm the kind of person that likes to be busy. I don't like to sit about.' She did, however, place great store by the routine of an afternoon nap while her husband looked after the house and children.

Marital and family relationships

Mrs Kevans felt her husband had adjusted well to his new situation, aided by his equitable temperament. 'He's not a cantankerous person or owt like that; he's really passive and laid back. I don't think I could do with a cantankerous one round my neck.' Only occasionally was there evidence of tension between them.

> There are odd times when she'll say, 'It's about time you got a job', because we're more or less together all the time and you do sometimes get on top of each other. And at other times,

conversations dry up whereas if you've been to work all day you've got something fresh to come home and talk about.

The Kevans benefited from a network of close, caring relationships in their large, extended family. Their children helped with shopping and gardening. Mrs Kevans was one of three sisters who shared the care of their invalid mother, while both she and her husband kept an eye on their elderly widowed neighbour. Every weekend, children and grandchildren congregated at the Kevans' house.

Stress and coping

Mrs Kevans claimed a relatively stress-free existence. Only the miners' strike seems to have caused her distress. Mr Kevans similarly regarded himself as unstressed. This was despite their mutual recognition of considerable differences of temperament.

> I confide, a lot of people don't. He's not very chatty altogether. He never worries you with anything. Anything that he worries about will come out in conversation with someone else. Some people find it easier to talk to strangers than their own.

> She reckons I don't talk things over as much as I should with her. . . . I don't see why I should trouble anybody else. She'll come home from work some days saying she's had enough but it soon blows over. I wouldn't say she's someone that dwells on it too long. I'll just buck her up and say, 'You know what they're like', and this, that and the other. That seems to help a bit.

Summary

Whilst conceding that he occasionally felt unsettled at being out of work, Mr Kevans was able, like Mr Dear, to cite ill health as a valid reason for his continuing unemployment. He had in any case been glad to get out of an industry changing beyond recognition. He took on a number of traditionally female functions with equanimity, especially as they made him feel useful. Mrs Kevans enjoyed the responsibility of her job. The support from her husband and children enabled her in turn to support her own mother. She liked to keep busy and she was. Their differences in temperament remained untested by his unemployment or her job and the extended family posed few problems. Coping here was a happy union of all these factors.

Case study 3: Mr and Mrs Mackintosh

Mr and Mrs Mackintosh were in their late forties with two sons, one at primary school, the other, 21, still living at home.

Redundancy, health and unemployment

Life seemed to hold few compensations for Mr Mackintosh, who had left the pit due to the onset of lymph cancer. Now apparently fully recovered, he was embittered by the rundown of the industry and the lack of viable employment alternatives. He was additionally sensitive to the attitudes of neighbours in the new estate on the periphery of the old pit village.

> I get depressed, I get fed up. I try, you keep yourself busy with things you do. . . . I used to have a sense of pride that everything I'd got I'd worked for. I feel guilty that I'm being paid for doing nothing. All right, my son will say, 'Well, dad, you paid enough in and, with what you've been through, you deserve it.' But I say, 'That's not the point.' To be honest, I feel like a bloody sponger. It gets me down. I go to the local club now and I suppose that some people could be looking at me and saying 'Look at that! The idle bugger's never worked since he left the pit.' They don't understand why: it's not through choice, it's because I refuse to work for two pounds an hour!

Women's employment and domestic labour

Mrs Mackintosh worked as a supermarket assistant, a job she regarded as severely stressful and patently unrewarding. On a three-week cycle, she was required to work 17.5 hours for the first two weeks and 39 hours for the third. Though she welcomed the independence of having a job, she was far from happy with the nature of her work:

> I like the independence . . . but your employers expect you to work harder for the same money. You're expected to do everything. They want more out of you all the time and they're push, push, push, and you feel like you're never going to

finish. What really annoys me is that I have to lift heavy boxes of soap powder and things like that, and I always think, 'I'm going into middle age and I shouldn't have to do this', and yet my employers are so tight-fisted it's more or less 'If you want the job, you work harder'. That annoys me. They shouldn't be allowed to take that attitude but they can because there's always someone there to take your job.

Mr Mackintosh was exasperated by this exploitation of his wife, which he was powerless to alter.

Given the chance, I think she'd leave tomorrow. She's having to work harder. I think that shop's getting away with bloody murder, to be honest, safety wise. These lasses are lifting great boxes of soap powder. . . . It's men's work that they're doing: they're actually lifting and loading wagons and stuff like that. It's scandalous! It's a source of strain to me because I know she'd like to finish there but she can't. She's stuck, the same as I was at the pit. . . . If I could get a decent paid job she could maybe leave and I want her to because I can see at times it gets her down. I want her to be able to come in and say, 'I don't like that job' and me to be able to say, 'Well, pack it in. We can manage on my wages.'

Mrs Mackintosh was tolerant of her husband's attempts at housework.

If I'm at work he will do the housework for me. He'll dust and wash the pots and when I come home he'll have me scrambled egg on toast or a sandwich made and he'll say, 'I've hoovered up and I've dusted and I've made the beds.' He is very good like that and he will do his little bit. It's not my standard, sort of thing, but you don't say anything about it, just 'Thank you, dear'.

She reckoned that in any case she did three-quarters of the housework.

Marital and family relationships

Mr Mackintosh explained how he would bridle if his wife mentioned his lack of work:

She slips up sometimes, comes out with something that she doesn't mean that way but she, like, covers it up in case I take it the wrong way. She'll say something like 'If you were working, we'd be able to', and then she says, 'I'm sorry, I don't mean it like that, love.' She knows how it gets me down and she'll say to me, 'Don't let it worry you,' and I say, 'Yes, but it does bother me because I can't see myself getting a job for years.'

Mr Mackintosh was all too well aware that he was something of a burden to his wife. 'She's taken a lot of crap I've dished out. I don't mean violence – I've never hit her – but whenever I've got moody or depressed, she's put up with it.'

The greatest source of tension was the intensity of his political beliefs.

His argument is, 'Get that bloody lot out! Stand them up against a wall and shoot them!' I'm one of those who think they should all get together and sort a way forward. . . . He gets very angry indeed. . . . I don't tend to say a lot because I know that makes him worse. I know deep down inside he's worrying about whether he'll ever get a job again and whether he'll be here next year. That's what he does worry about, so I don't say anything.

To make matters worse, Mrs Mackintosh seemed to find herself confronted by the ever-increasing demands of her family.

I've got less time now than I did have a few years ago because, when you're at work all day, you come home and sit for an hour and then think, 'I'm going to have to get up and get the ironing done and the bedrooms want tidying round', and you can't tend to sit like you used to do. Before, when I cleaned, I finished at twelve and had all the afternoon to myself to do just what I liked, but now I don't get enough time, really. I'm outnumbered for a start. The eldest one will come in and say, 'Haven't you done this?' and I say to him, 'I've been at work all day! You do it! If you were in a flat on your own, you'd have to do it!' And Len will agree with me but then turn round and say, 'Will you do so and so?' and I just can't win. I do get a bit annoyed. Sometimes I don't mind but it just depends. Sometimes it's all down to work and what kind of a day you've had.

Conflict between father and son was rife, since Mr Mackintosh could not accept his son's decision to leave school after achieving ten O levels. Mrs Mackintosh respected her son's decision but felt obliged to intercede in periodic arguments.

Both partners had little support from their extended families, though for rather different reasons, as Mrs Mackintosh explained.

> I've never really had a good relationship with my mother, ever. I tend to tolerate her only because she's my mother. I know it sounds awful but it's true. . . . I get on ever so well with my brother and I always have done. . . . Len has always stuck to family as well. He'd go out with his brothers and his uncle and his dad, but when Len had cancer it tended to split his family and his younger brother in particular turned against him because of his cancer.

Nor were there any friends to provide support.

> No, not really. I never have what you call bosom friends because I always find some friends soon become enemies. . . . I more or less keep to myself. I have friends at work and odd neighbours but I'm not really involved.

Mrs Mackintosh's comments on friends were matched by those of Mr Mackintosh on neighbours.

> Most people round here are actually Conservative. I don't know what we're doing living here. There were quite a number of people during the strike who said, 'They ought to shut the bloody pit, that would serve them right!' It makes you all the more determined.

Stress and coping

Mr Mackintosh recognized that he was stressed by his ill health and unemployment. Having appeared to survive one bout of cancer, he had suffered not one but two relapses.

> I had this lymph cancer again and it's the anger. Why me? Why again? That's every two years: three times I've had this! Then you've got this hopelessness of ever being able to get another job and sometimes just small things stress you up.

Mrs Mackintosh had to cope with her husband's emotional vola-
tility, depressive tendencies and acute sense of boredom and
isolation.

> Sometimes it can be hard work, really hard work. I took him
> away the other weekend for his birthday. We had three nights
> away and I think that upset him a little bit, and he said, 'You
> shouldn't be doing this, I should be doing this.' And all I say
> is, 'Look at the years you've kept me. All we've done is changed
> over for a while until things pick up.' I think he sometimes gets a
> little bit jealous that I'm working and he isn't.

But such occasional treats did little to ward off his bouts of
depression.

> When he's just had a bad day and he's got up in a bad mood to
> start with, he's not himself and you can see he's going to have a
> bad day and he's fed up. . . . Then, of course, when he's like that
> and I go out to work, it's on my mind all the time at work, so I've
> got that there at the back of my mind. He's going to have one of
> his off days and I'm not there, and you sort of go to work all
> jumbled up to start with, so that doesn't help and then you get
> to work and you have the few odd customers and your super-
> visor's there and you've got to do this and that and it all
> builds up.

Her symptoms of stress included sweating, breathlessness and irrit-
able bowel syndrome. Some of her remedies were unorthodox, like
sessions in the bath with a book, a cigarette and a cup of tea. She
provided a graphic account of when her stress had been at its
highest and her capacity to cope at its lowest.

> When he was ill, I lost quite a lot of weight. It wasn't only
> chemotherapy and all his treatment, it was all the talk about
> the pit shutting down as well. And, of course, Len didn't know
> whether to go for redundancy. I didn't confide a lot actually.
> I did it on my own because I couldn't talk to anybody without fill-
> ing up. . . . It took a couple of months and then I went to pieces.
> I used to find I'd go and get the bottle of whisky out to make me
> sleep. . . . I used to get tearful at work and have to go to the loo
> quite a lot. I would fill up ever such a lot. I used to cry into my
> whisky. . . . Both sides of the family got so upset they used to
> make me feel ill and I used to avoid them as much as possible.

They used to be telling me on the phone how they felt and I used to think, 'Bloody hell, what are you telling me for? Don't you think I've got enough?' And there was me having to go to the hospital every day and it didn't matter what mood he was in I had to cope with it. . . . When we found out he was clear, that was when I sort of went to pieces. . . . I'd managed to get all through that bad period without breaking up once and that's when it all came to a head in a final release. But I'd got a little boy to see to and you can't fall apart when you've got a little one to see to. You've got to pick yourself up for them. So I had to straighten myself out.

Summary

Mr Mackintosh harboured deep and permanent bitterness at the government's decision to close most of the mines. To this political resentment was added the guilt and shame at not being able to find a job and becoming financially dependent on his wife. The enduring fear that his cancer would return compounded matters, rendering him moody and depressed. His wife's ability to cope with his emotions was handicapped by the unsatisfying nature of her job, the tensions between father and son and the lack of support from relatives or friends. Thus the Mackintoshes experienced more stressors and had fewer coping resources than either of the other two couples. They were always vulnerable to any one source of stress; in the face of multiple sources, they barely survived.

DISCUSSION

The nine theses presented earlier provide a useful framework for collating our case-study findings. We cannot, on the basis of three case studies, generalize; neither would we seek to. Rather, we are interested in refining our understanding of how and under what conditions such generalizations might hold. For while the theses, and the largely quantitative studies which support them, have established the basic psychological structure of the effects of unemployment, they have been less concerned with the social and psychological processes involved.

The majority of the theses cited earlier proved valid for our case studies but only at a very high level of abstraction. For example, we did find that male involvement in domestic labour increased only marginally but there was great variation in the way this outcome was accomplished. The wife might forbid, tolerate or welcome male involvement and it appeared to be her opinion which counted. Similarly, in general families did seek to maintain rather than alter existing patterns of behaviour, though this might involve quite considerable change in male responsibility for childcare. There is no doubt that in our case studies the wife's psychological reaction to her husband's unemployment was conditioned by his psychological reaction, though men in objectively similar circumstances actually reacted quite differently. Thus the psychologically harmful effects of unemployment were evident in the case of Mr Mackintosh but less so in those of Mr Dear or Mr Kevans, largely because of the way they rationalized their unemployed status. The latter two also evolved strategies for coping which fit the category of 'constructive adaptation' to unemployment, though Mr Mackintosh is less easily placed in the alternative category of 'resigned adaptation'. His response would be better termed 'resentful maladaptation'. Mr Mackintosh was also the only one to resent the loss of his social identity as a miner. Neither Mr Dear nor Mr Kevans seem to have had difficulty in forsaking their occupational identity, suggesting that identification with it may be a matter of degree.

Women's capacity to cope with an unemployed husband was, in two of the cases, clearly enhanced by both enjoyment of their own jobs and social support from relatives, just as in the third case dislike of the job and the lack of social support proved to be handicaps. Our cases were almost polarized along these lines, so we could not consider a situation where positive social support was combined with negative experience of work or lack of social support with an enjoyable job. It is thus difficult to tease out the possible implications of the idea that one sphere of life can compensate for another.

Finally, in terms of the nine theses, the one for which we found least direct support (and the one which is most tenuously supported by the literature) is the claim that unemployed men may be hostile to their wives' paid employment. None of our three men evinced such hostility. However, its potential was tempered by the fact that the women worked part-time in low-paid occupations, so that their earning capacity was limited. There was also evidence of self-conscious claims by the men that their financial contribution to the household had not diminished, despite their unemployment.

It would appear that the acceptance of the wife's employment is conditional upon the form and magnitude of the threat it poses to the male role as breadwinner.

Examination of the applicability of the nine theses to our case studies has suggested the need to pay attention to the fine details of how unemployed men and their wives manage or fail to cope, especially the nature of the transactions between husband and wife in the context of specific cultural assumptions about gender. These are the basis for our concluding comments.

CONCLUSION

In our study we have attempted to follow Jackson and Walsh in developing a 'framework for understanding unemployment as a *family* experience rather than as a *solitary* event' (1987: 195; original emphasis) – a framework which can structure the analysis of 'the psychological processes involved in intra-family and family–environment dynamics brought about by unemployment' (1987: 196).

Our interest has not been in causal factors or mediating variables of a kind which might be identified in a large-scale survey. Rather, we have used detailed case studies in order to identify the interpretative or cognitive processes which appear important for the degree and nature of coping with job loss, which, as Jackson and Walsh emphasize, threatens both the man's identity, personal and social, and the social organization of t e family.

What we wish to identify are ..ae issues which require resolution and the interpretative strategies available. Both issues and interpretations are heavily structured by gender relations (the established norms in mining communities) and gender relationships – how these are mobilized and adapted within any particular marriage. We shall suggest that this negotiation is not an equal one and its implicitly defined purpose is the protection of a revised role of the male within the family.

Our micro-analysis is consonant with the views of Liem and Liem (1988, 1990) that the man sets the agenda: it is his interpretation of and reaction to unemployment with which the wife had to cope. He lays down the terms in which the couple have to renegotiate their relationship. This coping through negotiation is constrained or enabled by his interpretation of four issues.

First, there is the man's perception of the reasons for his unemployment. In the case of mining, this related to views of the politics and economics of the coal industry and whether miners had been victimized. Second, there is the way in which ill health and unemployment are related to each other. Ill health can be seen as an external factor causing unemployment about which nothing can be done, or it can be experienced as compounding feelings of personal failure and victimization. Third, there is his perception of the effect of unemployment on his function as provider, whether he feels he has 'failed' his family or whether he is able to accept a reduced economic role and contribute to the household in other ways. Finally, there is the question of whether the man can find a substitute for the purposive structure of paid work, the construction of a routine around hobbies or childcare vying with lethargy and despair.

It should be noted that in each of these issues the most successful adaptations are not necessarily linked to the most 'valid interpretation'. The view of mine closures as an act of political vengeance, for example, seems at least as legitimate as one which accepts the historical inevitability of their closure. But the latter seems to lead to less resentment and stress. Anger about the random nature of illness is no less valid than acceptance of disability but is psychologically destabilizing. Thus for the wife, coping meant negotiating with her husband's interpretations of the significance and meaning of his unemployment and ill health. The main way in which she could immediately affect such interpretations was to reach some agreement about his involvement in housework. Generally, some contribution was agreed without any substantial implications for the traditional division of domestic labour, in which the woman had as heavy an investment as the man – if only because it salvaged some semblance of routine. In this as in other issues, the woman's coping seemed to be directed at sustaining her husband's male identity in the absence of paid employment.

From our case studies, we can identify at least three stratagems to achieve this goal. The first is to endorse *rationalizations* for the state of affairs, each of which rescues the man from any blame: that the husband has kept the wife for years, so that now she's paying him back; that she doesn't expect him to work for low wages; that his health doesn't allow him to do much. As Jackson and Walsh (1987: 211) have noted, the sick role absolves the individual of responsibility to meet conventional obligations. The second strategy is a *revalidation* of a revised male role, so that the husband contributes to the family in some other way than as main breadwinner: that his projects may make some money; that he looks after the children; that he helps about the house. A third strategy is the *ruse*, maintaining an illusion of male contribution: he pays what he has always paid, he does his best with the housework. These are not mutually exclusive stratagems; indeed, it is their combination which seems most productive.

All this is hard work for the woman and its effectiveness appears to be conditioned by a number of factors. The sensitivity of his feelings will shape the nature of her response. The prior nature of the marital relationship will provide mechanisms for conflict resolution or escalation. The woman's resources in coping also depend upon factors outside the couple. A rewarding job will sustain the woman's efforts, but an unrewarding one will undermine them. Other resources of support may be a help or a hindrance. As Jackson and Walsh (1987: 207) comment, the wives of unemployed men feel an obligation to reassure and support their husbands but no one necessarily reassures the wives.

What is therefore important is the extent to which other members of the immediate and extended family, and the community as a whole, support the woman in her efforts. Where there is already tension in the immediate family – for example, between husband and son – coping with unemployment is more difficult, since resentment becomes projected on to what is already a difficult relationship, so that the woman's role as mediator is under strain. Grown-up children can be supportive in practical and emotional ways or they can unintentionally compound stress where they present problems of their own. Ageing parents requiring care can be yet another source of strain or a welcome opportunity to keep busy. Finally, the community at large may offer a view of unemployment which supports or undermines attempts to preserve a sense of male identity.

There is, then, no single coping strategy which is likely to be effective in response to male unemployment following voluntary redundancy as a result of ill health. As others have noted:

> understanding how a family handles an assault like unemployment requires not so much the correct classification of its relational or coping style. Instead, it entails the concrete exploration of the family's ongoing exchange with the relevant surround-

ing context, whether that be the kin network, the neighbourhood or the workplace.

(Liem and Liem, 1990: 202)

We have here highlighted the factors which seem important in shaping the outcome of male redundancy for the family: the man's perception of his situation, the wife's stratagems and resources in supporting him. But what we have referred to as a process of coping through negotiation cannot be undertaken by individuals outside the cultural context which defines the terms in which they must operate. In mining, and indeed other traditional working-class communities, coping with unemployment requires the re-casting of the male presence within the family within the parameters of established male identity. As McKee and Bell found, even among the families of unemployed men, there remained an ideal of the male breadwinner and the female homemaker as the 'right, natural and proper order which supported conventional ideas about masculinity, authority, identity, marital stability and pride' (1985: 394).

In seeking to understand reactions to unemployment it is apparent that idealizations of gender roles are evident in the words of those experiencing unemployment. Gender roles also appear central to our analysis. A working definition of gender roles might be a set of expectations and prescriptions which are culturally transmitted and reproduced. Although individuals may re-create and negotiate their own particular versions of the prevailing norms, they are unlikely to alter them radically. It could even be argued that unemployment lays bare the vulnerability of these roles, to which the reaction is to rescue and restore rather than revise them. Hence the overriding need is to re-negotiate a sustainable version of male identity without the major breadwinner role which traditionally validated it. But this has to be undertaken within the given prescriptions about gender roles, a process Morris calls 'a re-negotiation of certain details of everyday life within the household . . . distinct from any serious negotiation of underlying principles' (1985: 414). Thus what the woman has to do is to protect established male identity in renegotiated terms which allow him to feel that he is still a real man, husband and father, even though his role as principal breadwinner has gone. If this can be accomplished, the potential strain on each partner, the relationship and the family as a whole can be ameliorated. If it cannot, then all those involved will exhibit signs of stress. The trouble with men then becomes the trouble for women.

How well women cope depends upon a wide range of factors, over many of which – especially her husband's interpretation of his situation – she has little or no control. In this situation of relative powerlessness, the woman must use what resources she has. These include her general skill in handling her husband, the stratagems to which she can resort, any strength she can draw from her own job and, most importantly, the support she receives from her close family. Since this kinship network is maintained by women, it becomes the female responsibility to bolster male identity when it is threatened by external circumstances. In conditions of adversity, it is women who restore male self-respect; through gender relationships they reproduce gender relations and thus their own roles as protectors of male identity.

ACKNOWLEDGEMENTS

The research reported on in this chapter was funded by the ESRC (Project ref X206252004) as part of the Management of Personal Welfare Research Programme.

REFERENCES

Baruch, G.K., Biener, L. and Barnett, R.C. (1987) 'Women and gender in research on work and family stress', *American Psychologist*, 42: 130–6.

Binns, D. and Mars, G. (1984) 'Family, community and unemployment: a study in change', *Sociological Review*, 32(1): 662–95.

Brown, G.W. and Harris, T. (1978) *Social Origins of Depression*, London: Tavistock.

Critcher, C., Dicks, B. and Waddington, D. (1992) 'Portrait of despair', *New Statesman and Society*, (23 October): 16–17.

Dew, M.A., Bromet, E.J. and Schulberg, H.C. (1987) 'A comparative analysis of two community stressors' long-term health effects', *American Journal of Community Psychology*, 15: 167–84.

Dicks, B., Waddington, D. and Critcher, C. (1993) 'The quiet disintegration of closure communities', *Town and Country Planning*, 62(7): 174–6.

Farmer, V. (1986) 'Broken heartland', *Psychology Today*, 20(4): 54–62.

Jackson, P.R. and Walsh, S. (1987) 'Unemployment and the family', in D. Fryer and P. Ullah (eds) *Unemployed People: Social and Psychological Perspectives*, Milton Keynes: Open University Press.

Joelson, L. and Wahlquist, L. (1987) 'The psychological meaning of job insecurity and job loss: results of a longitudinal study', *Social Science and Medicine*, 15(12): 179–82.

Laite, J. and Halfpenny, F. (1987) 'Employment, unemployment and the domestic division of labour', in D. Fryer and P. Ullah (eds) *Unemployed People: Social and Psychological Perspectives*, Milton Keynes: Open University Press.

Lennon, M.C. and Rosenfield, S. (1992) 'Women and mental health: the interaction of job and family conditions', *Journal of Health and Social Behaviour*, 33: 316–27.

Liem, R. and Liem, J.H. (1988) 'Psychological effects of unemployment on workers and their families', *Journal of Social Issues*, 44(4): 87–105.

—— (1990) 'Understanding the individual and family effect of unemployment', in J. Eckenrode and S. Gore (eds) *Stress between Work and Family*, New York: Plenum Press.

McKee, L. and Bell, C. (1985) 'Marital and family relations in times of male unemployment', in B. Roberts, R. Finnegan and D. Gallie (eds) *New Approaches to Economic Life*, Manchester: Manchester University Press.

—— (1986) 'His unemployment, her problem: the domestic and marital consequences of male unemployment', in S. Allen, A. Waton, K. Purcell and S. Woods (eds) *The Experience of Unemployment*, Basingstoke: Macmillan.

Morris, L. (1985) 'Renegotiation of the domestic division of labour in the context of male redundancy', in B. Roberts, R. Finnegan and D. Gallie (eds) *New Approaches to Economic Life*, Manchester: Manchester University Press.

—— (1988) 'Employment, the household and social networks', in D. Gallie (ed.) *Employment in Britain*, Oxford: Basil Blackwell.

—— (1992) 'Domestic labour and employment status among married couples: a case study in Hartlepool', *Capital and Class*, 49.

Nathanson, C. A. (1975) 'Illness and the feminine role: a theoretical review', *Social Science and Medicine*, 9: 57–62.

Parry, G. (1986) 'Paid employment, life events, social support and mental health in working-class mothers', *Journal of Health and Social Behaviour*, 27: 193–208.

Penkower, L., Bromet, E. and Dew, M.A. (1988) 'Husbands' layoff and wives' mental health', *Archives of General Psychiatry*, 45: 994–1000.

Ross, C.E. and Mirowsky, J. (1988) 'Child care and emotional adjustment to wives' employment', *Journal of Health and Social Behaviour*, 29: 127–38.

Van Hooke, M. (1990) 'Family responses to the farm crisis: a study in coping', *Social Work*, 35(5): 425–31.

Waddington, D.P., Dicks, B. and Critcher, C. (1994) 'Community responses to pit closure in the post-strike era', *Community Development Journal*, 29(2): 141–50.

Waddington, D.P., Wykes, M. and Critcher, C. (1991) *Split at the Seams? Community, Continuity and Change after the 1984–5 Coal Dispute*, Milton Keynes: Open University Press.

Warr, P. (1985) 'Twelve questions about unemployment and health', in B. Roberts, R. Finnegan and D. Gallie (eds) *New Approaches to Economic Life*, Manchester: Manchester University Press.

Warr, P.B. and Jackson, P.R. (1987) 'Adapting to the unemployed role: a longitudinal investigation', *Social Science and Medicine*, 25: 1219–24.

Wass, V. (1989) 'Redundancy and re-employment: effects and prospects following colliery closures', *Coalfield Communities Campaign Working Papers*, 5: 3–21.

—— (1991) 'The psychological effects of redundancy and worklessness: a case study from the coalfields', Paper presented at the Coal, Culture and Community Conference, Sheffield City Polytechnic (September).

Wright, S.E. and Rosenblatt, P.C. (1987) 'Isolation and farm loss: why neighbours may not be supportive', *Family Relations*, 36: 391–5.

Part III
Service providers, men and welfare

Chapter 10

Screening out men
Or 'Has Mum changed her washing powder recently?'

Jeanette Edwards

SETTING THE SCENE

The absence of men in studies of the social welfare and health of women and children is noticeable. They may be cited as one of the problems facing women caring for children, but are rarely mooted as a solution. The responsibility for caring for children continues to be placed squarely on the shoulders of women, as does the responsibility when things go wrong. There has been a tension in much feminist debate, as well as that concerned with social policy, between deploring the absence of men as fathers and supporting the role of women as mothers. Men are perceived to pose difficulties both when they are present and when they are absent. As Sara Ruddick points out:

> the official story cannot conceal the fact that, as Gertrude Stein remarked, 'fathers are depressing'. . . . Some fathers are literally lost or gone; others can be located but will not, except under rarely effective legal pressure, offer cash or services. Fathers who provide materially for their children as best they can, rarely assume a full share of the emotional work and responsibility of childcare.
>
> (Ruddick, 1990: 223)

And further on:

> If an absent father is depressingly disappointing, a present father can be dangerous. . . . Whatever his personal tendencies . . . temptations toward excessive, judgmental control will be exacerbated by his sense that he is entitled to rule over women and children.
>
> (Ruddick, 1990: 223–4)

Depressing indeed! Moreover, these comments portray an ambivalence about the role of men in the home: trouble if they're there and trouble if they're not. This chapter identifies a similar ambivalence in ways in which providers of community health and social services perceive the role of men as fathers. Workers perceive a lack of support from male partners as a major problem facing many of the women with whom they work, but at the same time they appear unable or unwilling to include men within the ambit of their work, unless they are the sole carers of children. Thus while the service providers in this chapter generally express a wish for men to be more active in the care of their children and more supportive of their female partners, they provide services geared predominantly towards women. And while men may, and many do, absent themselves from childcare, I argue that they are also *made* absent. There is a process whereby, through the language and practice of workers, men are screened out: they are not only excluded from discussion about the welfare of their children but are also, thereby, absolved from responsibility. Furthermore, the needs of men as fathers are perceived quite differently from the needs of women as mothers.

This chapter identifies a tension between the stated aims of service providers who work with families deemed to be 'in need', and their attitudes towards men as carers. I do not wish to downplay nor undermine service-provider experiences and understandings of the extent of violence – physical, sexual and emotional – perpetrated by men in some of the homes they visit; community health and social service workers – particularly social workers – are faced daily with its effects on the women and children with whom they work. A conflict of interest between women and children and men in their lives who are abusive, to greater or lesser degrees and in more or less explicit ways, may provide a good reason why the workers in this study rarely see their role as providing health and social services to men. At the same time, however, there is evidence that when workers interact directly with men as fathers, particularly when they deal with men as sole carers of children, they base their assessment of needs on a different set of assumptions and premises than when assessing the needs of women as mothers.

There has been an increasing emphasis in policy discussion and government White Papers on the way in which parents might become more 'responsible' for their children's physical and mental health (Graham, 1979, 1982). The Children Act of 1989 placed an emphasis on 'parental responsibility' and sought to broaden the net of responsibility to include 'putative fathers' and 'unmarried fathers' under the rubric of parent (Chapter 2, this volume; and see Community Care, 1990).[1] At the same time it also declared it the duty of local authorities to inform absent fathers of child protection and care proceedings.[2] More recent legislation makes an attempt at placing fathers back where, it is assumed, they belong – as the financial providers in families. Hence the Child Support Act of 1991 aimed to enforce the responsibility of absent fathers for their children by assessing and demanding a financial contribution. While this, in principle, may be no bad thing, in reality, as many commentators have noted, it has resulted in further hardship and has increased conflict between separated parents. At worst, it further impoverishes poor women caring for their children and limits benefits going directly to children from absent fathers; while at best it changes not one iota the financial well-being of sole parent families (Chapter 2, this volume; Boden and Childs, 1996).

While there is a common perception that men are increasingly absenting themselves from 'families', they are at the same time increasingly present at the birth of their children (Chapter 3, this volume; Oakley, 1993). During the past two decades, expectant fathers have taken and been given a place in the delivery room. Social analysis of this presence is again marked by ambivalence. For example, Mira Crouch and Lenore Manderson (1993) argue that the trend acts to affirm the values of heterosexual parenting in the face of uncertainty over the role of men as financial providers. They warn of the dubious benefits this may bring to women, and in particular of the danger that women will be required to be as responsible for the well-being of men inside the labour room as they normally are elsewhere. Men's presence in the delivery room and their involvement in the process and procedures of childbirth provokes, from this perspective, unease: will not men demand the same kind of attention during the birth of their children which they demand and are accustomed to receiving in most other spheres of daily life?[3]

The past decade has witnessed relentless media and political attention on 'the evils' of single parenthood; female lone parents are held responsible for no end of social ills: 'juvenile delinquency', 'truancy', 'eating disorders', 'suicide', 'low educational standards' and all manner of other 'anti-social behaviour' have been identified as 'consequences' of lone parenthood (Edwards, 1995; see Mullings (1995) for a discussion of the same in the United States). Social commentators in this tirade against single parents have all too often disregarded the role and responsibility of men, both those who are present as much as those who are absent, for the health and welfare of their children.

Politicians and the media may have attempted, however unhelpfully at times, to redefine and re-emphasize the place and role of men as fathers, but in the realm of social policy, and where responsibility for the welfare of children is allocated, men are noticeably absent. Judith Milner (1993) has analysed, from the perspective of social services, the way in which child protection referrals systematically deal with mothers and fathers differently, to the extent that '[f]athers not only disappear from the system but they are frequently excluded by the terms of the initial enquiry' (1993: 52; see also Marsh, 1987). She writes candidly and in retrospect from the position of a practising social worker: 'Whilst I was consciously aware that I was conspiring with a system which scrutinized mothering, I was not as aware of my complicity in a process which avoids scrutinizing fathering' (Milner, 1993: 59).

BANTON AND TARROW

The study on which this chapter is based was carried out in two areas of Greater Manchester during 1991 and 1992. It confirms Milner's experience of a reluctance to scrutinize men as partners and parents. The aim of the study was to explore 'social support' from the perspective of community health and social service workers, particularly those working with families containing pre-school-age children. Hence, community midwives, health visitors, social service staff and voluntary sector workers were interviewed.[4] The two localities, 'Banton' and 'Tarrow',[5] each have a population of about 12,000 people. The majority of residents in both are white and working class, and are identified as having large numbers of materially disadvantaged residents marked by a reliance on fixed state benefits or low wages. Both are dominated by large local authority housing estates, and poor housing is identified as a major problem in both areas. Although adjacent geographically, each comes under the jurisdiction of different health and local authorities.

Banton and Tarrow are both infamous neighbourhoods within two different cities. They are both associated with high crime rates, particularly among young men. Many workers said of each place that it 'has a bad name', although some argue that its reputation is unwarranted. One health visitor explained that the reputation of Banton preceded residents but that, in reality, it is no different from many other places: 'The estate has a reputation, but the fathers that I visit there have got no extraordinary problems.' Workers also point out that the appearance of Banton and Tarrow is deceptive: both are on the outskirts of the urban conurbation and they appear more spacious and rural than many inner urban areas but, it is argued, they have similar kinds of problems to those recognized to be features of 'inner cities' and with the additional difficulty of inadequate and expensive public transport.

Social workers point out that the families with whom social services usually work are not representative of the area as a whole. A social worker in Tarrow explained it this way:

> Certainly the ones we look at are low income, generally poor educational attainment, unemployment and family breakdown, partner breakdown, domestic violence, disharmony – without making a sort of global statement. We don't know it's any worse than it is anywhere else.

Taking seriously the point made by this social worker that their caseloads comprise families facing particularly dire sets of circumstances, the remainder of this chapter will focus more on the views of health visitors and community midwives than social workers. I add the caveat, however, that for both community health and social service providers 'problem families' loom larger in their perception of these two areas than numbers alone might suggest. This is also likely to be an artefact of the research itself which was designed to look at 'social support' from the perspective of health and social service providers working with families deemed to be 'at risk'.

MEN: USEFUL TO HAVE AROUND?

Service providers in Banton and Tarrow, when thinking about difficulties facing young children and their carers, invariably point to the high number of single parents in the two areas. In response to questions which asked them to identify the major problems facing families with young children in these two areas, the majority of workers mentioned poverty, poor housing and unemployment, all of which they associated with lone parenthood. Many workers made a chain of connections: unable to work due to lack of affordable childcare and adequately paid jobs, lone mothers have to rely on inadequate and fixed state benefits and rented local authority accommodation which all too often is in poor state of repair. Nearly all the workers we interviewed said they thought it was useful or beneficial to work with both parents if both were involved in the care of their children. Those respondents who elaborated on this question suggested it was better both for children and mothers if men were involved in childcare. Arguments were often put forward that children benefit from having *two* parents around and that women benefit from having the support of men. The prevailing opinion was that if men wish to play a part in the care of their children, then service providers should encourage them to do so. However, several workers suggested that health and social service professionals deliberately excluded men, and while they argued that there might be good reason for doing so, they also pointed out that it was not necessarily in the interest of children. As one social worker put it:

> I think fathers get the rough end of the stick really, and I think if they are willing, if they want to be part of their child's life, then it's good to be able to include them in that. Give them a lot of support. . . . Yeah, I think it is important for the children to have the father around.

When both parents take part in the care of children, workers think it generally beneficial to deal directly with both. It is illuminating, however, to unpack the reasons for this. As mentioned earlier, the workers in this study emphasized the fact that men's participation in childcare benefits both mothers and children: it lessens the burden on women and provides children with extra or substitute care and attention. Moreover, workers suggest – albeit implicitly – that the presence of fathers is helpful to them in their work. Workers were more or less explicit about the potential for men to aid them in their work. Some suggest that if a 'good relationship' is forged between fathers and workers, fathers can be called upon to reinforce the instructions and advice that workers give to mothers. Fathers might also provide supplementary or cor-

roborating information. A health visitor explored the reasons for
dealing directly with men, as follows:

> and if you want to leave a specific instruction for the mum then
> the dad's there anyway and he'll hear it first hand off us . . . so it's
> very beneficial if he's there. And sometimes you get more infor-
> mation from him as well as from the girl herself, and if you need
> extra, if you need extra help from the dad, then you're talking to
> him there, in front of – you know – in front of his partner.

A number of other workers pointed out that they would contact
men, or speak directly with them, *if* they were worried about the
women in their care. One midwife explained how she might 'interview' a father before discharging a woman and baby in order to
assess the kind of support or help available at home.

Emerging from the interviews and conversations with workers
are three interlinked ways in which men are perceived to be potentially helpful – to workers. First, they may heed the advice of
workers and follow instructions, especially if that advice is given
them directly. In this context, fathers are more likely to follow
instructions if those instructions are received 'face-to-face' from
the worker rather than 'second-hand' through the mother.
Second, men may reinforce messages that workers give to women.
To put it bluntly, and not in the words of workers themselves,
they can ensure that women do as workers suggest. Third, men
can provide women with the 'extra' support they may require; in
this context, fathers may act as a substitute for workers, or for
kin. Fathers are perceived, in other words, as filling a gap. This is
how one midwife explained it:

> Well, because we are seeking the support of the husbands, or say
> the partners, more and more. There are a few of these girls whom
> we as midwives feel they need extra support,[6] and you will find
> the girls that are not really that mature they need their partners
> other than – you know, more than – say, their mums and dads.[7]

This worker suggests that for those (young) women who are perceived to need 'extra support', it is often more useful for workers
to elicit the support of partners than parents.

In none of these three interlinked reasons for eliciting the support
of men is there a sense that workers feel the need to deal with men
as co-parents; as equally responsible and mindful carers of their
children. Workers are evidently not resistant to dealing directly

with men as fathers. They point out that men's help can be harnessed in a variety of ways. But it seems, to this observer at least, that the work of men in caring for children, while perceived to be valuable, is conceptualized as supplementary – as an additional benefit.[8] Men may either help workers, or support their partners, or both, but they are rarely perceived as solely, or even equally, responsible for the care of their children.[9]

MEN: ABSENT OR ABSENTED?

During the interviews, workers highlighted the absence of men as fathers in both Banton and Tarrow, yet accompanying workers during their working day, I was struck by the number of men with whom we came in contact.[10] Their presence could not have been predicted from the interviews alone, nor from what workers were saying prior and during fieldwork. The kind of information generated by different research methods has been well documented (see, for example, Chapter 1, this volume) and this is not the place to embark on a discussion of methodology. However, it is worth noting that interviews, structured, unstructured or semi-structured, are more often than not particular social events, carried out in a place marked for that particular purpose, after more or less detailed explanations of the aims of the research (as far as they are known). The question–answer format has its own rules and its own outcomes. Interview questions invite respondents to generalize, to theorize from what they already know from a variety of sources. Service providers in this study made sense of the questions posed by the researcher, not only through their direct experience with clients over time, but also through comparison and analogy with what they know from other domains of social life, which might also include their own experience of kinship and parenthood. In addressing topics to do with the practices of parents, and the relationship between parents and children, they also draw, inevitably, on culturally specific ideas of what constitutes appropriate child-rearing practices, as well as what constitutes ideal child-rearing units.

In the interviews, many workers observed that there are, in the words of at least one worker, 'a lot of single parents' in Banton and Tarrow. In the words of another, 'men are just not around', and of another, 'there are not many fathers in these parts'. 'A father', in this context, appears to be synonymous with husband or cohabitee; to be 'a father' requires a residential relationship. The workers in this study rarely comment on the role of non-resident fathers.[11] From the perspective of these service providers, 'stability' and 'consistency' are central to the well-being of children. As one midwife explained:

> There's not a lot of continuity. A lot of the families, a lot of the girls we meet, their parents have split up . . . or they've got problems and they're not actually communicating with their parents . . . and they tend to change partners quite frequently, so they'll come back again with the next pregnancy and then with a different partner again. So there's no real stability.

It is the continued *presence* of men, in whatever shape or form, that workers identify as a positive influence on the lives of women and children (see Chapters 3 and 12, this volume). In the words of another midwife:

> Quite a lot of them are, maybe, on their own with one, maybe two, maybe three [children] so obviously – well I feel they don't perhaps cope quite as well as somebody who's in a stable relationship, getting support from a partner.

Workers' emphasis on 'stability' screens out the possibility of supportive relationships that are neither residential nor permanent. It also begs the question of what men actually *do* in households; it is clear that there are many residential relationships which are not supportive of women. But stability is often conflated with support. While it would be presumptuous of me to deny the possibility that long-term, heterosexual relationships forge deep and insightful understandings of mutual needs, it cannot be assumed. We need to ask what is it about continuity and stability that might axiomatically benefit women and children.[12] It could also be argued that to jettison an unsupportive male partner, despite the longevity of a relationship, might enhance the well-being of a woman and her children. But providers of community health and social services in this study tended to focus on what they perceived to be the primacy of stability. A health visitor in Tarrow commented:

> I think there's a lot of change-over in partners. There's a lot of different names, you know we've got families with three or four children in the same family with different names, and I wonder if that doesn't affect the children.

Whether this health visitor is concerned about the stigma attached to families that do not conform to an ideal child-rearing unit, which includes a heterosexual couple and their biological off-spring, or about the psychological effects on children of having siblings who do not share the same patronym, is difficult to discern from this quote alone. However, both are identified as potential difficulties and again I would argue that neither can be assumed. Concomitant with a notion that single women are less likely to be in supportive relationships than married women, is an idea that change in household composition is automatically detrimental to the well-being of children. Health and social service providers assess the welfare of the families they serve with reference to normative ideas about appropriate child-rearing units, which in this case ideally combines marriage and co-residence with biological *and* social parenthood.

It might be useful at this point to look a little closer at the way in which workers draw on the idiom of 'stability' and the way in which 'unstable' is, on occasion, synonymous with 'chaotic'. Workers sometimes speak of either 'chaotic households' or 'chaotic families', particularly where there is concern about the welfare of children. The term 'chaotic', when applied to families, evokes a sense of constant movement, of impermanence and disorder. These are households perceived to be in constant flux: relationships within them are said to change frequently (often formulated in terms of men 'coming and going'); houses, general practitioners and schools are also frequently changed. If we unpack the notion of 'chaotic' further, it includes ideas about child-rearing practices, and in particular a lack of 'consistency' and/or 'routine'.[13]

It is women as mothers who are more often than not perceived to be responsible for the chaos of their families; it is they who are blamed for being neither 'consistent' in their child-rearing practices nor providing the 'routines' upon which infants are said to thrive. Furthermore, when workers define the needs of children in terms of 'stability', they often describe women as if they were in control of the whereabouts and activities of men. The choices that men exercise over where and with whom they live, their part in what workers are describing as 'instability', the decisions they make to move their household, or to leave partners and children, and to move in with new partners and children, are screened out of the discussion. It is in just such a way that I argue men are *made* invisible.[14]

A further reason workers give for seeing and speaking with mothers rather than fathers is that men are neither interested, nor forthcoming, in issues to do with childcare. One health visitor in Tarrow listed the reasons why she rarely worked with men as fathers: 'Because they [the women] are usually the carers, and more often than not they're single parents, and because the father's perception of childcare is that it is women's work.' Another health visitor, this time in Banton, explained why she worked predominantly with women: 'The majority of men will go out of a room, or whatever, when a health visitor comes . . . children are seen as women's work . . . it's probably one of the main reasons.' From the perspective of workers, men are either not there or, when they are, are uninterested. Again, men are seen as culpable. Workers' views of how men make sense of the domestic scene are often couched in terms of social class. The quotation that follows is from a health visitor in Tarrow:

> And also with it being a very settled community and working class, the men very often feel it's the woman's role to look after the children. Full stop. The men don't really have a lot to do with the children. And, therefore, when the children don't do things that the men think they should, they criticize or probably attack both the wife, for not sorting the children out, and the children, for not doing what the father thinks [they] should be doing.

Comments, such as men 'traditionally' do not take care of children, or that men are 'traditionally' authoritarian, while ostensibly referring to the past, are also idioms of class definition. 'Tradition', in this context, evokes a notion of a 'tight-knit' gendered and raced community with a strict sexual division of labour. An implicit comparison is made with a 'modern', middle-class diaspora where, instead of a pre-given division of labour based on sex, choices are made and strategic decisions taken. The vestiges of a former rigid definition of gender roles, which allocated women to childcare, and men to paid labour, are said to be still in force in places like Banton and Tarrow. One voluntary sector worker explained how she would like to work more closely with men, but perceives the problem as inhering in *their* own old-fashioned perception of fatherhood:

> It's very difficult, I think, to engage the men in – in and around – childcare concerns. I think that the staff would generally hold the

view that that's to do with the role of the traditional – of the traditional roles of men.

For service providers, then, the way in which men perceive their role as fathers is unhelpful. 'Traditional' male roles, which include asserting authority and ownership, while not participating in the day-to-day care of children, are said to persist in Banton and Tarrow. This leads to problems in the relationship between fathers and those providing health and social services, especially when fathers do not appear to value the input of professionals. As one social worker explained:

> I think a lot, not in every case, I think . . . sometimes the man probably doesn't *believe* in social services, doesn't *believe* in health workers and it's hard to work with that. But I think if the male wants to be actively involved then you should encourage that and it's good for everyone really [emphasis added].

Most of the service providers in the study felt that it was their job to encourage and work with men who are interested, and who *want* to play a part in the care of their children. However, the initiative, it would seem, has to come from men themselves. Workers point out that most men in Banton and Tarrow think that childcare is the preserve of women. They also talk about this as a given – as a product of class, custom and history. In conceptualizing men's lack of interest in childcare in terms of class or perhaps 'cultural' differences, service providers abrogate their role in working with men as fathers. This in turn confirms and reinforces the view that childcare is solely a matter for women.

From the perspective of many service providers in this study, residents of Banton and Tarrow were somehow 'behind the times'. While we have no reason to doubt that many men play a highly selective role in domestic work across all sectors of British society, health and social workers' ideas about men in Banton and Tarrow draw on generalizations about the interests of men, and more precisely on stereotypes of working-class, male preoccupations. There is an implicit comparison between working-class and middle-class men in the views of workers. But we need to look carefully at the suggestion that working-class men take *less* responsibility for childcare than middle-class men. Such a statement reveals as much about the relationship between professionals and clients as it does about the relationship between men and women.[15] A health visitor, who had earlier in the interview said she never saw men in Tarrow because they were not interested in issues of childcare, spoke thus about her caseload:

> I do visit quite a few where I do see men and they are very responsible and they take on a very similar role to a lot of women and the interest is the same. But I'd say, on the whole, that wasn't too often where I would see [men]. . . . And you tend also, particularly if it's a working family, you tend to see the man in the first couple of weeks and then that's obviously it if he's gone back to work.

From the perspective of service providers in this study, some men as fathers are present and take an interest (in the work of, for example, midwives and health visitors) but they are few and far between;[16] some men are absent because they are employed; and some men absent themselves predominantly because they do not see it as their place. I want to suggest that in many cases service providers understand the absence of men due to employment as legitimate; these men, in other words, are not willfully absenting themselves from childcare and, furthermore, when they are around, they take the kind of interest of which workers approve. I want to argue that there is a tendency, albeit subtle, for workers to make connections between employment and marriage which congeal into a moral perspective. Hence, unmarried and unemployed fathers are more likely to be associated with the, in this context, *negative* values of 'tradition': that is, 'traditional' male roles which do not include childcare.

I began this section by commenting on a discrepancy between the views of workers in interviews and their experience during a working day. An example from fieldwork will illustrate my point. One Saturday morning I accompanied a community midwife on her home visits, nine in all. Towards the end of the morning I commented that there seemed to be a lot of interested fathers around. The midwife agreed:

> Yes, even girls living on their own in flats – there's only a few that don't have any contact with partners. Even if they're single they still have a partner around. They like to be there when the midwife is there – see what she's up to.

This midwife remarks not only on the presence of men, who do not necessarily live with women and their babies, but also on their curiosity.

In an interview with this same midwife several months before, she had impressed on me the fact that there was a dearth of fathers in these parts. This example might be used to highlight the different occupational niches occupied by midwives and health visitors. It could be argued that midwives, who visit daily for the first ten days after the birth of a child (including weekends) are more likely to come into contact with new fathers than, say, health visitors who, with a much larger caseload, not only visit individual families much less frequently but also visit at a stage when for men the novelty of a new baby has worn off. Similarly, the specific role of social services in child protection, in assessment and in surveillance and policing, will influence the way in which parents welcome, or not, the intervention of social workers. But rather than use this example to explore differences between occupational groups, I wish to draw attention again to the different kinds of data generated through either interviews or conversations during everyday working lives. Workers see men in the abstract as a category of person neither present, nor interested. Individual examples which present evidence contrary to this assumption emerge in response to different questions, in different contexts.

From the perspective of service providers who wish for more appropriate and consistent support for women in the difficult task of tending children and homes, it is men who absent themselves from both parenting itself and from services that focus on the welfare of children. While that might be the case, I have argued that there is also a process in operation whereby men are *made* absent. Workers reiterate that it is beneficial for women and children, as well as for workers, if men are involved in the care of their children. Yet there appears to be no concerted effort to involve them.

I am not advocating, necessarily, that community health and social service providers *should* be working with men, but I am suggesting that we need to look at why, if service providers think it so important to work with men, they do not. The enormous responsibility shouldered by women in the care of families, in Britain at least, means that it is *they* who should influence and inform appropriate and relevant services, and it may be the case that women do not *want* men included – that, instead, they want specialized professional services relevant and appropriate to their needs as mothers.

Indeed, we need look no further than the extent of domestic violence, child abuse and emotional cruelty perpetrated by men in
families for a clear indication that it is crucial for women and children to have access to confidential and safe services. But service
providers are not basing their practice on the explicit needs of
their clients, but rather on assumptions about the division of
labour in households and, significantly, on what they perceive to
be the role of men. For the most part, they are not emphasizing
the fact that women need exclusive and specialized services, but
they are saying that men should be more active in the care of
their children. The two are not, of course, mutually exclusive.
One worker, a community midwife, did speak in interview of her
reservations about the presence of men in antenatal and postnatal
clinics. In answer to the question about whether she saw both
parents, she replied candidly:

> Antenatally? It varies. It varies. I'm almost suspicious if a part-
> ner comes with – this is an awful thing to say – but I have a lot of
> cynicism about a young couple in Banton where the partner
> comes [with her] for a physical. I feel it's an infringement on
> her freedom. . . . I don't see it as . . . say the upper middle-
> class partner attending – has the – it's got the same philosophy
> behind it. Do you know what I mean?
>
> I mean, women never speak openly if they've got the male
> there. Never. They're not as honest.

This midwife identifies the need for services orientated to women,
and what is no doubt the real possibility of men monitoring, or inhibiting, the interactions of their partners. The question is whether
it is proper to attribute such a factor especially – even solely – to the
working classes, and furthermore whether the provision of community health and social services to families ought to be premised on
that possibility. Most other workers talked of the advantages,
rather than disadvantages, of men being present at clinics and meetings with health and social service providers; they also suggest that
it is men who, for a variety of reasons, absent themselves.

This section has explored the view of community health and
social service providers that men as fathers, in two areas of Greater
Manchester, do not consider themselves to be responsible for childcare. They believe, however, that men's commitment to the care of
their children benefits mothers and infants as well as aiding them in
their work. Before going on to look at what happens when service

providers do come into contact with men as fathers, I want to look briefly at the language of child protection. I will suggest that this language again screens out men. It disguises the responsibility of men, on the one hand, for the distress of some women and children and, on the other, for alleviating it.

THE LANGUAGE OF CHILD PROTECTION

In two of the quotations presented above, women as mothers are referred to as 'girls'. There is evidence from the study on which this chapter is based that women are more likely to be referred to as 'girls' if they are single and live on council estates in Banton and Tarrow, than if they are married and live in owner-occupied houses. An explicit example was provided by a community midwife who talked of her concern that the women she felt would benefit most from parentcraft classes were those who did not attend. 'The girls in Tarrow', she argued, are more likely to need parent-craft classes than 'the mothers in Heaton'.[17] Comments often heard from both health visitors and midwives focus on the 'type of girl' who is not motivated to attend clinics or classes.[18] The label 'defaulter' carries with it a number of judgements and assumptions that go beyond the mere non-attendance at clinic – in the same way that a 'beltin' mum', an expression of affirmation I heard on more than one occasion, carries with it the sense of 'good mothers' who heed advice, ask questions and use the services provided appropriately.

I have found the concept of infantilization useful in thinking about the use of 'girls' and 'mums' to refer to women as mothers (Hockey and James, 1993). It is striking, but perhaps not surprising, that young men as fathers are rarely referred to as boys. Numerous examples of the way in which infantilization works through the use of language and through particular forms of communication emerged in this study. Three brief examples, taken from fieldwork, will serve to exemplify the process.

The first finds us in an ante natal clinic held at a GP's surgery. A woman, visibly pregnant, is lying on the couch in the surgery, the midwife has already written on her records her weight and blood pressure. She has palpated the women's abdomen, and asked her how she has been feeling. A male doctor enters the room and greets the woman without looking at her. He is reading her records;

he ignores the midwife. The doctor, without looking up, remarks on her weight gain. He meets her eye for the first time, wags his finger and says, 'You've been a bit naughty.' In the second example, we accompany a health visitor on a home visit. She is trying to elicit whether her client, who has recently given birth, is getting enough rest: 'Are you behaving yourself?' she asks the woman. The woman averts her eyes, looks sheepish, perhaps there is defiance in her shrug. The third example could be taken from any one of a number of postnatal visits, carried out by any one of a number of community midwives: 'I'm just going to check your tummy,' explains the midwife before palpating, with assuredness, the abdomen of a women who has recently given birth.

Ongoing communicative practice is complex: the choice of idioms, tone of voice and pattern of intonation communicate a variety of meanings and can be interpreted in a number of ways. There is no one-to-one correlation between a communicative act and a meaning. Rather than as processes of infantilization, wagging fingers, questions about behaviour and words like 'tummies' might be interpreted as part of a attempts to reject formality and as part of a process of forging intimate relationships between carer and cared for. I presented some of these thoughts back to workers who participated in the study and several workers, on different occasions, challenged my interpretation. One health visitor argued that the use of 'girls' is a term of affection which connotes familiarity. She gave the example of her own use of the expression, and suggested that I, likewise, would say things like 'going out with the girls'.[19] Other workers pointed out that reference to 'mums', as in 'one of my mums', or 'she's a beltin' mum', connotes informality and, again, familiarity. Similarly, 'ladies' is used in preference to 'women', which is thought to be too harsh, too distant and too formal. Although this is not the place to explore these linguistic and semantic complexities further, it is worth noting that a term of reference, or address, is but one element in a cluster of interlinked ideas that construct a composite person. And while 'girls' is most certainly used in those ways that workers suggest, 'girls' also incorporate ideas about age, marital status and social class.

The protection of children, of course, consists of much more than a particular discourse. There are children who are mistreated and suffer at the hands of their carers, both within institutions of the family and of the state. I confine my discussion here, however, to the language of 'child protection', and focus on the way in which, as in the example of terms of reference discussed above, idioms of 'child protection' are also marked by ambivalence.

In the initial stage of an investigation of child abuse, it is vital, argued one social worker, to support the 'non-abusing parent'. The prognosis for the child, as well as for the relationship between the child and 'non-abusing parent', is thought to be much better if support is provided from professionals right from the start. Broadly speaking, support in this context means helping the parent come to terms and deal with the allegations. Scarce resources, however, mean that such support is rarely forthcoming. In fact 'non-abusing parents' are more often than not part of the investigation. Whereas most sexual, and much physical, abuse of children is perpetrated by men, assessments are continually made of the ability and capability of women 'to protect' their children. The tension between 'support' and 'blame' is palpable. One social worker explained she was 'not into' blaming women for the sexual abuse of children, a view reiterated by several other workers, but many workers did express the view, more or less explicitly, that women fail to protect their children (see also Graham, 1979; Marsh, 1987; Milner, 1993). This is not the place to explore, in the detail it deserves, the difficult and complex assessments made by professionals in child protection procedures, and while I do not wish to play down the very real difficulties and dilemmas of social workers who are faced daily with the effects of cruelty and violence towards children, it is salutary to look at the discourse of child protection. I present a number of key features of this discourse in the form of a list. The list is crude and by no means exhaustive. I present it to indicate some of the commonly used idioms of social service providers in this study which, I argue, screen out men.

1 While there needs to be a balance between the *rights* of parents and children, ultimately the responsibility of social services is to the child; it is the child who is the *client*.
2 Mothers *abandon* or *reject* their children. Fathers leave, or are just 'not around'.
3 There are features which typify *sex-abusing families*.
4 A *family assessment* needs to be carried in order to assess, among other things, *parenting skills*.
5 One aim of social services is to *rehabilitate families*.

Idioms of family, like those of parent, are gender neutral. Perhaps they are meant to flag relationships rather than individuals, and perhaps they are meant to draw our attention to child-rearing units as systems,[20] but, at the same time, they divert attention away from the fact that much physical, and most sexual, abuse of children is carried out by men. As Marilyn French poignantly comments, language is used to obscure, on the one hand, who is actually taking care of children and, on the other, who is responsible for their impoverishment (1992: 139). I want to argue that ideas about 'sex-abusing families' or 'family rehabilitation' are part of the process whereby men are made absent. In the pursuit of gender-neutral language, the role of men is minimized. At the same time, men receive messages from health and social service workers, predominantly women, that the domain of childcare is not theirs, a message which may, or may not, resonate with what they already assume. What happens, then, when the message is at odds with what men do? What happens when men *are* actively concerned in the care of children?

MOTHERS AND FATHERS: DIFFERENT NEEDS

The health visitors in Tarrow run a clinic once a week in the health centre in which they are based. The clinic is held in a warm, light, colourful room. Mobiles hang from the ceiling, and friezes line the walls. One afternoon, with one health visitor on duty and a community medical officer (CMO) available in a different room, twenty-two infants were brought to the clinic and duly weighed and measured. Two babies were accompanied by their fathers only, and four by both parents. One man accompanied his partner as far as the door, and said he would return later; one woman came with her mother, and another with a friend. The remaining babies were brought to the clinic by unaccompanied mothers. Conversations between the health visitor and carers centred predominantly on three themes: feeding, rashes and teething. Babies are undressed and dressed again, some are taken to see the CMO, all have their weight recorded in parent-held records.

One of the unaccompanied fathers explains to the health visitor: 'I'm worried; no, I want to *ask* about this rash'. The rash is on his baby's stomach. The health visitor studies the rash, and asks him: 'Has mum changed her washing powder recently?'. He shrugs. He thinks. He cannot answer the question. 'How the hell should I know?' he asks loudly, brashly, for the benefit of the audience, thereby, retrieving his dignity. The health visitor explains about dry skin and eczema, that many babies get it and most outgrow it.

Would it be too far-fetched to imagine that this man left the clinic with the impression that, somehow, the clinic and its workings are the domain of women, rather than men? This incident serves to illustrate the way in which men constantly receive messages from health and social service professionals that childcare and housework are not primarily their concern. When service providers do come across men who are active in the domestic sphere, they commonly joke with them to the effect that their partners have got them 'well trained'.

Talking to me, workers were positive about fathers they knew. They commented in glowing terms about men who show concern about and interest in their children: qualities which go unremarked when exhibited by women. I draw on three examples from fieldwork to show how the needs of women as mothers and of men as fathers are perceived differently by workers.

Accompanying a health visitor in Tarrow on her home visits, I visited the home of a man whose wife was in hospital, diagnosed with severe postnatal depression. He was temporarily caring for his two children and young baby alone. The health visitor asked him about the children, how he was coping with the baby, and if he needed anything. She had told me before the visit that he had refused the offer of home-care services. Before we left, the health visitor asked the man if he was 'managing' with the washing and ironing; the implication being that, if not, she would arrange for help. He continued to maintain that he was fine: he needed nothing and was coping well.

In this study at least, such a question was rarely, if ever, addressed to a woman. Indeed, a woman's capability as a mother and a person is assessed through her work in the home, which includes washing and ironing clothes. In interview, workers were invited to choose those things that they thought might improve the welfare of children in Banton or Tarrow. They were presented with a list that included nursery provision, meeting places, public transport, and help with housework. Not one of the service providers interviewed selected 'help with housework' from this list. They were then asked if any were *not* relevant in Banton or Tarrow. While the majority of respondents said that all the items on the list would benefit families with young children, those who did identify one or more as irrelevant invariably pointed to 'help with housework'. The ambiguity of the question may be partly responsible for such a response; for example, several workers pointed out that housework is not something that *directly* affects the health and welfare of children.[21] Many service providers appeared to be making a distinction between those things they perceive as having a direct effect on children and those things which might be helpful, but are not crucial. Some offered comments such as 'You don't *have* to do your housework, do you?', or 'I don't think housework makes much difference: better not be or mine's very deprived', which underlines the ambiguity of the question. Other remarks, however, suggest that workers think the carers of children (that is, women) *ought* to do their own housework, and that to provide help with it is not necessarily useful. During the interviews, comments such as 'maybe you could help to teach them how to do it, [but] not to do it for them', '[w]e'd *all* like help with housework', and 'I don't think anybody needs help with that unless they are lazy', were recorded. There is evidence, then, that from some service-provider perspectives, housework is not only the preserve of women but also an activity that is a compulsory part of their motherhood on which moral assessments are made. For men housework is optional; they can be offered help with housework without it reflecting on their abilities as a father, or indeed as a person.

The second example comes from the work of a voluntary organization which attaches individual volunteers to families deemed to be 'in need' of support. One of the major roles of volunteers is to 'befriend' clients, and the recruitment campaign of the organization is obviously aimed at women as mothers. Organizers attempt to match volunteers and clients from the information they have of each. The perceived needs of clients, as well as what clients and volunteers are perceived to have in common – for example, age and gender, and the types of households in which they live – are criteria used to match volunteers to clients.

During fieldwork, I was able to attend the training sessions held for new volunteers, and at that time there was one male and six female trainees. During the period of training, trainee volunteers were matched with 'families'. The one man had been attached by the organizers to the father of two young children whose wife had died the year before. Several months after the training sessions, I spoke with him at length about his work with the family. He was still visiting them, but less often than initially. He explained that the man had never really talked to him, nor used him as a confidant, which is what he had expected his role to be. Instead, he baby-sat one evening a week, and sometimes for an hour or two during the day while the man went shopping. None of the female volunteers, as far as I am aware, provided a similar service to the mothers they visited. Female volunteers did take children out. In one case, where a mother of five children was in hospital, the volunteer took the children to the park on Saturday mornings to allow the father to catch up with the housework. A different volunteer, attached to a lone-parent family where the mother worked, looked after the child one or two afternoons a week, while she worked. Volunteers, as noted above, are predominantly married women, some with young and others adult children, and the services they can offer are, as might be supposed, constrained by their own domestic responsibilities (Edwards and Popay, forthcoming). Hence it is not necessarily possible for them to offer to babysit in the evening, but I think we miss the point if we only focus on the pragmatics of the relationship. Practical concerns are not the only considerations brought into play when the needs of clients are assessed and negotiated. The organizers and volunteers make assessments not only of the kind of services that individual clients require, but also of what women as mothers ought to expect. Child-minding may be perceived as a legitimate request, but it has to be for legitimate reasons, such as, in the examples just cited, during crises and for work. It is not considered legitimate for women to request child-minding for shopping or pleasure.

This is exemplified further in the next example taken from a meeting of the panel responsible for allocating local authority nursery places. The meeting was organized by social services and attended by nursery staff as well as a social worker and a health visitor. It is held regularly to discuss and make decisions about the applications for nursery places. Demand for local authority nursery places is far greater than the places available; in the words of one panel member: 'to supply the need in this area we would need another couple of nurseries'. Given the discrepancy between the demand for nursery places and their availability, criteria are constantly being drawn upon to distinguish between those 'in need' of a nursery place and those not. While workers recognize the arbitrary nature of such criteria, in that they realize there are many more young children in Banton who would benefit from nursery places than at present do, they are nevertheless required to impose some priority on the various applications. A criterion for decision made explicit in the meeting I attended was that decisions should be based on the needs of the child rather than the parent; in other words, places should be offered to *children* who might benefit from time spent at the nursery, rather than to *parents* who might benefit. Hence children who were deemed to be 'in need' of 'stimulation', or with identifiable and diagnosed 'special needs', or those diagnosed as 'failing to thrive', were clear candidates for a place at the nursery. It was less clear whether places should be offered to allow lone mothers to work or to offer lone mothers some respite. Perhaps if lone mothers were ill they could be offered a temporary nursery place for their child until the crisis had passed.

The panel discussed an application by a lone father for a nursery place for his 2-year-old daughter. The social worker had been instrumental in helping the man gain custody of his child. She voiced her concern that he should not be given preferential treatment merely because he was a man, and the ensuing discussion focused on whether a child, in similar circumstances (also adequately cared for) but living with her mother rather than her father, would be offered a place. The consensus was that she would not. The social worker argued that the man does not need a nursery place but does need 'a babysitter now and again, so he can go out for a pint'. Such a need was rarely, if ever, presented as a priority for women as mothers. Although several members of the social service team in Banton were concerned with the lack of babysitting facilities for mothers, such concern was mostly couched in terms which focused on the well-being of the child; for example, a fear was often expressed that without appropriate babysitting services, children were being left alone, or with under-age babysitters, and were consequently 'at risk'. In discussing the needs of women who live alone with children, a babysitting service, although not totally irrelevant from the perspective of service providers, is low on a list of priorities. Higher on the list are issues such as parenting skills (see Edwards, 1995; Edwards and Popay, 1994). To put it crudely, men may be better parents for having time out, and women for learning more about the management and development of children.

ENDNOTE

Service providers in this study argue that men should take a more active part in the care of their children. The provision of community health and social services has – understandably, given that women are usually the primary carers – been directed and geared towards women as mothers. Workers argue that men are unwilling to involve themselves in childcare, which includes interacting with community health and welfare services. However, this chapter has argued that when men do interact with service providers, they are often presented with messages that reinforce and reiterate the idea that the care of children is best and more appropriately carried out by women. It is clearly the case that women as mothers should have, and in some contexts need, access to confidential and caring welfare services, but it is also clear that many women would like the fathers of their children (whether married, cohabiting or neither) to play a part in their children's upbringing. This is unlikely to develop, given men's proved reluctance in the field, unless services are also sensitive to that need and actively promote communication with men. This chapter contends that there is a need in late-twentieth-century Britain to take seriously gendered relationships in the provision of health and social services and, furthermore, to dwell on the constraints and pressures that women as workers face when dealing with men as clients.

From this study, it is clear that we need further research on what men want, *vis-à-vis* fatherhood. We need to know more about the differences that class, employment and marital status have on the roles and practices of men as fathers, and consequently to find ways – if this is what men and women want as parents – of including them as co-parents and as equally responsible as women for the welfare of their children. A tension to which we keep returning, and which lies at the heart of this chapter and at the root of the ambivalence expressed about men by the service providers in this study, is expressed thus by Ann Snitow: 'On the one hand, *sacred* motherhood. On the other, a wish – variously expressed – for this special identity to wither away' (Snitow, 1990: 35). There is a tension between providing services which are sensitive to the specific needs of women, and services which aim to shift a dominant and inhibiting attitude that childcare is, and ought to be, the exclusive domain of women. Perhaps that tension is necessary, and there is a need for services to look both ways. If this is the case, then more attention must be paid to the ways in which men are to be included as co-parents and equally responsible for the well-being of children and family relationships.

ACKNOWLEDGEMENTS

I am very grateful to the workers who tolerated my presence and questions, gave me their time and patience, and taught me much more than this chapter reveals. My thanks also to Jennie Popay, Cathy Pratt, Patty Peach and Patrick Crozier for their help and support at different times during this project.

NOTES

1 Both the Child Support and the Children Act underline the physiological basis of fatherhood.

2 I observed the impact of this ruling just after the Act was implemented. I accompanied to court a social worker who was aiming to place an emergency care order on three children. A man, the father of one of the children, had been informed of the court proceedings. The mother of the child had not been told that he had been notified. On seeing her ex-partner for the first time in ten years, she assumed he must be in court for a different reason. She was shocked to see him again in these circumstances. Meanwhile, he told the social worker later that he had attended court because he had understood the notification as a court order demanding his presence. Both the man and woman were extremely uncomfortable and unhappy to be in each other's presence at what was already an extremely stressful time, particularly for the woman.

3 This is again a rather gloomy analysis and might look different were it to contain the voices of new parents themselves. Nevertheless, a first draft of this chapter was written during the time of the Vauxhall (or was it the Peugeot?) 'new man', who shows his sensitivity and fatherly devotion by taking the new baby for a ride in the new car in the early hours of the new day.

4 Semi-structured interviews with 84 workers were conducted and followed by a period of ethnographic fieldwork with each of the occupational groups in the study. The researcher spent between four and seven weeks with members of each organization, accompanying individual workers during their working day and sometimes at the end of it: hence time was spent with workers in, for example, their offices and cars, in clinics, courts and pubs, as well as in the homes of their clients.

5 The place names are disguised following conventions of confidentiality.

6 Use of the term 'girls' in this context is, of course, significant, and will be returned to later (see also Edwards, 1995; Edwards and Popay, 1994).

7 This midwife recognizes the difficulty entailed in assuming that young women have the support of their parents. Janet Finch (1989) has demonstrated clearly the way in which help and aid from kin cannot be predicted.

8 I am reminded of the way in which the ex-miners quoted in Chapter 9, this volume, describe housework as 'helping out' their wives, and the way in which the women describe the helpfulness, or not, of their husbands.

9 Unless they are single fathers; but then, as we shall see, the needs of single fathers are perceived to be different from the needs of single mothers.

10 Although men may be involved in the care of their children it is not necessarily in the financial interest of women with unemployed partners and reliant on state benefits and local authority housing to cohabit. An extremely interesting and evocative ethnographic study of caring and coping among poor African-American families in the United States in the 1970s illuminates this point despite its focus on an earlier decade and a different continent (Stack 1974).

11 There has been little research exploring the role of non-cohabiting fathers.

12 I am reminded, here, of the priority placed recently on 'continuity of care' in maternity services, which begs the question of how the 'continuity' of what women perceive as poor care can be beneficial.

13 'Consistency' and 'routine' are things which many service providers identify as qualities of child-rearing which children need if they are to 'thrive'.

14 It would, of course, be patronizing, as well as incorrect, to portray women with whom the service providers in this study work as either passive or lacking in autonomy. The choices and decisions that women make, whether poor or wealthy, about sexual relationships and cohabitation are complex, and this is neither the place nor am I the person to attempt an analysis of them. However, from the perspective of women as mothers, while it may be in their and their children's interest to change partners, or GPs, or homes, their decisions are not made in a vacuum. Notable and extensive research has identified some of the constraints under which many women with young children live and which influences the decisions they make (see, for example, Oakley, 1980a, 1980b; Graham, 1982).

15 It seems to me that research on men and childcare which looks carefully at class, race, sexuality and age is long overdue.

16 There is an assumption in these views that communication with health professionals is a good indication of the level of support men give women and their interest or involvement in childcare.

17 Heaton is a pseudonym for a relatively affluent area of the city consisting mostly of owner-occupied houses.

18 This is a highly contentious and intriguing observation which requires further research, especially in the light of comments from several workers in this study that they, when pregnant or with young children, rarely attended maternity or child guidance clinics.

19 The example of 'going out with the girls' refers to socializing with peers, friends or colleagues: with those who are perceived, in a sense, to be equal.

20 Hilary Graham wrote, in 1979, of a DHSS paper entitled 'Reducing the risk: safer pregnancy and childbirth', that:

> [The] image of childrearing is reflected in the vocabulary employed: in the avoidance of sexually specific terms like 'mother' and 'father' and the introduction of the more androgynous concept of 'parent'. . . . However, when we look beyond the statements of principle and consider the proposed strategies, a rather different – and atavistic – picture emerges. The father, far from being a co-partner in childrearing, fades back into his traditional role on the periphery of family life.

It is depressing to be writing of the same thing today, although it is to the credit of Graham that she drew attention to such phenomena sixteen years ago.

21 The only other item which emerged in reponse to this question was 'improved transport'; again, this reponse may be attributed to the ambiguity of the question.

REFERENCES

Boden, R. and Childs, M. (1996) 'Paying for procreation: child support arrangements in the UK', *Feminist Legal Studies*, 4(2): 130–57.

Community Care (1990) 'The guide to the Children Act 1989' (19 April).

Crouch, M. and Manderson, L. (1993) *New Motherhood: Cultural and Personal Transition in the 1980s*, Amsterdam: Gordon & Breach Science Publishers.

Edwards, J. (1995) '"Parenting skills": views of community health and social service providers about the needs of their "clients"', *Journal of Social Policy*, 24(2): 237–59.

Edwards, J. and Popay, J. (1994) 'Contradictions of support and self help: views from providers of community health and social services', *Health and Social Care*, 2: 31–40.

—— (forthcoming) 'Women, social support and the voluntary sector of health and social care'.

Finch, J. (1983) 'Dividing the rough and the respectable: working-class women and pre-school playgroups', in E. Gamarnikow, D. Morgan, J. Purvis and D. Taylorson (eds) *The Public and the Private*, Aldershot: Heinemann.

—— (1989) *Family Obligations and Social Change*, Cambridge: Polity Press.

French, M. (1992) *The War against Women*, London: Penguin.

Graham, H. (1979) '"Prevention and health: every mother's business", a comment on child health policies in the 1970s', in C. Harris (ed.) *The Sociology of the Family: New Directions for Britain, Sociological Review*, monograph 28.

—— (1982) 'Perceptions of parenthood' *Health Education Journal*, 41(4).

Hockey, J. and James, A. (1993) *Growing Up and Growing Old: Ageing and Dependency in the Life Course*, London: Sage.

Marsh, P. (1987) 'Social work and fathers – an exclusive practice', in C. Lewis and M. O'Brien (eds) *Reassessing Fatherhood: New Observations on Fathers and the Modern Family*, London: Sage.

Milner, J. (1993) 'A disappearing act: the different career paths of fathers and mothers in child protection investigations', *Critical Social Policy*, 38: 48–63.

Mullings, L. (1995) 'Households headed by women: the politics of race, class and gender', in F. Ginsburg and R. Rapp (eds) *Conceiving the New World Order: The Global Politics of Reproduction*, Berkeley: University of California Press.

Oakley, A. (1980a) *Women Confined: Towards a Sociology of Childbirth*, Oxford: Martin Robertson.

—— (1980b) *Becoming a Mother*, Oxford: Martin Robertson.

—— (1993) *Essays on Women, Medicine and Health*, Edinburgh: Edinburgh University Press.

O'Brien, M. and Lewis, C. (eds) (1987) *Reassessing Fatherhood: New Observations on Fathers and the Modern Family*, London: Sage.

Ruddick, S. (1990) 'Thinking about fathers', in M. Hirsch and E. Fox-Keller (eds) *Conflicts in Feminism*, London: Routledge.

Snitow, A. (1990) 'A gender diary', in M. Hirsch and E. Fox-Keller (eds) *Conflicts in Feminism*, London: Routledge.

Stack, C. (1974) *All our Kin: Strategies for Survival in a Black Community*, New York: Harper & Row.

Chapter 11

Redundant men and overburdened women
Local service providers and the construction of gender in ex-mining communities

Bella Dicks, David Waddington and Chas Critcher

'I remember the familiar smell of pit clothes. I recall clothes warming, spread round an open coal grate, always ready for the wearer. . . . My mother, always a slave to her men and the pit, washed and patched those clothes regularly, and just as often scrubbed the backs of daily washed bodies. 'My best suit', my father would announce, his eyes looking at me. He knew I hated those clothes, dulling the grate, dirtying the hearth. 'Best suit', he'd say, preparing to go to work, 'What do you say, Peg? For without these', and he paused so that his words could take effect 'without these clothes, there wouldn't be any others.'

(B. Walters, 1986)

This is how Barbara Walters, a miner's wife and daughter, and an activist in the 1986 strike in the South Wales Afan Valley, described her childhood memories as she contemplated the closure of the pit that had provided work for her husband, her father, and his father before that. The pit clothes lying beside the fire, worn by the men and maintained by the women, symbolized the provision of the family wage, at a time when the mines provided work for thousands of men, and the role of women was to service the family. In the present-day mining community, women continue to service the family, but under very different conditions. Since the end of the 1984/85 coal dispute, the vast majority of the country's deep-mine collieries have closed down, with the rump newly privatized. In South Yorkshire, a handful of coalfield communities still hung on to their pit at the time of our fieldwork, but, with workforces whittled down to a quarter of their pre-strike size in the run-up to privatization, the number of mining jobs available for men was already severely restricted. By the 1990s, to continue Barbara

Walters' metaphor, it seemed the pit clothes had been consigned to the rubbish bin.

The aim of this chapter is to consider how various health, welfare and education service providers comprehend mining communities as they are now constituted, and, in particular, how they view the question of gender relations in the context of the restructuring of the local labour market. Data from interviews conducted with a range of local teachers, education and welfare officers, health visitors, practice nurses, GPs, social workers and youth workers will be examined in order to illustrate how providers interpret the sources of stress and difficulty in the localities, and their understanding of what support is available.[1] These interviews took place in four communities: community A, where the pit had been closed for 18 months at the time of the research; community B, where it had been closed for 6 months; community C, where it was still open, but its future was threatened; and community D, where its future was at the time considered relatively safe. In all four communities, regardless of whether the local pit was open or closed, providers' observations pointed to the same set of concerns.[2] It will become clear that the starting point of analysis in providers' accounts is the fact of male job loss: from this phenomenon is seen to flow a river of social deprivation. The difficulties begin and end with men, since the communities' problems are perceived to stem from the loss of the 'family wage'. However, it is women who carry the burden of male joblessness, through their continued role as family carers and servicers. What providers see confronting them is largely a community of men as frustrated redundants and women as harassed housewives, with children caught in the middle of a family context characterized by confusion and dysfunction. In the midst of this bleak picture, providers look to the extended family as a source of support.

In the first section of this chapter, we look at providers' accounts of the sources of stress in the community, and how these are framed by a particular model of gender relations. This model, we shall argue, derives from providers' implicit endorsement of the traditional gender division of labour in the family, which they understand as functional in a number of ways. In the second section, we examine how providers conceptualize the informal support that exists in the community, and investigate further the effects of women's and men's traditional positioning within these networks. We shall offer support for the view – for example, Finch (1989) –

that welfare policy relies heavily on traditional feminine identity, through the unrewarded caring work performed by women in their traditional roles. While providers value these roles for their function in supporting the family, men are no longer assigned a role at all. Providers view masculine identity in terms of the bread-winner function; when that function can no longer be fulfilled, the position of men within the family is felt to be problematic. Although unable to provide the family wage, unemployed men are not yet understood as carers, so their presence in the home is evaluated negatively. Providers tend to channel their efforts to supporting women's caring roles, and identify a return to 'real' jobs (that is, for men) as the palliative the community requires.

SOURCES OF STRESS AND GENDER RELATIONS

Then and now

In 1975 the sociologist Martin Bulmer described the typical mining village as a place of 'communal social relationships' with 'a shared history of living and working in one place over a long period of time'. This produced a 'mutual aid characteristic in adversity and . . . [an] inward-looking focus on the locality, derived from occupational homogeneity and social and geographical isolation from the rest of society' (Bulmer, 1975: 88). This image of the mining community, particularly its focus on 'mutual aid', has proved extremely enduring in the popular mind, and was continu-ally evoked by providers as they contemplated the current situation facing the communities in which they worked. As one particularly nostalgic GP made especially clear, looking back with regret to his early days in community A, the major thread running through providers' accounts was an explicit comparison between the past and the present:

> I came here in 1966 when this was really an old-fashioned pit vil-lage, where the patients were miners and all the families were related, and there was a considerable family spirit. It was all very interesting. It was honest, working class people, their houses were clean and I was on first name terms with them. I had a very happy relationship with them.

Along with the 'clean houses' – maintained, of course, by an invisi-ble army of unpaid women like Barbara Walters' mother – came a vigorous community spirit of mutual aid, as a fellow GP in community B described:

> In the old days when the coal mine employed 2,000 people, most of the people down each street had at least one person in the household working down the pit, and sometimes two or three, and the generations before those had worked down the pit. So there were strong ties along the street – everybody more or less knew something about every house. It did give rise to a sense of community. Everybody knew each other and everybody helped each other, and everybody knew what was going on.

Now, however, times had changed for this doctor:

> There are now increasing social problems. As I say, we have all these unmarried mothers on the increase, which is partly a result of the benefit system because they're financially better off if they don't get married. It's creating problems for the future, because children who grow up not having a stable mother and father relationship – some cope very well, and others don't cope so well and the children become hooligans by the age of ten.

Underpinning this narrative of decline is a structured opposition between the current social profile of the community, and an 'ideal-type', rooted in the past, against which the present state of disintegration is measured. Although other service providers were perhaps less overtly nostalgic, the community of yesterday remained very much a reference point for their current assessments. In particular, as we shall see, providers' assessments of the decline in community well-being turned on the loss of the family wage, previously provided by men in their traditional breadwinner role. In what follows, we shall attempt to unravel some of the gender issues involved in these changes from the providers' points of view.

Male redundancy: the construction of men as workers and women as carers

Service providers identified the role of male job loss as the catalyst for a range of problems encountered among their client groups. Their concerns tended to cluster around two areas: an increase in poverty and its various effects both on families' material well-being and on community crime; and an increase in stress and psychological or behavioural problems in both children and adults. This chapter will focus on the latter. As much of the literature on the effects of unemployment has shown, its social consequences cannot be reduced to the single issue of material well-being. Instead, a range of features, such as lack of structured time, loss of status, loss of social networks and so on – have been shown to be significant elements in the widely noted increase in stress experienced by the unemployed – see Warr (1987) for a review of this extensive literature. Providers interviewed were, on the whole, very conscious of these extra dimensions, attributing to them a wide range of negative effects in their dealings with community members.

In their considerations of the effects of unemployment, providers were exclusively concerned with the ramifications of *male* job loss. To a certain extent, this preoccupation emerges from the terms of the project itself, in that the project's explicit agenda concerned the effects of restructuring in a male-dominated industry. However, service providers were dealing with a client group that was by no means confined to mining or ex-mining families, and interview questioning was deliberately not confined to the issue of mining redundancy *per se*. It was providers' understandings of the causes and nature of stress in general that questions sought to access. Yet the possible effects of female redundancy, or the rigours and demands of women's employment conditions on both women and their partners, were largely absent from the providers' accounts of the determinants of stress.

This neglect cannot be accounted for by the historic absence of women from the labour force in mining communities. In our survey of 400 miners, ex-miners and their partners, almost exactly 50 per cent of the women were in paid employment. More women with non-mining partners were in paid work than those whose partners were still in mining (57 per cent as opposed to 42 per cent), suggesting that more and more women turn to paid work as the mining industry declines.[3] The vast majority (71 per cent) of women in paid employment worked fewer than 31 hours per week, but this still leaves one-third who were in full-time employment. Of those who had been employed in the past, some had been made redundant (15 per cent), some had stopped due to illness (26 per cent) and others had left to look after young children (51 per cent). None of these, including, arguably, the last, should be considered a voluntary withdrawal from employment. Most of the paid work for women was concentrated in the service sector – particularly in

caring, catering and sales – but, even though these were jobs characterized by low pay and demanding conditions, it was clear from our
subsequent interview data that women were considerably attached
to them. What these data, in fact, show, is that women's employment experiences, both negative and positive, were significant factors in their own psychological well-being, and that redundancy
itself, however occasioned, could be just as stressful for women as
it was for men (cf. Coyle, 1984; Martin and Wallace, 1984).

However, as we have seen, neither women's redundancy and
unemployment nor their employment experiences figured significantly in providers' explanations for women's stress. On the other
hand, many noted that women were now increasingly in paid
employment, as a health visitor in community C observed: 'Quite
a few of the middle-aged women here work and their husbands
don't. It's a reversal of roles, actually. If anybody works in the
village, it's more the women who are working, and the husbands
haven't got jobs.' However, the increasing importance of the
female wage to the family did not lead providers to focus on
women as workers – whether redundant or employed. The providers we interviewed, of course, were predominantly concerned
with the issue of *family* welfare. We shall see in what follows that
providers' implicit understanding of the determinants of family
psychological health rests on a model of employed father and
non-employed mother. This may well divert attention away from
women as independent participants in the wider restructuring of
the labour market. Since the roots of family problems are identified
in the loss of the male wage, women tend to be seen as largely
passive recipients of stress from this single factor.

Male redundancy and the traditional model of masculinity

The almost exclusive focus on loss of the male wage can arguably
also be attributed to the nature of colliery work itself, which, in
relation to other manual jobs, is heavily imbued with connotations
of strength, danger, dignity, pride and the presence of strong union
activity, thereby constituting a source of considerable working-class
masculine status (Brown, 1985). Social workers in community B
observed the difference in the quality of jobs currently available:

SOCIAL WORKER 1   The work that is available is so obviously differ-
    ent from working in an industry like coal mining. You just can't

compare it – kind of supermarket jobs, driving jobs, that's the sort of thing that would be available, say, if you were prepared to move around the area. It's just completely different.

SOCIAL WORKER 2   They're nothing jobs, really. They could be here today and gone tomorrow. There's no sort of vocational tradition to it.

It is necessary to recognize that the loss of this specific 'vocation' is understood by providers not only in employment terms, but in cultural terms as well (we use the term 'culture' to interpret those aspects of providers' talk that indicate an acknowledgement of shared values and a particular way of life). The type of redundancy under discussion is one that comes pre-packaged, as it were, with a set of cultural meanings which belong to a traditional masculine paradigm, and thus providers tended to focus on the damage done to a whole *way of life* when the pit closes. This way of life is explicitly gendered, since it was understood to rest on a fundamental and sharply defined division of labour in the family between men's role as providers and women's role as servicers. Now that the family wage was no longer provided by men, the continuing cultural currency of the male breadwinner ethic was identified by providers as a major obstacle to adaptation, and one which specifically created problems for women. The health visitor quoted earlier goes on to say:

> You've got a tradition where the men work, the men are the breadwinners, and the wives stay at home, and I think there are going to be a lot of problems with men coming to terms with redundancy. The main point of tension is that the wife is going out to work and the man's at home, which is a real bash to his ego. They've been used to going out and having money, and then they're suddenly at home, and they don't know what to do.

The focus here is on the damage done to traditional masculine *self-esteem* when the redundancy occurs. This is felt to unleash a whole series of tensions in the family realm. This exchange between two workers from the childcare social work team in community B illustrates the nature of such tensions:

SOCIAL WORKER 1   From the point of view of families, the effect of losing the breadwinner could, in the short term, perhaps not show too much because of the redundancy money. But in the long term loss of breadwinner of the family is going to develop the sort of classic symptoms of changing the whole family dynamics.

SOCIAL WORKER 2   You see, the macho man will find it very hard to take on the role of maybe hoovering up and things like that while his wife works at the supermarket.

In this way, providers' interpretations of the effects of unemployment were consistently framed by one common-sense reference point: that family problems arise from the loss of men's role as family provider, and from the strain on women's caring roles induced by this. In this sense, then, 'redundancy' is seen by providers not only in terms of non-employment, but also in terms of masculine identity – the redundancy of the traditional male breadwinner role.

In general, then, in our providers' accounts, the question of male employment redundancy was equated with a wider cultural redundancy, involving profound repercussions for masculinity, and for the community as a whole. Because the source of masculine identity was located in the breadwinner role, men were understood to suffer a profound psychological *loss* on becoming unemployed. Men were stressed and frustrated not only because of the condition of unemployment per se, but also because of its attendant consequences for their masculine identity. Since women were seen as emotional carers in the family, men's redundancy was seen as a problem which women had to deal with, in terms of the indirect effects it exercised on their ability to perform their own traditional roles. In fact, as we pointed out at the beginning, the issue of male redundancy was seen by providers as being a problem for *women*, and one explanation for this certainly lay in providers' feelings that women were on the receiving end of a traumatized masculinity. In this sense, women were seen as having to cope with the difficulties imposed by men. The rest of this section will show the extent to which, to use the words of McKee and Bell (1985), *his* unemployment is seen as *her* problem (and a problem for children).

Male redundancy: a problem for women and children

Reduced income – a problem for women

First, women are understood to have responsibility for the family purchases. Men's own potential worries over finances were hardly mentioned in comparison with the anxiety women were felt to be under. One GP in community C expressed this in a rather blunt way:

> I envisage quite a few problems for younger miners who can't get jobs now. As I say, it will be the wives that will be trying to balance the books, and who'll be in this surgery wanting tranquillisers, and counselling and seeing the CPN [community psychiatric nurse].

The difficulties of balancing the family budget were seen as resulting in considerable stress for women, which providers saw manifesting itself in psychological problems such as heavy drinking. This account, from an education and welfare officer in community D makes explicit the point that it is women who are at the sharp end of money worries:

> It's really hard work to manage on benefits and to have any kind of life at all. It means whoever's dealing with the family budget has to really work at that and seek out cheaper things, and really work at preparing economical meals that will feed a family. . . . More often than not it's the women doing that. And more often than not the number of women who are heavy drinkers is very worrying.

The root of the problem in these accounts is that, after male redundancy, women's role as family servicers is made more difficult, as the practice nurse in community C describes:

> After redundancy, men still carry on their lives as before. They go out fishing and to the pubs. They do their own thing, and the wife is still left as they would have been if the husband had been working, but they just haven't got the finance. That is the added burden. They've got to try and make ends meet, but they haven't got the support there.

What these accounts suggest is that the problem is not so much that it is women's role to ensure that meals arrive on the table, but that women are carrying out this role in an impoverished situation.

Men's presence in the home – a problem for women

The second source of stress identified by providers was the transferral of male time from place of employment to the domestic sphere.

After redundancy, the traditional demarcation of time and space in the household was disrupted by the extended male presence in the home, and women's work in the home was made significantly more difficult. This is how one of the GPs in community A put it:

> Women do have the greater burden. It's partly because there is an attitude, particularly amongst some of the older miners, that the chap goes out to work and he earns his money, and the wife sits at home preparing the dinner, washing the clothes and looking after the kids. When the man comes home after a hard day's work deep underground where it's hot and sweaty, he then goes out for a drink at night, stays in the pub until 11 o'clock at night and then goes home. Some of the men who have taken redundancy have still got that attitude, except they stay in bed until 11 o'clock, and then they get under their wife's feet. This causes a lot of stress. It's not generally the women's fault, it's just the way the men have been brought up – he's been put into a situation that he's not familiar with. We get women coming in and saying that their husbands are forever picking things up and messing around and getting under their feet. They like to have their own time at home to get things sorted out.

Thus men's presence in the home is alien and disruptive, and, because the home is constituted as the woman's realm, it is women who suffer the consequences. At the same time, this informant clearly identifies traditional masculine values as problematic, given the current 'unfamiliar' labour-market conditions.

Men in the house all day – a problem for children

Aside from the view that the male presence in the household constituted a problem for women, there was also a widespread feeling that it impacted on children too, in that it negatively affected child-rearing practice. The following comments from members of the social work childcare team in community B describe what they felt happened:

SOCIAL WORKER 1   Men being at home all day does cause problems. A lot of the stuff that we deal with is to do with parents who don't co-operate with each other in terms of management of children's behaviour. That has a lot of effects on children.

Previously, perhaps the approach to discipline has been one where mum was a little bit soft perhaps but the threat that 'I'll tell dad' was still there. This tended to be a traditional and acceptable way of dealing with things, whereas when you've got two people always under the same roof, one of whom tends to be a bit soft on discipline, with the other perhaps taking a more authoritarian line – which does seem to typify some of the mining families – then the clashes that we've identified in terms of managing children's behaviour have actually been very difficult to deal with.

SOCIAL WORKER 2   Where there's only the one there, you have got consistency. There's a parent used to childrearing and the absent one gets used as a threat.

SOCIAL WORKER 1   The consistency gets lost. It may be that you don't approve of the line that's been taken, but the fact that at least it's consistent has some merit, whereas when you've got one parent saying one thing, and one saying another . . .

Again, in this account, we are presented with a perspective that sees the presence of both men and women in the home as problematic, in that there is no longer a sharply defined division between the parent-as-authority and the parent-as-carer. The introduction of 'dad' into the children's daily environment has the paradoxical effect of reducing authority, since the very essence of that authority is held to derive from men's daily absence from the home. The 'ideal' situation appears to be the traditional one, in which one parent stays at home and the other goes out to work, thereby maintaining the 'consistency' of the domestic environment.

Women's absence from the home – a problem for children

Whilst men's *presence* in the home is seen as largely negative in its effects on children, some providers tended to see women's *absence* from the home as problematic too. In several providers' accounts, the fact that women are increasingly employed outside the home is constructed as a problem for children's welfare. One of the headteachers in community A said:

When the mines were working, it was very important that when the miner got home there was a meal ready for them, a decent meal, and the net result was that a lot of the wives didn't go out to work. But, starting from the miners' strike and going on from there, the women have started to go out to work and to look for jobs, and, to some extent, it's been acceptable for them to undertake poorly paid jobs which have very serious unsocial hours. The net result is that we find quite a lot of the kids do come from families where the mother's going out to work at 6 o'clock in the morning, or where she's not getting back until 8 or 10 at night. The kids are being left then, obviously, to fend for themselves.

This account clearly identifies the transformation in the traditional gender division of labour as a prime source of disruption in the family, and reconfirms the absence of men as potential carers from many providers' way of thinking. It is as if men are written out of the family picture. Women's work outside the home is interpreted as problematic for children, by reference to an underlying narrative of deprivation whereby men's redundancy causes women to go out to work and thus children to be neglected. Although providers recognized that labour-market conditions had changed, many were still seeing masculinity in monolithic terms, continuing to position men as redundant workers rather than potential carers. There are many indications from our provider interviews that, while the negative effects of the traditional division of labour were acknowledged (in terms of the limitations it placed on women's freedom, for instance), nevertheless, the 'old' ways of distributing the respective responsibilities for childcare and the family wage were seen as functional for children's security and continuity. A common underlying theme was that at least in the past, when the men went out to work and the women stayed at home, there was a clarity of roles and expectations that produced positive effects. The current cause for concern stemmed from a feeling that families were being launched into a situation of confusion and uncertainty, whereby traditional gender roles were maintained in the family under labour-market conditions that no longer allowed them to function. This resulted in women being subject to increasing pressures, which would, it was felt, have negative consequences for childcare.[4]

Men's stress – a problem for women

A fifth way in which male redundancy was seen by our providers as problematic for women was through its effects on men's emotional well-being. What is striking from the providers' accounts of this process is that this stress was invariably perceived in terms of its effects on women and children. A practice nurse in community A said that a large amount of her work consisted of dealing with women's stress about men's stress:

> I do a lot of counselling. Mainly, it's on the women who come in with problems. They do come with other things first – they've got an ache somewhere – but then they do say that their husbands are out of work. . . . They're getting very stressed up with their marriages, mainly with their husbands being at home. . . . Some of them are concerned about how their husbands are coping with it, because they're not coping well either. They say their husbands are getting very depressed. They don't want to bother getting washed and changed, they're not bright and alert like they used to be. They're just having trouble finding jobs, and they can't cope with just sitting around. A lot of the wives just say that they can't cope with their husbands getting so depressed. They just don't know what to do with them.

There is a clear understanding in accounts such as this one that women are at the 'sharp end' of male stress. Since they are positioned as emotional carers, they 'feel responsible' for alleviating their partners' problems. The point is that service providers clearly conceptualized the problems of unemployment-related stress in terms of a linear relationship between the event or threat of male redundancy, its 'direct effects' on men and the subsequent 'indirect effects' on women and children. We thus have a model which moves from (1) male redundancy and job insecurity, to (2) men's responses to this, (3) women's responses to men's stress and (4) the effects of this on the family as a whole. As we can see, the origin of these difficulties is located in male labour-market experience. Men's reaction to the loss of employment is structured by a further loss to their masculine identity, causing their stress to 'erupt' in the domestic sphere. In this general sense, men are seen as introducing problems that women have to deal with.

Men's own stress, however, is curiously distant in providers' accounts. It is inferred from their observations of its effects on women and children, but rarely is it accessed directly through contact with providers. There seem to be two significant factors here. First, as other chapters in this book have pointed out, the structure of health, welfare and educational provision has tended to reproduce the terms of the traditional gender division of labour through its concentration on women as the primary carers of children. Therefore, service institutions and their practitioners have become habituated to dealing with women in matters relating to child welfare, and women have occupied the role carved out for them in terms of accessing practitioners. So, it is generally mothers who collect children from schools and talk to teachers, deal with the education and welfare officers, visit the doctor with sick children, engage with health visitors on the birth of a new baby, liaise with social workers and so on, just as it is women who form the bulk of health and welfare workers (see Davis and Brook, 1985). As a result, service providers have direct access to the signs of women's stress, whereas men's remains largely hidden. As one of the GPs interviewed said: 'On the whole, women consult doctors more than men consult doctors – perhaps the reason for that is that women tend to have more contact because of the children.' This creates a curiously self-sustaining paradox. Since, through the perpetuation of a female-dominated caring culture, potential evidence (if any exists) of men as carers is unlikely to become visible, practitioners will continue to frame men as workers *because* the carers they see are women, and attribute the caring role to women *because* men – almost by default – are constructed as workers.

The second factor may well be merely an effect of the first: that practitioners themselves tended to judge men as ill-equipped, for various reasons, to give voice to their own stress. In our research, the view that men are disabled from expressing emotional problems was voiced by several service providers. One of the root inhibiting factors identified as an obstacle to male disclosure was the issue of men's self-esteem. Providers felt that men are reluctant to articulate their own vulnerability and neediness. The stress therapist in community D pointed out:

> I'd say about 60 or 70% of the people I see are women. I think it's maybe easier for women to come. Also, GPs will more readily identify problems in women and refer them on. Men are reluctant to ask for help, especially when you've got a man who's got stress, and a lot of problems, resulting from losing his job and his perceived social standing – that reinforces his sense of failure. He already feels a failure, and thinks it's bad to have this problem with stress. To them, it's actually very difficult to accept the need for help.

In this account, attention is focused on the operation of a masculine code of self-sufficiency, which values work and devalues emotional vulnerability. Men's jobs are understood to involve the extra dimension of social standing, which means that men 'feel a failure' when they lose their jobs. Talking about stress is difficult because it is equated with 'failing' in the masculine ideal.

So far, we have seen how providers' understandings of the problems facing the communities are rooted in a concern over the loss of the breadwinner role. This loss is problematic because it threatens the provider/servicer dyad – taken to be the ideal arrangement for children's upbringing. As a result of financial deprivation, the male presence in the home and men's damaged self-esteem, women are no longer provided with the means by which to service the family in a stable, regular and well-resourced domestic environment. Instead, they bear the brunt of the strain of male unemployment, and are 'having' to resort to paid work – contributing to the neglect of children and home. Meanwhile, traditional working-class masculinity is seen as increasingly dysfunctional because it has been robbed of its functionality – to provide the family wage. It is because, therefore, of changes in the labour market that gender roles need to adjust, since the traditional division of labour is no longer functional for the family.

In turning, now, to the question of social support, we shall consider how providers evaluate the existing informal support networks that families can access. On the whole, we shall see that providers rely very heavily on an expectation of mutual aid for women through the extended family, although many are concerned that these networks may be threatened in the future. It will be argued that there is an inherent tension in the fact that providers see women as both bearing the major burden of male unemployment while simultaneously constituting the strength of the networks, and that providers may therefore underestimate the formal support that women need.

SOCIAL SUPPORT AND THE EXTENDED FAMILY

As we saw in the previous section, providers tended to look back to the past, when securely employed fathers provided the family wage and women looked after the family, as a time of relative material and social prosperity for the community. This buoyancy had been destroyed by the loss of male employment. On the other hand, the providers saw one aspect of the traditional mining community as still in place: the 'mutual aid' and closeness that characterized Bulmer's ideal-typical community. As the first section argued, the providers we interviewed were all in agreement that there were now immense pressures on women, and yet paradoxically, they tended to assume that the women were well supported by kinship networks – composed, also, of women.

When asked to describe the community they were working in, the vast majority of service providers focused immediately on features indicating community cohesion, self-sufficiency and mutual aid. The social workers in community B described it like this, in an exchange focusing on perceptions of the local community:

SOCIAL WORKER 1　People here in [community B] like to stay near their families. It's a close community isn't it?

SOCIAL WORKER 2　There's a lot of large, extended families there as well that have been very supportive.

SOCIAL WORKER 3　It really is a helpful sort of network, and I wonder if the lack of social amenities is to some extent compensated for by the actual closeness of the community that makes do. The demands aren't made for services, because what they're doing is getting help from the next-door neighbour or family.

This account shows the extent to which providers depended on the informal support provided by community networks as a means of reducing the burden on formal services. Providers were often explicit about the extent to which these networks facilitated their formal provision, as in this health visitor's account (community C), for instance, where the networks were seen as a good source of information:

The families themselves are pretty close knit because they don't tend to move away. So there's a good extended network there for families, for each other, and of course for friends – because they grow up together, go to school together, their children have children, so the village is quite intertwined. This is very helpful for us, because if they're not at home when you call, I usually know exactly where to find people. You get a lot of information that perhaps you don't even ask about.

'Helpfulness' is therefore seen by the providers as an enduring feature of mining communities, and it is clear that families who help one another are also 'helping' the providers. It is also clear, however, that the source of this 'mutual aid' is located in networks of women. Although providers often expressed their observations of the self-help culture in gender-neutral terms (as in the above use of the term 'people'), it was clear that it was women who were providing the informal services. This is apparent in the following account, from an education and welfare officer in community C:

> There is this huge sense of family here, which is fairly unique, I think, to mining villages. . . . You find that as well if there's a crisis: someone says 'our so-and-so's missing from home' and you'll go along to the house, and there'll be our so-and-so's family, and aunty thingy, and her from up the road – and they do congregate like that . . . I do think that without that family and friends network, there'd be an awful lot more trouble than there is now.

It is fairly clear that the 'people congregating together' are women: aunts, female neighbours and so on. Indeed, the officer goes on to say: 'I think other women are very heavily relied on. You see women picking up armfuls of kids. They're not child-minding them, they're just picking them up because mum's not there.'

Women, therefore, constitute a resource which prevents 'an awful lot more trouble' from occurring. From the providers' point of view, it is because women can be relied on to help one another out with children and family stress that the community is still able to hold together.

Indeed, there was a worry among providers that this source of support might decline as the effects of unemployment deepened. The ability of women to provide support to other women is clearly reduced where women are unsupported themselves, or are single parents having to cope single-handedly with their own immediate families. A feeling common to all providers' observations was that this traditional model was giving way to one in which the norm was single parenthood. The majority of the providers identified the number of unsupported mothers as a major problem for children's material and social welfare, although it was the GPs who were particularly blunt about the moral implications of the situation. The GP in community A estimated that 80 per cent of his antenatal patients were 'unmarried mothers', and his colleague in community D particularly singled out as a problem 'single-parent families with hygienic standards far below what we were

used to', adding that 'they've become a great user of medical services, and their demands on us are quite exceptional'. The GP in
community C specifically drew a comparison between the mining
families who were not high users of his services, and the newer
arrivals into the village:

> The council have tended to use [community C] as a dumping
> ground for people that they didn't want anywhere else. I'm
> lucky, from the point of view of my work load, because these
> are very high-demand patients and the miners were not, really.
> They were very grateful for what you did for them, and they
> were very considerate people. . . . I've still got the old families
> on my list, but we're certainly getting different people now
> with different attitudes. And different problems. The nature of
> people that are moving into the village now are people with
> big problems.

In this way, a clear distinction was drawn between the self-sufficient
mining families, and the 'new arrivals' who are seen as very
demanding of doctors' time. The rather condemnatory tone used
by the GPs in describing the single-parent families was not replicated by other providers, it must be stressed, yet the feeling that
mining families could be relied upon to look after themselves was
extremely widespread. A social worker from community C
summed up the general impression that the bulk of the community's
welfare demands came from outside of the traditional networks:

> I think in real terms people who've had a long-standing associa-
> tion with the mining industry in actual fact are the backbone of
> strength in the community. I wouldn't want to identify people
> from within the mining community as real users of services, or
> as making many demands on social services. I think in a sense
> we look to that community to offer us some sense of support
> and comfort. I think the point about the mining community
> having been the backbone of the community is particularly sig-
> nificant because it makes you wonder what happens to those
> people that really have been the strength when that industry
> and that sort of employment goes. That would suggest, to me,
> a rather gloomy future – they may leave the area.

This provider clearly distinguished between two communities: the
one composed of mining and ex-mining families, and the one that
would be left if the other disappeared. In many accounts, the dis-

tinction between the extended and the unsupported family emerged clearly as a question of resources, with the 'older' model seen as self-sufficient and the 'newer' one seen as bringing a high demand for services.

So, for the providers, where the extended family endured, it represented a resource that they could draw on. Yet many providers also had an ambivalent attitude towards kinship networks, since they were often seen as obstructing the interventions of formal services. This is expressed clearly in the following account from a health visitor in community B who came up against a contradiction between the community's self-sufficiency and its penetrability as far as formal services are concerned:

> Well, in terms of this community being a close one, I find it a rather difficult community to log into. I came from an industrial, modern sort of area, where they were all new people arriving into the area and they were more receptive to advice and education, whereas in a community that have lived here for the last I don't know how many generations, they're very resistant to change. I mean, you talk about the health divide, and trying to encourage healthy eating, it's very difficult here. It's because the power of grandparents and the extended family over child-rearing practice is incredible, and it's really hard to sort of replace granny.

We could interpret this difficulty in terms of a clash of two cultures. The traditional community is on the one hand endorsed for its mutuality, while on the other this same mutuality is seen as a barrier to the intervention of professional knowledge. In particular, the hold that older women, such as 'granny', exert over child-rearing practice is seen as problematic. What service providers seem to favour is a traditional-style community based on the extended family, where women are at the domestic helm, but have a 'modern' and 'open' approach to professional advice, and a receptiveness to welfare interventions.

To conclude this section, then, we can summarize service providers' working assumptions about men's and women's community 'functions' as follows. First, women occupy a rather contradictory position in this schema. On the one hand, because their difficulties are defined (and accessed) by providers through their positioning as carers, women are felt to be on the receiving end of a range of problems resulting from endemic male unemployment. On the other hand, the communities are felt, on the whole, to be well provided for in terms of informal social support – which is largely maintained by the same women. This suggests that, even though they are understood to produce stress, women's traditional roles in the community continue to be seen as a positive resource – provided that these do not work against the ability of service providers to intervene where necessary. Second, men's identity continues to be articulated to the productive public sphere. This is seen as a problem by practitioners only inasmuch as that sphere no longer provides the family wage. In this sense, men are seen as doubly redundant: unable to provide for the family materially, they are also culturally excluded from becoming carers due to the endurance of the breadwinner ethic. But the very fact that the providers are operating in a system that relies on women's unpaid labour means that this cultural exclusion is simply perpetuated. While traditional male roles are identified as a problem by providers, since they increase the burden on women without providing the family wage, traditional female roles, at least in terms of women's caring networks, are implicitly – if not explicitly – seen as the glue which continues to hold the community together.

In recent years, research evidence about the onerous nature of women's caring roles has been steadily accumulating, and our interview data with women and with men certainly confirm this. In some cases, men were doing significant amounts of caring, but on the whole the 'breadwinner ethic' was still firmly entrenched. However, the women and men we interviewed directly contradicted the picture of community closeness painted by providers. In general, with one or two exceptions, interviewees' opinions invariably focused on a *loss* of closeness, and, in particular, a loss of emotional and practical support for women. Our research shows that women may well be actively involved in extended support networks, but that these can be considerable sources of strain for them, as well as sources of support. It is women who are both needing and providing help, in a context where they are also often expending considerable energy in paid employment. In this context, where the male cultural 'taboo' on caring continues, female-sustained support networks can become vulnerable. At the same time, support for women as workers is virtually absent, which is linked in with another absence: the absence of support for men as carers. There is also a question mark over the extent to which these networks are necessarily support, as opposed to control, networks. Our research further suggests, and other studies have shown – for example, Binns and Mars (1984) – that extended family relations can be characterized more by resentment and avoidance than mutual aid and loving care, especially during unemployment (whether his or hers), where intergenerational conflict in particular may come to a head.

However, in welfare organizations, these difficulties are often submerged. That is not to say that they go unacknowledged; many of the providers we spoke to – especially those who were working very much 'on the ground' through regular contact with families in their own homes – were fully aware of the complex and often strained nature of both inter- and intra-family networks. However, these providers were operating within a welfare paradigm that has particular assumptions built into its very structure. For instance, the exclusion of men from providers' vistas on the subject of caring is reproduced in the wider structures of the benefit and taxation system (Land, 1978). It is very difficult for providers to step outside these social and cultural frameworks, and, since the rhythms of their work recur on a day-to-day basis, their working assumptions about gender continue in a relatively pragmatic way, so that internal inconsistencies and contradictions fail to surface. Many stated that the research interview had represented the only occasion where they had been able to discuss with one another the deeper issues involved in their work, at a general and overarching level that was not entangled with individual cases.

Rather, it is at the level of policy-making that the terms of the traditional gender division of labour are most effectively reproduced. It is fairly clear that the type of kinship system found in mining communities, which provides its own informal services for extended family members, is exactly the kind of community that Mrs Thatcher was urging the country to return to during the heyday of the New Right approach to welfare:

> We know the immense sacrifices people will make for the care of their near and dear – for elderly relatives, disabled children and so on, and the immense part which voluntary effort even outside the confines of the family has played in these fields. Once you give people the idea that all this can be done by the state . . . then you will begin to deprive human beings of one of the essential ingredients of humanity – personal moral responsibility.
>
> (Margaret Thatcher, quoted in Croft, 1986)

As sociologists have argued – for example, McDowell (1989) – this rhetoric of *personal* responsibility actually means *family* responsibility – which in practice means women's responsibility, since it is women who are positioned as carers in the family (Finch and Groves, 1982). At the same time as women are having to step in as carers to replace the state provision, they are also entering the labour market in increasing numbers.

CONCLUSION

In this chapter, we have tried to outline some of the approaches to gender relations that underpinned service providers' understandings of community problems and resources. It has been shown that service providers started with a particular ideal-type of community well-being, against which current conditions were measured. This ideal-type operated as a kind of shadow behind providers' assessments, and was characterized by a strict gender division of labour maintaining the male breadwinner role and networks of mutual aid sustained by women. It was seen as functional for children since it provided the secure, ordered and stable existence considered necessary for their development. It also left women free to operate effectively and autonomously in the domestic realm. In the current context of high unemployment, providers recognized that the traditional role of women to support and care for men and families was under increasing strain. This was the source of providers' anxieties, since they depended on the continued operation of the female role to 'keep things together'. This traditional role reached beyond the immediate family, to the care of neighbours' and friends' children, as well as to elderly relatives, in-laws and neighbours, and was thus essential for informal community support.

Unemployed men's traditional roles in the family, on the other hand, were felt to be problematic. Since it could no longer deliver the family wage, the endurance of a domestic gender division of labour subjected women to extra stress since men's unproductive presence in the home disrupted their traditional routines. In addition, men's deprival of the breadwinner role was felt to have profound consequences for their self-esteem and masculine identity, and, since women were responsible for emotional care in the family, the effects of this 'masculine loss' were largely their burden. We thus have a linear narrative of stress, whereby men lose their jobs and their masculine self-esteem, women's traditional roles are strained, and as a result, children suffer. The focus of providers' attention remained fixed on women because their family-based agenda privileged the traditional role of women as the crucial factor in preventing family disintegration. As a result, women's other roles, particularly as workers, were largely absent from the picture, and – crucially – potential strategies for supporting men as carers were similarly underdeveloped. In the current context of male redundancy and increased female labour-market participation, such assumptions can only add to the burden of the female 'dual role'.

The research presented here lends weight to the well-developed feminist critique of welfare provision that has shown how traditional models of gender relations, particularly through the extended family, have been useful for professional service providers, in that they have prevented too many demands being made on their services. Mary Langan (1985), for example, has shown how the 'unitary approach' to social work theory and practice, developed in the 1970s, depended on a functionalist view of the family and community as a basis for care and thereby ignored the exploitative relations that underpin family structures. Other feminist studies – for example, Land (1978); McIntosh (1981) – have shown that these principles also lie at the root of welfare state policy as a whole, whereby social security and other legislation is designed to depend on the unpaid labour of women in the home.

There is now a body of feminist work arguing that women's unrewarded caring work represents the supporting pillar of community care practice and legislation – for example, Parker (1990). Our data show that women's activity in extended family networks is secured at a high price. It means they are providing care for a range of different needs, and there is evidence of increasing stress as a result. This is particularly the case where so many women are also in full or part-time paid employment, and are less well-off financially due to partners' unemployment. The providers are certainly right to fear the effects of a breakdown in this female provisioning, since there is little evidence that men will simply step in to take over the responsibility for care, somehow tearing down a centuries-old masculine culture in one effortless transition. However, if welfare policy-makers were seriously to think through the long-term effects of current labour-market restructuring in areas dominated by traditional male sectors, then the transferral of wage earning from men to women would surely emerge as a crucial element. If providers were more ready to see women as workers as well as carers, then the case for formal childcare, improved benefits legislation and publicly resourced community care provision might be more effectively articulated. In the process, men's own entombment in the bread-winner ethic might even begin to crumble.

NOTES

1 Our project did not involve matching the users and providers of one particular service. Instead, we interviewed a range of different providers – wider than the ones represented here – in order to gain a general impression of how the communities as a whole were evaluated and assessed by professional workers operating within them. As such, we do not have a fixed constituency of users that providers will have accessed, and many of our community interviewees may have little or limited experience of the services we contacted.

2 The fact that providers from the different communities did not differ as to their assessments of community needs is not surprising, since each community had high levels of unemployment due to the run-down of the mining and related industries across the region as a whole. By the time the providers were interviewed, the government had announced its sweeping colliery closure programme of October 1992, and both com-munities C and D were told to expect the imminent closure or moth-balling of their pits.

3 Some recent literature on unemployment (see Cooke, 1987) suggests that women whose partners became unemployed were more likely to withdraw from paid work themselves, for various reasons, although there is still controversy about this. Our research sample is too limited to support or refute these claims; however, a substantial number of survey respondents were in partnerships where the man was unemployed and the woman was in part-time paid work. Unfortunately, several studies suggest that part-time work for women simply allows them to continue bearing the burden of unpaid caring and domestic work (Morris, 1992).

4 Women revealed a range of concerns over employment. Some of these centred on the satisfaction they derived from their work, and others on the strains that it involved. Several had been involved in lengthy disputes at work, where the issue of redundancy was a constant threat. Indeed, by the time the providers were interviewed, one of the major employers of women from communities A and B, a mushroom farm, had made eighty women redundant, sparking off a protracted and bitter dispute which involved the women in months of picketing and protest. During our (unsuccessful) attempts to secure an interview with the manage-ment, one of the local managers referred to his employees as 'Scargill's wives'.

REFERENCES

Binns, D. and Mars, G. (1984) 'Family, community and unemployment: a study in change', *The Sociological Review*, 32(4): 662–95.

Brown, R.K. (1985) 'Attitudes to work, occupational identity and industrial change', in B. Roberts, R. Finnegan and D. Gallie (eds) *New Approaches to Economic Life*, Manchester: Manchester University Press.

Bulmer, M. (1975) 'Sociological models of the mining community', *Sociological Review*, 23: 61–92.

Cooke, K. (1987) 'The withdrawal from paid work of the wives of unemployed men', *Journal of Social Policy*, 16: 371–82.

Coyle, A. (1984) *Redundant Women*, London: The Women's Press.

Croft, S. (1986) 'Women, caring and the re-casting of need – a feminist re-appraisal', *Critical Social Policy*, 6(1): 23–39.

Davis, A. and Brook, E. (1985) 'Women and social work', in E. Brook and A. Davis (eds) *Women, the Family and Social Work*, London: Tavistock.

Finch, J. (1989) *Family Obligations and Social Change*, Cambridge: Polity Press.

Finch, J. and Groves, D. (1982) *A Labour of Love*, London: Routledge & Kegan Paul.

Land, H. (1978) 'Sex-role stereotyping in the social security and income tax systems', in J. Chetwynd and O. Hartnett (eds) *The Sex-role System*, London: Routledge & Kegan Paul.

Langan, M. (1985) 'The unitary approach: a feminist critique', in E. Brook and A. Davis (eds) *Women, the Family and Social Work*, London: Tavistock.

McDowell, L. (1989) 'Gender divisions', in C. Hamnett, L. McDowell and P. Sarre (eds) *The Changing Social Structure*, London: Sage Publications in association with the Open University.

McIntosh, M. (1981) 'Feminism and social policy', *Critical Social Policy* 1(1): 32–42.

McKee, L. and Bell, C. (1986) 'His unemployment, her problem: the domestic and marital consequences of male unemployment', in S. Allen, A. Watson, K. Purcell and S. Wood (eds) *The Experience of Unemployment*, London: Macmillan.

Martin, R. and Wallace, J. (1984) *Working Women in Recession*, Oxford: Oxford University Press

Morris, L. (1992) 'Domestic labour and employment status among married couples: a case study in Hartlepool', *Capital and Class*, 49: 37–49.

Parker, G. (1990) *With Due Care and Attention*, Family Policy Studies Centre.

Walters, B. (1986) 'Best suit, the Afan Valley in 1969', in R. Samuel, B. Bloomfield and G. Boanas (eds) *The Enemy Within: Pit Villages and the Miners' Strike of 1984–5*, London: Routledge & Kegan Paul.

Warr, P.B. (1987) *Work, Unemployment and Mental Health*, Oxford: Clarendon Press.

Chapter 12

Men and childcare
Policy and practice

Keith Pringle

This chapter focuses on a central tension within British childcare discourse (both academic and practice-based). On the one hand, an emphasis on the importance of men in childcare and families is growing ever clearer, articulated by a diverse range of interest groups (see Chapter 3, this volume). At the same time, some commentators are pointing out that an uncritical advocacy of men's involvement in childcare entails considerable problems. I want to interrogate this tension and to suggest that, even though complete resolution may be unlikely, some creative and positive outcomes are possible.

Men engaged in childcare professionally and/or personally have a major responsibility *and* opportunity for challenging those many negative attitudes and practices pervading our society which, I will argue, are associated with some dominant forms of masculinity. Those dominant forms reflect the complex interplay of a range of sources of oppression including heterosexism, racism, disablism, ageism and classism as well as issues of gender. Thus the project advocated here for men engaged in childcare is broad in its anti-oppressive scope. At its heart remains the central objective of challenging men's violences.

WHAT DO WE MEAN BY CHILD CARE?

Most discussions about issues of men in childcare have focused on men either as professionals within the caring professions or as men in families, rarely both. There are reasons for this separation and some of them have validity. After all, it can be argued there are concerns attaching to formal childcare settings which are even more pressing than they are in the context of 'in home' care. I provide two examples. First, where people entrust their children to 'out of home' childcare services for whatever reason, it may be that they should expect those children to be at least as safe as (perhaps even safer than) when they are in their own homes. Observable standards of welfare and safety are, therefore, particularly required in such settings. Second, 'out of home' childcare settings often cater for a larger number of children, one way or another, than many 'in home' settings. As a result, a lack of welfare or safety in such settings may have negative consequences for much larger numbers of children. Once again, standards of welfare and safety are therefore at a particular premium in these environments.

This is not to deny the primacy of children's welfare in their own homes and the need to take action to promote it. Rather, it is to suggest that an argument can be constructed for taking even more rigorous action to promote children's welfare in 'out of home' situations. For that reason it may be legitimate to separate out discussions about children's welfare in formal settings from those pertaining to 'in home' ones. Consequently, later in this chapter I shall address issues of children's safety specifically in relation to formal settings. In other respects, however, it can be argued that it is legitimate to address issues of childcare across the board, bringing together the situations which exist in formal and less formal settings.

First, and most obviously, many (though not all) of the dilemmas relating to men's more active engagement in professional childcare are directly transferable to the situation where men are caring for children on an unpaid basis in their own, or indeed others', home setting. Partly this derives from the fact that power relations within welfare services are to some extent structured in ways that mirror the dynamics of oppression to be found in wider society (Pringle, 1995: 206). Especially relevant here is the point made by Harlow and her colleagues (1992: 134–5; see also Chapter 1, this volume) that welfare services can in some respects be regarded as private, domestic work made public. Consequently, it is hardly surprising that oppressive dynamics found in the private sphere should be replicated, or indeed reinforced, in the context of public welfare organizations.

Second, in many respects the division between formal and informal settings is increasingly being eroded. This reflects relatively long-term and more recent trends in childcare provision.

Particularly since the mid-1970s there has been a major shift in Britain from residential to family placement as substitute forms of care (Frost and Stein, 1989: 108–10; Bullock, 1993: 217). Family placement represents a spectrum of provision in terms of its 'professionalization', ranging from foster-carers with little training and no formal 'pay' through to 'professional' family placement workers in their own homes who often have training and pay commensurate with, or superior to, residential childcare staff. These developments illustrate the limitation of any simple dichotomy between formal/informal or 'in home'/'out of home'.

Further limitations are evident when we consider certain principles in current childcare practice. Governmental emphasis on the priority to be given to care of children by their families has been expressed in the Children Act, 1989 (DOH, 1989) and more recently echoed in the document 'Messages from research' (DOH, 1995). Many commentators see in the latter clear indications that the balance of policy is shifting to supportive social work services for families and away from removal of children to substitute care, albeit without the resources or the structures to achieve a satisfactory standard of care in that change (Parton, 1996a; Pringle, 1996b). If the primary form of state intervention in childcare for the future is to be direct family support, then the case for separating out formal and informal childcare settings becomes even weaker.

In some ways events are already moving ahead of these government policies, in that service users are increasingly providing childcare services for other users. A particularly clear example of this is the significant growth of user-centred, often user-led, groups providing help to child survivors of sexual abuse and their non-abusing parents as well as to adult survivors (Pringle, 1995: 196–200). As recent research in the North-east of England suggests, the development of such services provided by users may sometimes be in direct response to the perceived inadequacies of statutory service provision (Gray et al., 1996).

Thus, in discussing the situation of men in childcare, some considerations around safety may apply more urgently in formal as opposed to informal settings, even though many issues straddle this divide. Consequently, the remainder of this chapter reviews the role of men in childcare provision across the widest range of settings, formal and informal.

INCREASING MEN'S PARTICIPATION IN CHILDCARE PRACTICE

Calls for men's greater participation in family life have come from advocates representing a wide range of political and other perspectives. The right-wing 'think-tank' the Institute for Economic Affairs (IEA), for example, has issued a series of publications which attribute a broad spectrum of social ills to the growing absence of men in families – for example, Murray (1990); Dennis and Erdos (1992); Dennis (1993). Their specific arguments about the impact of fathers' absences have been widely critiqued, particularly by feminist and pro-feminist commentators – for instance, Cochrane (1993); Campbell (1993); Millar (1994); Chapter 3, this volume.

Similarly, commentators have noted the many ways in which government administrations since 1979 have maintained a wide spectrum of policies signalling their clear preference for families with men in them (Smith, 1994). These policies include the implementation of 'Section 28' (Richardson, 1996: 17) and the near exclusion of women lacking 'stable' relationships with men from NHS fertility treatments (Carabine, 1996: 63), reflecting what Jo VanEvery refers to as 'hegemonic heterosexuality' (1996: 40). Furthermore, the White Paper on Adoption (HMSO, 1993) was bold in its statement that

> [there] must . . . be a strong presumption in favour of adoption by married couples. . . . Some children, often with special needs, are successfully adopted by unmarried women, women who are no longer married or women widowed early. The devotion and care they can bring to children often rightly commands admiration.

It went on to say that apart from these and 'a small number of other exceptional circumstances . . . [t]he Government . . . does not propose that unmarried couples should be able to apply for adoption' (1993: 9). This position sits extremely uneasily with the clear evidence of successful lesbian/gay adoption and fostering (Rickford, 1992; Taylor, 1993).

For very different reasons, as we shall later see, many feminist and pro-feminist commentators also advocate men's greater participation in family life even if they are, to varying degrees, sceptical about the extent and speed of that participation (Segal, 1990; Campbell, 1993; Thompson, 1995). Much support for this position also comes from the European Commission (EC) which in its 1992 Recommendation (EC, 1992: 92/241/EEC, Article Six) makes clear that Member States should promote and encourage increased participation by men for the care and upbringing of children. The 1994 White Paper on European Social Policy, *A Way Forward for the Union* (EC, 1994), re-emphasizes the importance of this theme. The EC Network on Childcare has also carried it forward with great energy (EC Network on Childcare, 1993, 1996; Jensen, 1996) – albeit with very little concrete impact on the British government (Moss, 1994), and despite the fact that the Network's co-ordinator was British and based in one of the country's leading social research units funded by the Department of Health.

In Britain a series of documents and articles have advocated more inclusion of men in statutory and non-statutory services for children (Ruxton, 1991; Holt, 1992; Chandler, 1993). Perhaps not surprisingly, many of these contributions also focus on men working in family centres, an area of welfare where the demarcation between formal and informal childcare becomes blurred for the variety of reasons already noted. The journal *Working with Men* provides an ongoing record of welfare initiatives by men around Britain directed at children and young people in a wide range of settings, such as community education, health projects, probation as well as day care. Interestingly, references in *Working with Men* to initiatives within the fieldwork of social services departments are few and far between, perhaps reflecting the increasingly crisis-driven nature of childcare work there (Pringle, 1995).

So, in Britain there has been no shortage of calls for men's greater inclusion in childcare or 'the family'. However, as indicated earlier, the motives of these advocates vary, in some cases quite dramatically. For instance, the IEA and the former government clearly regarded men's inclusion in families as a nostrum for a moral and social decline in Britain which most of the other commentators mentioned above would almost certainly attribute to other causes than the absence of men – see, for instance Campbell (1993), especially Chapter 17.

Moreover, unlike the other commentators mentioned above, the IEA and official documents are largely silent about what men should actually *do* in families. It is almost as though the very physical *presence* of men in families is enough in itself for right-wing advocates, regardless of men's precise role there. Yet, as Campbell makes clear (1993: 310), in the allegedly golden past to which right-wing theorists appeal, men were often emotionally absent from their families even if they were there physically. The underlying message of Campbell's analysis 'seems to be that masculinity does not need bolstering: it needs changing'. It is such changes that are the focus of anti-sexist advocates of men in childcare – precisely what men should be doing in childcare and the ways in which men engaged there should express their masculinity in a positive fashion.

MEN'S GREATER PARTICIPATION IN CHILDCARE: THE ANTI-SEXIST CASE

The anti-sexist – that is, feminist and pro-feminist – case for men's greater participation in childcare stands on arguments relating to benefits to children, benefits to women and benefits to men (EC Network on Childcare, 1993; Chandler, 1993; Thompson, 1995). While there is much of value in these arguments, we need to beware of over-simple analyses. Also, the value they promise can only be achieved by placing men's greater childcare engagement within a broader model of men's practices, which centres on issues of men's power and is grounded in the materiality of women's and men's lived experience.

THE BENEFITS TO CHILDREN

Much research has demonstrated that, generally speaking, men can perform parenting perfectly adequately. The problem is that for various structural and/or personal reasons many men choose not to fulfil that potential or only fulfil it in selective and very partial ways (Segal, 1990: 37–46; Marsiglio, 1995). That men on the whole can indeed provide successful nurturance to children is borne out by more recent research in both Britain (Barker, 1994) and the United States (Marsiglio, 1995). Moreover, there is every reason to believe that the potential capacity of men to nurture is also applicable to those who work in more formal childcare settings (Ruxton, 1991; Chandler, 1993).

However, the analysis of men as childcarers becomes over-simple when claims are made that men's presence in formal and informal settings is a *necessity*. We can begin to deconstruct such deterministic claims by referring to studies on the developmental progress of children in lesbian households (for example, Golombok et al.,

1983; Patterson, 1992). No one would deny that more research on this issue is required both to broaden the evidence and to deepen it longitudinally. However, there is an impressive consistency in the data we do possess. The children in these households seem to develop emotionally and physically just as well as children brought up in heterosexual ones. We are also increasingly aware that, as children develop into adults, the processes by which they shape their identities are far from simple. A theme which sometimes occurs in advocacy of men's being engaged in childcare is that boys will not be able to learn how to be fathers themselves unless they too have father models. While one would not deny that children may well benefit from emotional proximity to adults of both genders, there is a danger of being too crude and prescriptive in analysing this. For instance, it is increasingly apparent from research in the United States (Daly, 1995) and in the United Kingdom (Heward, 1996) that men's construction of their masculinity, and in particular those aspects related to fatherhood, are heavily influenced in complex ways by significant female figures, not least mothers.

As Heward (1996: 480) has argued

> individuals construct their masculinities actively within complex and changing family and other contexts constrained by gendered structural power relations. . . . Women and relations between men and women are a potent source of change in intimate relations. . . . Theories which transcend the tired oppositional gender categories and identifications are needed to understand intra and interfamily gender relations within their structural contexts. This would permit a wider variety of outcomes to be envisaged and make mothers integral rather than peripheral to the process of constructing masculinities in families.

One can add to this sophisticated perspective the conclusions of feminist and pro-feminist analyses of the alleged need for a male figure at the *centre* of children's (and in particular boys') lives (Phillips, 1993: 143–98; Pringle, 1995: 60–77). For instance, Phillips (1993) states:

> While boys need to learn about the male world, they can manage without a resident male, provided that their mother can provide a safe enough base from which they can explore. It is a great help

if the mother has some emotional back-up but that doesn't have to come from a man.

The same logic can be applied to the alleged necessity for men's presence in more formalized childcare provision (Jensen, 1996). Of course many men will have much to offer as workers in childcare services. However, there seems to be no valid argument to support the contention that male workers must always be present in more formal childcare settings for the benefit of children (Pringle, 1992, 1993).

So far in reviewing this debate, we have dwelt on the extent to which men's positive contributions to childcare are essential to children's welfare. It is time to introduce another vital factor into the argument: the violence of some men towards children. In fact, many commentators fail sufficiently to take into account the potential 'down-side' of men's presence in childcare. For instance, the EC Network on Childcare, in strongly advocating men's greater participation, mentions that 'taking more responsibility for children must also involve men taking more responsibility in other areas. . . . They must acknowledge, take responsibility for and deal with negative male behaviour – family violence and abuse, sexual harassment, etc.' (1993: 14). However, this important theme is not expanded upon and it sits stranded within a text which otherwise extols the virtues of men as carers of children. Similarly Jensen (1996: 23), whose whole focus is the issue of men working in childcare services, devotes only one and a half pages to the topic of men and sexual abuse in a document which is fifty-five pages long.

Another example of this disparity of attention between the pros and cons of men in childcare can be found in the US literature on fatherhood. Recently William Marsiglio has edited what is in almost all respects a comprehensive text on fatherhood drawing together much of the available research around the topic (Marsiglio, 1995). Yet in this otherwise comprehensive survey, what is striking is the almost total absence of any reference to the massive issue of emotional, physical or sexual damage which some paternal figures may inflict directly or indirectly upon their children.

A recent comment by Jeff Hearn about work on men by men, which he has made specifically in relation to women's oppression at the hands of men, is equally applicable to the situation of children (1996a: 22):

the majority of this work, and particularly that which has come to be known as 'men's studies' (especially in the United States), has generally not explored the question of men's violence to any large extent. . . . It is partly for this reason that more critical studies on men and masculinities are being developed.

Elsewhere, I have reviewed in detail the place of men in social welfare including childcare (Pringle, 1995). Suffice it to say here that, whilst not denying the abuse of power which women may exercise over children (Hanks and Saradjian, 1991; Elliott, 1993; Kelly, 1991, 1996), men's violences present a considerably larger threat in many respects. This is particularly true in relation to sexual violences both inside and outside the home (Pringle, 1995: 39–52, 169–203). However, we should not underestimate the extent to which men perpetrate other forms of oppression against children, including physical assault (Andrews, 1994), even if the preponderance of men in that form of abuse is not quite so striking as it is with sexual abuse. Furthermore, recent attention has been focused on the emotional, physical and sexual abuse of children which may accompany men's oppression of female partners (O'Hara, 1993; Mullender and Morley, 1994; Saunders, 1994). Finally, we should bear in mind the point made by Beatrix Campbell about the saturation of our society by masculinized images of brutality and domination (see also Hearn, 1990, and McCollum *et al.*, 1994).

Men's potentially positive contribution has to be framed within a set of practices which guard against the negative impact (including abuse) which some men may have on the welfare of children. Later in this chapter I will outline a strategy for limiting the scope of potential abuse by men in childcare. In summary, as I have argued elsewhere (Pringle, 1995: 75–6):

> The overall evidence seems to suggest that families do not need fathers. That is not at all the same as saying that men should not be in families. . . . The question is not really whether men should or should not be in families. The question is what kind of a man, what kind of masculinity, has most to offer to other human beings, including women and children.

This places in sharp focus the critical issue of how to assist men to express themselves, as men and as human beings, in ways that are positive rather than negative for those people around them, a topic returned to later in the chapter. At this point, however, we turn to those arguments which validate men's involvement in child-care by reference to the benefits for women.

THE BENEFITS TO WOMEN

Many of the relevant issues here parallel those broached in the previous section. Once again, there is considerable validity in some of the arguments put forward. For instance, Thompson (1995: 471) is no doubt correct in regarding men's greater involvement in child-rearing and the consequent erosion of gender stereotyping around 'caring' as, at one level, a potential move towards social justice. However, when taken in isolation from other measures, this kind of approach can become over-simple.

It is not at all clear whether or not men's shift to childcare functions, either in families or in more formal settings, would *necessarily* result in benefits to women. For such benefits to occur, the wider social contexts in which that shift takes place must also be the object of positive anti-oppressive change. For instance, Hilary Graham (1983, 1993) has explored the ways in which caring has come to profoundly underwrite a sense of self-identity and self-worth for many women in the same way as achieving goals for one-self may play a major role in underwriting the self-identity of many men (Baldwin and Twigg, 1991).

It may well be that if some gender shift in childcare is to be attained, then alternative ways of achieving self-identity and self-worth for women need also to be developed. The welfare services provide a good illustration of this point. If more men do enter child-care work, there is every indication at present, given the gender profile of social work management (Grimwood and Popplestone, 1993; Pringle, 1995), that one major result will be more men occupying management posts in that sector. Similarly, as Chapter 8 illustrates, the greater entry of men to home-based childcare does not *necessarily* result in an erosion of unequal power relations between women and men.

Any shift of men into childcare needs to be placed within the wider context of patriarchal relations, as illustrated by the issue of parenthood itself (see Chapters 3 and 8, this volume). Recently VanEvery (1996: 47) has considered whether too much emphasis is placed on parenthood as a factor in the gendering of power relations within the home. She indicates that motherhood may well be one process by which gender is constituted, but she also goes on to suggest that many social practices are involved in constituting gender there (1996: 52). Moreover, she adds that 'femininities and masculinities are usually constructed as complementary dyads – as heterosexual – and those dyads are usually unequal'.

Evidence of the massive problem of men's violence (emotional/financial/physical/sexual) towards women they know is more than well established (Pringle, 1995: 91–104; Hester *et al.*, 1996; Hanmer, 1996; Hearn, 1996a, 1996b). Changes in gender patterns regarding childcare involvement cannot be taken in isolation from the centrality of men's violences towards women any more than those towards children. The strictures of Hearn (1996a: 22) regarding the relative lack of attention paid by men in their writing on masculinity to the centrality of men's violences clearly applies here too. Recently, Victoria Robinson (1996: 120) has made a similar point in relation to the wider issue of men's power. She expresses a feminist concern about men's recent theorizations of masculinity:

> the current notion of emphasizing changing masculinities should not ignore or minimize men's continuing power at both a structural and personal level. For example, compulsory heterosexuality may be a reality for women and men but their experiences of it and the power and the privilege that accompany it are different.

The importance of looking beyond the immediate impact of men's greater entry into childcare towards the wider, gendered social and material relations within which that development occurs is reinforced by some of Jeff Hearn's recent work. He casts doubt, for example, on the continuing usefulness of the concepts 'masculinity/masculinities' as tools in developing an effective praxis for men (Hearn, 1996c). His reasons are multiple and complex but two of his concerns about the direction of men's writing about men are relevant here. First, he believes that the usage of the concepts in some hands (particularly the 'men's studies' school) tends to deny the relational dimension to gender analysis: in other words, too narrow a focus on the issue of 'masculinity/masculinities' may exclude the critical issue of men's relations with women (Hearn, 1996c: 203). Second, in the reification of 'masculinity/masculinities', he asks what has happened to men's material practices:

Not only do most versions of masculinity fail to address that question, but more fundamentally, they tend to divert attention away from material practices, whether in work, sexuality, violence or elsewhere, and away from a materialist or materially-based analysis of gendered power relations.

(1996c: 208)

Hearn's analysis is central to the conclusions to be drawn from the material presented in this section. If men are serious about challenging those relations of power which are oppressive to women, then greater participation in childcare by them must occur within the framework of much broader anti-oppressive practices. These include strategies by which men find more positive ways of expressing themselves in the lived experience of their relations with women, children and other men.

THE BENEFITS TO MEN

Research on men as carers of children makes clear that many men do enjoy that activity, whether in the home (Barker, 1994; Marsiglio, 1995) or at work (Ruxton, 1991). Whilst men should not be deprived of the opportunity to gain that satisfaction, this has to be balanced against the needs of both children and women.

This seems an appropriate point at which to foreground a particularly contentious issue. How can men's involvement in childcare within formal settings be combined with a policy which maximizes the safety of children there? One very particular context for this concern which we have already addressed is the clear preponderance of men as perpetrators of sexual violence against children.

A brief résumé of the main issues is provided here – these are dealt with at length elsewhere (Pringle, 1992, 1993, 1995). It is clear from all the relevant research that the large majority of men working in formal childcare settings will not sexually abuse the children in their care. However, there are indications (mainly from American studies) that a significant minority of men in those settings may do so (for example, Finkelhor et al., 1986; Fanshell, 1990; Rosenthal et al., 1991; Benedict et al., 1994), particularly as it is increasingly apparent that some men may target such work precisely because it gives ready access to large numbers of children (for example, see Hunt, 1994). What massively compounds the problem is that there appears to be no reliable way of vetting potential and actual sexual abusers out of the system (HMSO, 1992). Of course, statutory checks on prospective employees may 'weed out' people with some record of previous abusive behaviour. However, we know that only a very tiny minority of sexual abusers are ever dealt with by statutory authorities (see Hallett, 1995), so the effectiveness of formal checks is bound to be severely limited though they are of course still worth carrying out. Other measures which have been regularly recommended in inquiry after inquiry report appear to have minimal value in practice – for example, interviewing potential job applicants about their sexuality, and more training for staff managers (Pringle, 1993, 1995).

Additional strategies based on a gender analysis have been advocated (Pringle, 1995: 185–92). Though these will not eliminate the problem of sexual abuse in formal care settings (after all, a minority of such abuse *is* perpetrated by women), they ought to reduce it significantly. Those strategies centre on a spectrum of limitations on men's professional practice, ranging from the relatively minimal (for example, men avoiding touch as far as possible in communicating with children) to, at the other extreme, excluding men from some areas of childcare work. It should be emphasized that the number of situations where the risks to children would warrant the latter strategy will be very small indeed. A number of criteria have also been identified by which each particular care situation can be assessed in order to determine what level of restriction on men's professional practice is appropriate.

It is important to add, finally, that such strategies will not only have a protective function for children but also for staff. It is relatively rare for children to make deliberate false allegations of sexual abuse. However, it may be more frequent for children who have already endured sexual abuse at some other time in their lives genuinely to misinterpret the actions of staff as having an abusive purpose. Often this will be due to the patterns of 'grooming' that abusers may have imposed on them in the past. Hence the protection which, I argue, is also afforded to staff by the strategies put forward here primarily for the safety of children.

The direct danger of sexual abuse to children is not the only issue relevant to the question of limitations on men's practice in this field. A research project in the North-east of England compared statutory services available to child and adult survivors of sexual abuse with those services preferred by service users (Gray *et al.*, 1996). One interesting set of findings related to users' preferences regarding who should provide them with therapy. The issue of gender figured very prominently (Gray *et al.*, 1996: 194). The vast majority of users in the survey indicated a clear preference for women therapists; a minority expressed no preference either way; no one expressed a preference for a man. The preference for women extended to men respondents and included the small minority who had been abused jointly by a man and a woman. No respondents reported sexual abuse perpetrated by a lone female. Such a preference across the board could, of course, be interpreted as a manifestation of gender stereotyping on the part of respondents in relation to care and counselling – and indeed that may have been a factor. However, we also feel that the preference of respondents should be taken at face value: that is, as expressing unease about accepting help from men. We would not, of course, consider drawing any firm conclusions from this one piece of research. Nevertheless, it adds material to the debate about how far we *unreservedly* accede to men's desire to work across the whole range of child welfare settings.

A second reason put forward for suggesting that men's greater engagement in childcare will be of benefit to men themselves is that this will assist men to re-create positively the way they express themselves as men. In other words, nurturing children may be a central route by which men re-evaluate their general behaviour, as men, in their dealings with other people. The general idea behind this argument should not be discounted. Elsewhere (Pringle, 1995: 209) I have suggested that particularly significant life experiences may initiate in some men both an awareness of more caring/nurturing aspects of themselves and the motivation to demonstrate these aspects in their behaviour. In some cases this may have a generalizing effect, creating a similarly positive change in many of the behaviours by which men relate to other people, and indeed, to themselves. Perhaps the sudden dependence upon them of a parent, child or partner may act as such an initiating occurrence, as discussed in relation to male carers in Chapter 7, although such an event may also bring into stark, personal relief the destructive potential of dominant forms of masculinity.

Whatever the route, men need to take positive action to change oppressive power relations within a broad practice framework if the benefits which engagement in childcare work is alleged to bring are to be realized. This complements the conclusions drawn in the two earlier sections on benefits to the children and to women. My central argument is that men's more extensive engagement in childcare activities, formally and informally, may indeed offer potential benefits to children, women and men themselves, but *only* if that engagement involves men challenging dominant relations of power in the family, welfare services and society more generally. If such a broader practice is not implemented, then men's greater engagement in childcare by itself may simply result in replication of oppressive power relations in one form or another, annexation or colonization of initiatives developed by/for women; diversion of resources away from other initiatives promoting the well-being of women and/or children; sometimes perhaps even abuse of women and/or children (Pringle, 1995).

The greater engagement of men in childcare activities cannot be understood in isolation from wider considerations of men's power. The necessity for a coherent and concerted approach in the challenging by men of oppressive power relations is a theme which has run constantly throughout this chapter. In the next section I draw on my previous work to outline the form of such a comprehensive practice framework for men (Pringle, 1995: 204–19).

CHALLENGING OPPRESSIVE GENDER POWER RELATIONS: A PRACTICE FRAMEWORK FOR MEN

The principles of a framework for social welfare practice have to deal with some tensions which exist when addressing the complex issue of masculinities in the context of gendered power relations. These include the following:

1 how to maintain a focus on the core concern of the relations between women and men rather than simply on men alone (Hanmer, 1990: 34; Hearn, 1996c: 203; Robinson, 1996: 117);
2 how to interrogate the complexities of masculinity formation whilst grounding these in the materiality of men's actual practices (Hearn, 1996c: 204);
3 how to maintain at the centre of one's analysis of men's practices the issue of power and, in particular, of men's violences (Hanmer, 1990: 34; Hearn, 1996a: 22; Robinson, 1996: 117).

My method builds upon a theoretical model of gender relations developed by Connell (1987, 1995), explicitly tested out against empirical data (drawn largely from the field of social psychology –

for example, Archer, 1994) concerning men's violences and power (Pringle, 1995: 78–105, 175–80).

Connell's model of gender relations is not beyond critique on a number of grounds (see, for instance, Cornwall and Lindisfarne, 1994; Richardson, 1996). Nevertheless, it has particular salience in relation to the field of social welfare on several counts. In particular, Connell's overt acknowledgement of the complex interrelationship between issues of gender and other forms of oppressive power relations such as 'race', class and sexuality is closely aligned to models of anti-discriminatory (ADP) and anti-oppressive practice (AOP), which in recent years have become central to social and other welfare work (Thompson, 1993; Ali, 1996).

The framework requires those men practising within it to monitor constantly their own and others' anti-oppressive activity against the following oppressive possibilities:

1 colluding with oppressive practices of other men;
2 colonizing/annexing anti-oppressive initiatives of women;
3 diverting resources away from women's initiatives or other anti-oppressive activities;
4 using positions gained via anti-oppressive practice to abuse other people in whatever fashion, inadvertently or deliberately.

If men are seriously going to challenge oppressive gender relations, we need to act as far as possible in a concerted manner at all the 'levels' within society where such relations operate, ranging from our own individual behaviour, at one level, to the structural relations which operate at a societal level – and all points in between (Pringle, 1995: 213).

There is necessarily a theoretical and practical tension between a conceptualization of power which is postmodern/poststructual and the structural approach which underpins much of my analysis here. Nevertheless, I suggest that the relations of power operating at each level of anti-oppressive practice can be usefully viewed through a Foucauldian lens (Hekman, 1990; Sawicki, 1991; Pringle, 1995: 138–9). They can also be regarded as interacting between levels in a complex fashion: sometimes in conflict, sometimes in concert. Such complexity in practice always allows 'spaces' within which co-ordinated subversion of dominant structures may be achieved – indeed that is the object of the anti-oppressive project advocated here.

The image of 'levels' is meant only to act as a conceptual tool: any image seeking to represent the complexity of gender relations is bound to be crude and inadequate to the task. The dynamics of relations of power do not conform to any neat picture of levels (Connell, 1987, 1995). Adams (1996) suggests a similar scheme, based on the concept of 'domains' rather than 'levels'. This is perhaps a more appropriate way of talking about these issues, and this terminology is used here.

There are five domains of action in which men's concerted anti-oppressive practice should operate. These are described with some examples relevant to the issue of childcare. The first is work with, and upon, one's own personal and political oppressive behaviour in order to challenge it. One particularly obvious example might be that those men who may abuse children need to challenge their propensity to do so, otherwise their entry into childcare will seriously oppress, rather than benefit, children.

The second domain is individual work with other men and boys to promote mutual challenge of oppressive behaviours. For instance, if more men enter into paid work at family centres and nurseries, it is possible that this could lead to more sexual exploitation of women working there, unless men challenge their own and one another's behaviour.

The third domain is groupwork among/with men/boys for the purpose of mutually challenging oppressive behaviour, and strategic networking to challenge structural forms of oppression. For instance, groupwork among fathers at a family centre might be facilitated by a man worker who may, or may not, be a father himself. The focus of such groupwork might be how to parent one's children in such a way as to actively promote anti-oppressive attitudes and behaviour. Without concerted efforts in this direction, the entry of more men into child-rearing alone may simply replicate the inculcation of oppressive attitudes and behaviour in children, particularly boys. Just because a father engages in more child-rearing clearly does not guarantee that the model he presents to his child will be anti-oppressive. Quite the opposite may sometimes be the case.

Whether facilitators of individual or group menswork or boys-work need to be men is a complex issue (Pringle, 1995: 143–4, 214–18). Men have a responsibility to work with other men to counter the 'patriarchal dividend' (Connell, 1995: 79) which to a greater or less extent they share. In saying this, it is important to recognize that gender and other dynamics of oppression, around such issues as sexuality or 'race', are mutually mediating so that some forms of masculinity are subject to marginalization and/or subordination more than others (Connell, 1995: 80). The rationale for men working with men is also clearly supported by arguments against expecting women to work as facilitators for service users who are men, particularly where those men are abusers (Dominelli, 1991). Certainly, it seems to me that no woman should ever be obliged to undertake menswork or boyswork.

On the other hand, where work with men or boys is facilitated by men, potential problems may exist, particularly collusion with, and/ or abuse of, service users. Partly for these reasons, some feminist commentators advocate a clear place for women in pushing forward anti-sexist work with men and boys (Cavanagh and Cree, 1996). Co-working with a women may offer some counter to problems of collusion/abuse by men workers, and it is a way of operating I have generally found helpful for that very reason. In addition, women/men co-working is sometimes advocated as providing a useful model to group participants or in couple therapy. This argument is much less convincing partly because the underlying assumption appears to be deeply heterosexist (Christie, 1996:12).

Women/men co-work with men also has its own problems. From where will the female worker draw her support? Will she be oppressed by group participants and/or her male colleague? What structures need to be built in to avoid this? How strong does the relationship between the co-workers need to be? Clearly, there are no easy answers to these questions, and to some extent one has to fall back on taking each case as it comes. Salisbury and Jackson (1996: 6) seem largely to favour the model of men working with boys for their school-based programmes rather than woman/man co-working. On the whole, my own preference for ideal facilitation in most situations is co-working with a woman partner who is well aware of the problematics in gender relations, with, wherever possible, an additional video-linked consultancy team consisting mainly of women colleagues also well-versed in the problematics of gender relations.

The fourth domain concerns the creation of positive and structural change in agencies/institutions/localities/communities. For instance, men working in an agency can individually and collectively seek to have implemented effective harassment policies or recruitment policies which avoid discriminatory practices (Pringle, 1995: 198–200).

The final domain involves contributing to strategies of structural change at a societal level. For instance, men engaged with childcare in formal or informal settings could seek to organize regional or national initiatives designed to respond positively to the campaigns of the Zero Tolerance Trust (see Pringle, 1995: 165–6).

The examples I have given are simply illustrative. My aim here has been to set out some principles for practice. The potential applications of the framework will, in fact, be numerous and extensive. Wherever men are working with children and young people, and indeed adults – for instance, schools, community projects, nurseries, family centres, health projects, social work settings, probation and, last but not least, in their own homes – these wider considerations must enter into their practice. I am not suggesting that each man can be fully active in working anti-oppressively in all five domains. Nevertheless, whatever specific actions a man engages in directly, he should bear the wider context in mind and, as far as possible, network with men (and women) challenging oppressive gender relations in other domains of practice – see, for example, Salisbury and Jackson (1996).

In this chapter I am speaking in terms of my own personal social work practice. I am highly conscious of the plentiful evidence around abuse of women by men therapists (Pringle, 1995: 128–30). I am also deeply aware of the massive number of female service users who will, inevitably, have profound experiences of one or more forms of abuse by men in their lives, given the level of such abuse in society (Pringle, 1995: 40–1, 92–4). I am therefore alert to the negative meanings that therapy from a man may have for many women. For these reasons, I would rarely work with women users, either individually or in groups and then only in a female/male co-working context.

One final point is that in any setting such anti-oppressive action by men should be carried out only with the agreement of women who may also be working for the transformation of gender relations there. Active collaboration between women and men may be possible in some circumstances, though its form needs to be considered carefully lest oppressive gender relations come to structure the collaboration itself (Pringle, 1990). This applies not only to individuals working together, but also to collective collaboration.

CONCLUSIONS

In this chapter I have attempted to address what is becoming one of the most contested and contentious debates in social welfare: the place of men in childcare. In some respects elements of that debate are reflected in other issues of current controversy: for instance, the perceived shift in public policy away from child protection towards more emphasis on family support (Dartington Social Research Unit, 1995; Parton, 1996a; Pringle, 1996b). In both cases there are uncertainties about how to broaden and support parenthood. These in turn are partly a reflection of contradictory discourses around the issue of risk which pervade a wide range of social welfare systems at the moment (Parton, 1996b).

A further level of complexity to the debate about men in childcare is the transnational. The European Network on Childcare became a major influence in this debate. Its perspective on men in professional childcare, based on some Continental models orientated towards family support, seems to reflect a less intense focus on child protection (especially in relation to sexual abuse) than is the case in Britain (Pringle, 1996b). On the one hand, there is considerable cause to doubt whether levels of sexual abuse are actually less in Continental Europe than in the United Kingdom (Finkelhor, 1991). On the other hand, it is vital to avoid engaging in intellectual imperialism: one should not assume that in other countries social problems, such as sexual violence, manifest themselves to the same extent or in the same way as they appear to do in Britain.

Public policy on men's involvement in professional childcare may well be at a crossroads. Unfortunately, that debate might develop into a polarized argument on whether more men or fewer men should be in childcare work. This is, however, the wrong question. Instead, the real question is: what strategies can we devise to involve men in childcare in ways that will also maximize the safety of children, and indeed women? I have argued that men's greater involvement in childcare activities does have a real and vital anti-oppressive potential, with possible benefits for children, women and men themselves. However, if such positive outcomes are to be achieved, men's practice in this field has to be grounded in a broad anti-oppressive framework which places issues of their power and violence centre-stage.

REFERENCES

Adams, R. (1996) *Social Work and Empowerment*, 2nd edn, London: Macmillan.

Ali, S. (1996) 'Anti-oppressive practice in social work education', Paper presented at the Conference on Racism and Welfare, University of Central Lancashire (April).

Andrews, B. (1994) 'Family violence in a social context: factors relating to male abuse of children', in J. Archer (ed.) *Male Violence*, London: Routledge, pp. 195–209.

Archer, J. (ed.) (1994) *Male Violence*, London: Routledge.

Baldwin, S. and Twigg, J. (1991) 'Women and community care – reflections on a debate', in M. MacLean and D. Groves (eds) *Women's Issues in Social Policy*, London: Routledge, pp. 117–35.

Barker, R.W. (1994) *Lone Fathers and Masculinities*, Aldershot: Avebury.

Benedict, M.I., Zuravin, S. Brandt, D. and Abbey, H. (1994) 'Types and frequency of child maltreatment by family foster care providers in an urban population', *Child Abuse and Neglect*, 18: 577–85.

Bullock, R. (1993) 'The United Kingdom', in M.J. Colton and W. Hellinckx (eds) *Child Care in the EC*, Aldershot: Arena, pp. 212–31.

Campbell, B. (1993) *Goliath: Britain's Dangerous Places*, London: Methuen.

Carabine, J. (1996) 'Heterosexuality and social policy', in D. Richardson (ed.) *Theorising Heterosexuality: Telling It Straight*, Buckingham: Open University Press, pp. 55–74.

Cavanagh, K. and Cree, V.E. (1996) *Working with Men: Feminism and Social Work*, London: Routledge.

Chandler, T. (1993) 'Working with fathers in a family centre', *Working with Men*, 4: 11–13

Christie, A. (1996) 'Men social workers – balancing a non-traditional job', Paper presented to BSA Conference, University of Reading (April).

Cochrane, A. (1993) 'The problem of poverty', in R. Dallos and E. McLaughlin (eds) *Social Problems and the Family*, London: Sage, pp. 189–226.

Connell, R.W. (1987) *Gender and Power: Society, the Person and Sexual Politics*, Cambridge: Polity Press.

—— (1995) *Masculinities*, Cambridge: Polity Press.

Cornwall, A. and Lindisfarne, N. (eds) (1994) *Dislocating Masculinity: Comparative Ethnographies*, London: Routledge.

Dallos, R. and McLaughlin, E. (eds) (1993) *Social Problems and the Family*, London: Sage Publications.

Daly, K.J. (1995) 'Reshaping fatherhood: finding the models', in W. Marsiglio (ed.) *Fatherhood: Contemporary Theory, Research and Social Policy*, Thousand Oaks, CA: Sage, pp. 21–40.

Dartington Social Research Unit (1995) *Child Protection: Messages from Research*, London: HMSO.

Dennis, N. (1993) *Rising Crime and the Dismembered Family*, London: Institute for Economic Affairs.

Dennis, N. and Erdos, G. (1992) *Families without Fatherhood*. London: Institute for Economic Affairs.

DOH (1989) *Children Act 1989*, London: HMSO.
—— (1995) *Child Protection: Messages from Research*, London: HMSO.
Dominelli, L. (1991) *Gender, Sex Offenders and Probation Practice*, Norwich: Novata Press.
Dominelli, L. and McLeod, E. (1989) *Feminist Social Work*, London: Macmillan.
EC (1992) Council Recommendation (92/241/EEC), Brussels: European Commission.
—— (1994) 'A way forward for the Union: the White Paper on European social policy', Brussels: European Commission.
—— Network on Childcare (1993) *Men as Carers*, Brussels: European Commission.
—— (1996) *A Review of Services for Young Children in the European Union 1990–1995*, Brussels: European Commission.
Elliott, M. (ed.) (1993) *Female Sexual Abuse of Children: The Ultimate Taboo*, Harlow: Longman.
Fanshell, D. (1990) *Foster Children in Life Course Perspective*, New York: Columbia University Press.
Fawcett, B., Featherstone, B., Hearn, J. and Toft, C. (eds) (1996) *Violence and Gender Relations: Theories and Interventions*, London: Sage.
Ferguson, H., Gilligan, R. and Torode, R. (eds) (1993) *Surviving Childhood Adversity*, Dublin: Social Studies Press.
Finkelhor, D. (1991) 'The scope of the problem', in K. Murray and D.A. Gough (eds) *Intervening in Child Sexual Abuse*, Edinburgh: Edinburgh University Press, pp. 9–17.
Finkelhor, D., Araji, S., Baron, L., Brown, A., Peters, D. and Wyatt, G.E. (1986) *A Source Book on Child Sexual Abuse*, Los Angeles: Sage.
Finkelhor, D., Williams, L.M. and Burns, N. (1988) *Nursery Crimes: Sexual Abuse in Day Care*, Newbury Park, CA: Sage Publications.
Frost, N. and Stein, M. (1989) *The Politics of Child Welfare*, Hemel Hempstead: Harvester Wheatsheaf.
Gillan, C. (1996) Speech delivered at the Conference on Men in Child Care Services, Sheffield Old Town Hall (29 June).
Golombok, S., Spencer, A. and Rutter, M. (1983) 'Children in lesbian and single parent households: psychosexual and psychiatric appraisal', *Journal of Child Psychology and Psychiatry*, 24: 551–72.
Graham, H. (1983) 'Caring: a labour of love', in J. Finch and D. Groves (eds) *A Labour of Love: Women, Work and Caring*, London: Routledge & Kegan Paul, pp. 13–30.
—— (1993) 'Social divisions in caring', *Women's Studies International Forum*, 16: 461–70.
Gray, S., Higgs, M. and Pringle, K. (1996) 'Services for people who have been sexually abused', in L. McKie (ed.) *Researching Women's Health: Methods and Process*, Salisbury: Quay Books, pp. 177–200.
Grimwood, C. and Poppplestone, R. (1993) *Women, Management and Care*, London: Macmillan.
Hallett, C. (1995) 'Child abuse: an academic overview', in P. Kingston and B. Pehale (eds) *Family Violence and the Caring Professions*, London: Macmillan, pp. 23–49.

Hanks, H. and Saradjian, J. (1991) 'Women who abuse children sexually: characteristics of sexual abuse of children by women', *Human Systems: The Journal of Systemic Consultation and Management*, 2: 247–62.

Hanmer, J. (1990) 'Men, power and the exploitation of women', in J. Hearn and D. Morgan (eds) *Men, Masculinities and Social Theory*, London: Unwin Hyman, pp. 21–42.

—— (1996) 'Women and violence: commonalities and diversities', in B. Fawcett, B. Featherstone, J. Hearn and C. Toft (eds) *Violence and Gender Relations: Theories and Interventions*, London: Sage, pp. 7–21.

Hanmer, J. and Statham, D. (1988) *Women and Social Work: Towards a Woman-centred Practice*, London: Macmillan.

Harlow, E., Hearn, J. and Parkin, W. (1992) 'Sexuality and social work organisations', in P. Carter, T. Jeffs and M.K. Smith (eds) *Changing Social Work and Welfare*, Buckingham, England: Open University Press, pp. 131–43.

Hearn, J. (1990) '"Child abuse" and men's violence', in Violence Against Children Study Group (eds) *Taking Child Abuse Seriously*, London: Unwin Hyman, pp. 63–85.

—— (1996a) 'Men's violence to known women: historical, everyday and theoretical constructions by men', in B. Fawcett, B. Featherstone, J. Hearn and C. Toft (eds) *Violence and Gender Relations: Theories and Interventions*, London: Sage, pp. 22–37.

—— (1996b) 'Men's violence to known women: men's accounts and men's policy developments', in B. Fawcett, B. Featherstone and C. Toft (eds) *Violence and Gender Relations: Theories and Interventions*, London: Sage, pp. 99–114.

—— (1996c) 'Is masculinity dead? A critique of the concept of masculinity/ masculinities', in M. Mac an Ghaill (ed.) *Understanding Masculinities*, Buckingham: Open University Press, pp. 202–7.

Hearn, J. and Morgan, D. (eds) (1990) *Men, Masculinities and Social Theory*, London: Unwin Hyman.

Hearn, J. and Parkin, W. (1995) *'Sex' at 'work': The Power and Paradox or Organisation Sexuality*, London: Harvester Wheatsheaf/Prentice-Hall.

Hekman, S.J. (1990) *Gender and Knowledge: Elements of a Postmodern Feminism*, Cambridge: Polity Press.

Hester, M., Kelly, L. and Radford, J. (eds) (1996) *Women, Violence and Male Power*, Buckingham: Open University Press.

Heward, C. (1996) 'Masculinities and families', in M. Mac an Ghaill (ed.) *Understanding Masculinities*, Buckingham: Open University Press, pp. 35–49.

HMSO (1992) *Choosing with Care: The Report of the Committee of Inquiry into the Selection, Development and Management of Staff in Children's Homes*, London: HMSO.

—— (1993) *Adoption: The Future*, London: HMSO.

Holt, C. (1992) 'Developing effective work with men in family centres', Mimeograph, Barkingside: Barnado's.

Hunt, P. (1994) *Report of the Independent Inquiry into Multiple Abuse in Nursery Classes in Newcastle upon Tyne*, Newcastle upon Tyne: City Council of Newcastle upon Tyne.

Jensen, J.J. (1996) *Men as Workers in Childcare Services*, Brussels: European Commission.

Kelly, L. (1991) 'Unspeakable acts: women who abuse', *Trouble and Strife*, 21: 13–20.

—— (1996) 'When does the speaking profit us? Reflections on the challenges of developing feminist perspectives on abuse and violence by women', in M. Hester, L. Kelly and J. Radford (eds) *Women, Violence and Male Power*, Buckingham: Open University Press, pp. 34–49.

Mac an Ghaill, M. (ed.) (1996) *Understanding Masculinities*, Buckingham: Open University Press.

McCollum, H., Kelly, L. and Radford, J. (1994) 'Wars Against Women', *Trouble and Strife*, 28: 12–18.

McFadden, E.J. (1984) *Preventing Abuse in Foster Care*, Ypsilanti, MI: Eastern Michigan University.

McFadden, E.J. and Ryan, P. (1991) 'Maltreatment in family foster homes: dynamics and dimensions', *Child and Youth Services*, 15: 209–31.

Marsiglio, W. (1995) *Fatherhood: Contemporary Theory, Research and Social Policy*, Thousand Oaks, CA: Sage.

Millar, J. (1994) 'State, family and personal responsibility: the changing balance for lone mothers in the United Kingdom', *Feminist Review*, 48: 24–39.

Moss, P. (1994) 'Father, dear father', *Community Care* (October/November).

Mullender, A. and Morley, R. (eds) (1994) *Children Living with Domestic Violence: Putting Men's Abuse of Women on the Childcare Agenda*, London: Whitting & Birch.

Murray, C. (1990) *The Emerging British Underclass*, London: Institute for Economic Affairs.

O'Hara, M. (1993) 'Child protection in the context of domestic violence', in H. Ferguson, R. Gilligan and R. Torode (eds) *Surviving Childhood Adversity*, Dublin: Social Studies Press, pp. 126–33.

O'Neill, S. (1990) 'Men and social work: is there an anti-sexist practice?' Master's degree in social work thesis, University of Sussex.

Parkin, W. (1989) 'Private experiences in the public domain: sexuality and residential care organisations', in J. Hearn, D.L. Sheppard, P. Tancred-Sheriff and G. Burrell (eds), *The Sexuality of Organisation*, London: Sage Publications, pp. 110–25.

Parton, N. (1996a) 'Child protection, family support and social work', *Child and Family Social Work*, 1(1): 3–11.

—— (1996b) 'Social work, risk and the blaming system', in N. Parton (ed) *Social Theory, Social Change and Social Work*, London: Routledge.

Patterson, C.J. (1992) 'Children of lesbian and gay parents', *Child Development*, 63: 1025–42.

Phillips, A. (1993) *The Trouble with Boys: Parenting the Men of the Future*, London: Pandora.

Pringle, K. (1990) *Managing to Survive*, Barkingside: Barnados.

—— (1992) 'Child sexual abuse perpetrated by welfare personnel and the problem of men', *Critical Social Policy*, 36: 4–19.

—— (1993a) 'Gender issues in child sexual abuse committed by foster carers: a case study for the welfare services?' in H. Ferguson, R. Gilligan and R. Torode (eds) *Surviving childhood adversity*, Dublin: Social Studies Press, pp. 245–56.

—— (1995) *Men, Masculinities and Social Welfare*, London: UCL Press.

—— (1996a) University of Sunderland/University of Goteborg Joint Research Project: Summary of Findings, Centre for Social Research and Practice, University of Sunderland, unpublished.

—— (1996b) 'Protecting children against sexual abuse: a third way?' Paper presented at conference on Human Services in Crisis: National and International Issues, Fitzwilliam College, University of Cambridge (September).

Richardson, D. (ed.) (1996) *Theorising Heterosexuality: Telling It Straight*, Buckingham: Open University Press.

Rickford, F. (1992) 'Fostering with pride', *Social Work Today*, 28 (May): 12–13.

Robinson, V. (1996) 'Heterosexuality and masculinity: theorising male power or the male wounded psyche?' in D. Richardson (ed.) *Theorising Heterosexuality: Telling It Straight*, Buckingham, Open University Press, pp. 109–24.

Rosenthal, J.A., Motz, J.K., Edmonson, D.A. and Groze, V. (1991) 'A descriptive study of abuse and neglect', *Child Abuse and Neglect*, 15: 249–60.

Ruxton, S. (1991) '"What's *he* doing at the family centre?": the dilemmas of men who care for children', MA dissertation, Polytechnic of North London.

Salisbury, J. and Jackson, D. (1996) *Challenging Macho Values*, London: Falmer Press.

Saunders, D.G. (1994) 'Child custody decisions in families experiencing woman abuse', *Social Work*, 9: 51–9.

Sawicki, J. (1991) *Disciplining Foucault: Feminism, Power and the Body*, New York: Routledge, Chapman & Hall.

Segal, L. (1990) *Slow Motion: Changing Masculinities, Changing Men*. London: Virago Press.

Smith, A.M. (1994) *New Right Discourse on Race and Sexuality: Britain, 1968–1990*, Cambridge: Cambridge University Press.

Taylor, G. (1993) 'Challenges from the margins', in J. Clarke (ed.) *A Crisis in Care? Challenges to Social Work*, London: Sage, pp. 105–49.

Thompson, N. (1993) *Anti-discriminatory Practice*, London: Macmillan.

—— (1995) 'Men and anti-sexism', *British Journal of Social Work*, 25: 459–75.

VanEvery, J. (1996) 'Heterosexuality and domestic life', in D. Richardson (ed.) *Theorising Heterosexuality: Telling It Straight*, Buckingham: Open University Press, pp. 39–54.

Violence Against Children Study Group (eds) (1990) *Taking Child Abuse Seriously: Contemporary Issues in Child Protection Theory and Practice*, London: Unwin Hyman.

Index

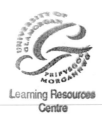

Learning Resources
Centre